Psychiatric–Mental Health Nurse Practitioner

4th Edition

CONTINUING EDUCATION SOURCE

NURSING CERTIFICATION REVIEW MANUAL

CLINICAL PRACTICE RESOURCE

Published by American Nurses Credentialing Center

Kathryn Johnson, MSN, PMHNP-BC, PMHCNS-BC
Dawn Vanderhoef, PhD, DNP, PMHNP-BC, PMHCNS-BC

**NURSING
KNOWLEDGE
CENTER**

Library of Congress Cataloging-in-Publication Data

Names: Johnson, Kathryn, 1947-, author. | Vanderhoef, Dawn, author. |
   Nursing Knowledge Center, publisher.
Title: Psychiatric-mental health nurse practitioner review and resource
   manual / Kathryn Johnson, Dawn Vanderhoe.
Other titles: Psychiatric-mental health nurse practitioner review manual
Description: 4th edition. | Silver Spring, MD : Nursing Knowledge Center,
   American Nurses Association, 2016. | Preceded by Psychiatric-mental health
   nurse practitioner review manual / by Kathryn Johnson and Dawn Vanderhoef.
   3rd edition. 2013. | Includes bibliographical references and index.
Identifiers: LCCN 2016012871| ISBN 9781935213796 (pbk.) | ISBN 9781935213802
   (ePub) | ISBN 9781935213819 (prc) | ISBN 9781935213826 (epdf)
Subjects: | MESH: Psychiatric Nursing--methods | Education, Nursing,
   Continuing
Classification: LCC RC438 | NLM WY 18.5 | DDC 616.89/0231--dc23 LC record available at
http://lccn.loc.gov/2016012871

The American Nurses Association (ANA) is the only full-service professional organization representing the interests of the nation's 3.1 million registered nurses through its constituent/ state nurses associations and its organizational affiliates. The ANA advances the nursing profession by fostering high standards of nursing practice, promoting the rights of nurses in the workplace, projecting a positive and realistic view of nursing, and lobbying the Congress and regulatory agencies on healthcare issues affecting nurses and the public.

CONTENTS

INSTRUCTIONS FOR OBTAINING CONTINUING EDUCATION CREDIT XI

CHAPTER 1. Taking The Certification Examination 1

General Suggestions for Preparing for the Exam   1

About the Certification Exams   8

Internet Resources   9

CHAPTER 2. Psychiatric–Mental Health Nurse Practitioner Role, Scope of Practice, and Regulatory Process 11

Nurse Practitioner Advanced Practice Core Content   11

Nurse Practitioner Advanced Practice Specialized Content   12

History of the NP Role   13

Professional Role Responsibilities   16

Roles of the PMHNP   22

Culturally Competent Care and Special Populations   23

Case Study 1   29

Case Study 2   29

Answers to Case Study Discussion Questions   31

References and Resources   32

CHAPTER 3. Theoretical Basis of Care 37

Biopsychosocial Framework of Care   37

Classification of Psychiatric Disorders: DSM-5   38

Therapeutic Relationship   38

Developmental Theories   40

Foundational Theories Supporting PMHNP Role   41

Nursing Theories   47

Case Study 1   48

Case Study 2   48

Answers to Case Study Discussion Questions   49

References and Resources   49

CHAPTER 4.   **Psychiatric–Mental Health Nurse Practitioner Professional Role and Health Policy: Leadership, Quality Improvement and Safety, Practice Inquiry, and Health Policy** 51

Leadership   51

Quality Improvement   55

Just Culture of Safety   55

Health Delivery Systems   56

Conflict of Interest   57

Rights of Clients   58

Health Policy Development   58

Case Study   59

Answers to Case Study Discussion Questions   60

References and Resources   60

CHAPTER 5.   **Neuroanatomy, Neurophysiology, and Behavior** . .63

The Nervous System   63

Neuroanatomy and the Brain   64

Neurophysiology and the Brain   68

Neuroimaging Assessment and Diagnostic Procedures   71

Genomics   73

Case Study 1   76

Case Study 2   76

Answers to Case Study Discussion Questions   77

References and Resources   77

CHAPTER 6.   Advanced Health and Physical Health Assessment . . 79

Physical Exam   79

Neurological Exam   80

Disease Prevention Activities   97

Gender-Based Medical Testing and Screening
Recommendations for the General Public   99

Health Behavior Guidelines   101

Public Health Principles   103

Case Study 1   105

Case Study 2   105

Answers to Case Study Discussion Questions   107

References and Resources   107

CHAPTER 7.   Pharmacological Principles 111

Concepts in Pharmacological Management   111

PMHNP Pharmacological Management Role   114

Case Study 1   120

Case Study 2   120

Case Study 3   120

Answers to Case Study Discussion Questions   122

References and Resources   123

CHAPTER 8.   Nonpharmacological Treatment 125

Individual Therapy   125

Group Therapy   127

Family Therapies   129

Complementary and Alternative Therapies (CATs)   132

Case Study   136

Answers to Case Study Discussion Questions   137

References and Resources   137

CHAPTER 9.   Depressive Disorders and Bipolar Disorders.....139

Sadness as a Common Emotional State   139

Major Depressive Disorder (MDD)   140

Persistent Depressive Disorder (Dysthymia)   166

Grief and Bereavement   169

Premenstrual Dysphoric Disorder   173

Bipolar (BP) Disorder   173

Stevens Johnson Syndrome (SJS)   184

Cyclothymic Disorder   186

Case Study   189

Answers to Case Study Discussion Questions   191

References and Resources   191

CHAPTER 10.   Anxiety Disorders, Obsessive–Compulsive Disorder, and Trauma- and Stressor-Related Disorders.....195

Anxiety Disorders   196

Panic Disorder   207

Agoraphobia   210

Specific Phobias (Simple Phobias)   211

Social Anxiety (Phobia) Disorder   214

Generalized Anxiety Disorder (GAD)   215

Separation Anxiety Disorder   218

Obsessive–Compulsive Disorder (OCD)   218

Posttraumatic Stress Disorder (PTSD)   222

Dissociative Disorders   225

Body Dysmorphic Disorder   226

Hoarding Disorder   226

Trichotillomania   226

Excoriation Disorder   226

Case Study   227

Answers to Case Study Discussion Questions   230

References and Resources   230

CHAPTER 11.   Schizophrenia Spectrum and Other Psychotic
Disorders. 233

General Description of Psychotic Disorders   233

Schizophrenia   235

Schizophreniform Disorder   258

Schizoaffective Disorder   260

Delusional Disorder   262

Brief Psychotic Disorder   264

Shared Psychotic Disorder (Folie á Deux)   266

Case Study   268

Answers to Case Study Discussion Questions   269

References and Resources   269

CHAPTER 12.   Neurocognitive Disorders .271

Cognitive Disorders   271

Delirium   271

Dementia   277

Major or Minor Neurocognitive Disorder Due to
Traumatic Brain Injury   285

Case Study   291

Answers to Case Study Discussion Questions   292

References and Resources   292

CHAPTER 13. Substance-Related and Addictive Disorders 293

Substance-Related Disorders   293

Case Study   308

Answers to Case Study Discussion Questions   310

References and Resources   310

CHAPTER 14. Personality Disorders. 313

Personality   313

Personality Disorders   314

Case Study   324

Answers to Case Study Discussion Questions   325

References and Resources   325

CHAPTER 15. Disorders of Childhood and Adolescence 327

Assessment and Care Planning for Children and
Adolescents   327

Oppositional Defiant Disorder (ODD)   329

Conduct Disorder   332

Attention-Deficit Hyperactivity Disorder (ADHD)   335

Autism Spectrum Disorder   340

Rett Syndrome   343

Eating Disorders   346

Intellectual Disability   351

Disruptive Mood dysRegulation Disorder   355

Case Study   357

Answers to Case Study Discussion Questions   358

References and Resources   358

CHAPTER 16. Sleep 361

General Considerations   361

Insomnia   362

Case Study 1   369

Case Study 2   369

Case Study 3   369

Answers to Case Study Discussion Questions   370

References and Resources   371

CHAPTER 17. Violence. 373

Intimate Partner Violence (IPV)   373

Assessment   375

Sexual Assault and Abuse   376

Lethality Assessment   379

Violence in School   380

Suicide Assessment   380

Homicide: Early Warning Signs   381

Threats of Violence   381

Case Study   383

Answers to Case Study Discussion Questions   384

References and Resources   384

APPENDIX A. Review Questions. 385

APPENDIX B. Review Question Answers. 409

INDEX 417

INSTRUCTIONS FOR OBTAINING CONTINUING EDUCATION CREDIT FOR STUDY OF THE PSYCHIATRIC–MENTAL HEALTH NURSE PRACTITIONER REVIEW AND RESOURCE MANUAL, 4TH EDITION

The Nursing Knowledge Center offers continuing nursing education contact hours (CE) to those who review and study this manual and successfully complete an online module. To obtain CE credit you must purchase and review the manual, pay required fees to enroll in the online module, and complete all module components by the published CE expiration date including disclosures, pre- and posttests, and the course evaluation. The continuing nursing education contact hours online module can be completed at any time prior to the published CE expiration date and a certificate can be printed from the online learning management system immediately after successful completion of the online module. To purchase the online module for this manual visit the Nursing Knowledge Center's online catalog at https://learn.ana-nursingknowledge.org/. Please contact online support with any questions about the CE or module.

Inquiries or Comments

If you have any questions about the content of the manual please e-mail revmanuals@ana.org. You may also mail any comments to Editorial Project Manager at the address listed below.

> Nursing Knowledge Center
>
> Attn: Editorial Project Manager
>
> 8515 Georgia Avenue, Suite 400
>
> Silver Spring, MD 20910-3492
>
> Fax: (301) 628-5342

CE Provider Information

ANA's Center for Continuing Education and Professional Development is accredited as a provider of continuing nursing education by the American Nurses Credentialing Center's Commission on Accreditation.

> ANCC Provider Number 0023.
>
> ANA is approved by the California Board of Registered Nursing, Provider Number CEP6178.

Disclaimer

Review and study of this manual and successful completion of the online module do not guarantee success on a certification examination. Purchase of this manual and completion of the online module are not required to obtain certification.

CHAPTER 1

TAKING THE CERTIFICATION EXAMINATION

When you sign up to take a national certification exam, you will be instructed to go on-line and review the testing and review handbook (http://www.nursecredentialing.org/ GeneralTestingRenewalHandbook). Review it carefully and be sure to bookmark the site so you can refer to it frequently. It contains information on test content and sample questions. This is critical information; it will give you insight into the nature of the test. The agency will send you information about the test site; keep this in a safe place until needed.

GENERAL SUGGESTIONS FOR PREPARING FOR THE EXAM

Step One: Control Your Anxiety

Everyone experiences anxiety when faced with taking the certification exam.

▶ Remember, your program was designed to prepare you to take this exam.

▶ Your instructors took a similar exam, and have probably talked to students who took exams more recently, so they know how to help you prepare.

▶ Taking a review course or setting up your own study plan will help you feel more confident about taking the exam.

Step Two: Do Not Listen to Gossip About the Exam

A large volume of information exists about the tests based on reports from people who have taken the exams in the past. Because information from the testing facilities is limited, it is hard to ignore this gossip.

▶ Remember that gossip about the exam that you hear from others is not verifiable.

▶ Because this gossip is based on the imperfect memory of people in a stressful situation, it may not be very accurate.

▶ People tend to remember those items testing content with which they are less comfortable; for instance, those with a limited background in women's health may say that the exam was "all women's health." In fact, the exam blueprint ensures that the exam covers multiple content areas without overemphasizing any one.

Step Three: Set Reasonable Expectations for Yourself

▶ Do not expect to know everything.

▶ Do not try to know everything in great detail.

▶ You do not need a perfect score to pass the exam.

▶ The exam is designed for a beginner level—it is testing readiness for *entry-level* practice.

▶ Learn the general rules, not the exceptions.

▶ The most likely diagnoses will be on the exam, not questions on rare diseases or atypical cases.

▶ Think about the most likely presentation and most common therapy.

Step Four: Prepare Mentally and Physically

▶ While you are getting ready to take the exam, take good physical care of yourself.

▶ Get plenty of sleep and exercise, and eat well while preparing for the exam.

▶ These things are especially important while you are studying and immediately before you take the exam.

Step Five: Access Current Knowledge

General Content

You will be given a list of general topics that will be on the exam when you register to take the exam. In addition, examine the table of contents of this book and the test content outline, available at http://nursecredentialing.org/FamilyPsychMentalHealthNP.

▶ What content do you need to know?

▶ How well do you know these subjects?

Take a Review Course

▶ Taking a review course is an excellent way to assess your knowledge of the content that will be included in the exam.

▶ If you plan to take a review course, take it well before the exam so you will have plenty of time to master any areas of weakness the course uncovers.

▶ If you are prepared for the exam, you will not hear anything new in the course. You will be familiar with everything that is taught.

▶ If some topics in the review course are new to you, concentrate on these in your studies.

▶ People have a tendency to study what they know; it is rewarding to study something and feel a mastery of it! Unfortunately, this will not help you master unfamiliar content. Be sure to use a review course to identify your areas of strength and weakness, then concentrate on the weaknesses.

Depth of Knowledge

How much do you need to know about a subject?

▶ You cannot know everything about a topic.

▶ Remember that the depth of knowledge required to pass the exam is for entry-level performance.

▶ Study the information sent to you from the testing agency, what you were taught in school, what is covered in this text, and the general guidelines given in this chapter.

▶ Look at practice tests designed for the exam. Practice tests for other exams will not be helpful.

▶ Consult your class notes or clinical diagnosis and management textbook for the major points about a disease. Additional reference books can be found online at http://nursecredentialing.org/PsychNP-TestReferenceList.

▶ For example, with regard to medications, know the drug categories and the major medications in each. Assume all drugs in a category are generally alike, and then focus on the differences among common drugs. Know the most important indications, contraindications, and side effects. Emphasize safety. The questions usually do not require you to know the exact dosage of a drug.

Step Six: Institute a Systematic Study Plan

Develop Your Study Plan

▶ Write up a formal plan of study.

▷ Include topics for study, timetable, resources, and methods of study that work for you.

▷ Decide whether you want to organize a study group or work alone.

▷ Schedule regular times to study.

▷ Avoid cramming; it is counterproductive. Try to schedule your study periods in 1-hour increments.

▶ Identify resources to use for studying. To prepare for the examination, you should have the following materials on your shelf:

▷ A good pathophysiology text.

▷ This review book.

▷ A physical assessment text.

▷ Your class notes.

▷ Other important sources, including: information from the testing facility, a clinical diagnosis textbook, favorite journal articles, notes from a review course, and practice tests.

▷ Know the important national standards of care for major illnesses.

▷ Consult the bibliography on the test blueprint. When studying less familiar material, it is helpful to study using the same references that the testing center uses.

▶ Study the body systems from head to toe.

▶ The exams emphasize health promotion, assessment, differential diagnosis, and plan of care for common problems.

▶ You will need to know facts and be able to interpret and analyze this information utilizing critical thinking.

Personalize Your Study Plan

▶ How do you learn best?

▷ If you learn best by listening or talking, attend a review course or discuss topics with a colleague.

▶ Read everything the test facility sends you as soon as you receive it and several times during your preparation period. It will give you valuable information to help guide your study.

▶ Have a specific place with good lighting set aside for studying. Find a quiet place with no distractions. Assemble your study materials.

Implement Your Study Plan

You must have basic content knowledge. In addition, you must be able to use this information to think critically and make decisions based on facts.

▶ Refer to your study plan regularly.

▶ Stick to your schedule.

▶ Take breaks when you get tired.

▶ If you start procrastinating, get help from a friend or reorganize your study plan.

▶ It is not necessary to follow your plan rigidly. Adjust as you learn where you need to spend more time.

▶ Memorize the basics of the content areas you will be required to know.

Focus on General Material

▶ Most of what you need to know is basic material that does not require constant updating.

▶ You do not need to worry about the latest information being published as you are studying for the exam. Remember, it can take 6 to 12 months for new information to be incorporated into test questions.

Pace Your Studying

▶ Stop studying for the examination when you are starting to feel overwhelmed and look at what is bothering you. Then make changes.

▶ Break overwhelming tasks into smaller tasks that you know you can do.

▶ Stop and take breaks while studying.

Work With Others

▶ Talk with classmates about your preparation for the exam.

▶ Keep in touch with classmates, and help each other stick to your study plans.

▶ If your classmates become anxious, do not let their anxiety affect you. Walk away if you need to.

▶ Do not believe bad stories you hear about other people's experiences with previous exams.

▶ Remember, you know as much as anyone about what will be on the next exam!

Consider a Study Group

▶ Study groups can provide practice in analyzing cases, interpreting questions, and critical thinking.

▶ You can discuss a topic and take turns presenting cases for the group to analyze.

▶ Study groups can also provide moral support and help you continue studying.

Step Seven: Strategies Immediately Before the Exam

Final Preparation Suggestions

▶ Use practice exams when studying to get accustomed to the exam format and time restrictions.

▷ Many books that are labeled as review books are simply a collection of examination questions.

▷ If you have test anxiety, such practice tests may help alleviate the anxiety.

▷ Practice tests can help you learn to judge the time it should take you to complete the exam.

▷ Practice tests are useful for gaining experience in analyzing questions.

▷ Books of questions may not uncover the gaps in your knowledge that a more systematic content review text will reveal.

▷ If you feel that you don't know enough about a topic, refer to a text to learn more. After you feel that you have learned the topic, practice questions are a wonderful tool to help improve your test-taking skill.

▶ Know your test-taking style.

▷ Do you rush through the exam without reading the questions thoroughly?

▷ Do you get stuck and dwell on a question for a long time?

▷ You should spend about 45 to 60 seconds per question and finish with time to review the questions you were not sure about.

▷ Be sure to read the question completely, including all four answer choices. Choice "a" may be good, but "d" may be best.

The Night Before the Exam

▶ Be prepared to get to the exam on time.

▷ Know the test site location and how long it takes to get there.

▷ Take a "dry run" beforehand to make sure you know how to get to the testing site, if necessary.

▷ Get a good night's sleep.

▷ Eat sensibly.

▷ Avoid alcohol the night before.

▷ Assemble the required material—two forms of identification, admission card, pencil, and watch. Both IDs must match the name on the application, and one photo ID is preferred.

▷ Know the exam room rules.

> ▶ You will be given scratch paper, which will be collected at the end of the exam.

> ▶ Nothing else is allowed in the exam room.

> ▶ You will be required to put papers, backpacks, etc., in a corner of the room or in a locker.

> ▶ No water or food will be allowed.

> ▶ You will be allowed to walk to a water fountain and go to the bathroom one at a time.

The Day of the Exam

▶ Get there early. You must arrive to the test center at least 15 minutes before your scheduled appointment time. If you are late, you may not be admitted.

▶ Think positively. You have studied hard and are well-prepared.

▶ Remember your anxiety reduction strategies.

Specific Tips for Dealing With Anxiety

Test anxiety is a specific type of anxiety. Symptoms include upset stomach, sweaty palms, tachycardia, trouble concentrating, and a feeling of dread. But there are ways to cope with test anxiety.

▶ There is no substitute for being well-prepared.

▶ Practice relaxation techniques.

▶ Avoid alcohol, excess coffee, caffeine, and any new medications that might sedate you, dull your senses, or make you feel agitated.

▶ Take a few deep breaths and concentrate on the task at hand.

Focus on Specific Test-Taking Skills

To do well on the exam, you need good test-taking skills in addition to knowledge of the content and ability to use critical thinking.

All Certification Exams Are Multiple Choice

▶ Multiple-choice tests have specific rules for test construction.

▶ A multiple-choice question consists of three parts: the information (or stem), the question, and the four possible answers (one correct and three distracters).

▶ Careful analysis of each part is necessary. Read the entire question before answering.

▶ Practice your test-taking skills by analyzing the practice questions in this book and on the ANCC website.

Analyze the Information Given

▶ Do not assume you have more information than is given.

▶ Do not overanalyze.

▶ Remember, the writer of the question assumes this is all of the information needed to answer the question.

▶ If information is not given, it is not relevant and will not affect the answer.

▶ Do not make the question more complicated than it is.

What Kind of Question Is Asked?

▶ Are you supposed to recall a fact, apply facts to a situation, or understand and differentiate between options?

▷ Read the question thinking about what the writer is asking.

▷ Look for key words or phrases that lead you (see Figure 1–1). These help determine what kind of answer the question requires.

Read All of the Answers

▶ If you are absolutely certain that answer "a" is correct as you read it, mark it, but read the rest of the question so you do not trick yourself into missing a better answer.

▶ If you are absolutely sure answer "a" is wrong, cross it off or make a note on your scratch paper and continue reading the question.

▶ After reading the entire question, go back, analyze the question, and select the best answer.

▶ Do not jump ahead.

▶ If the question asks you for an assessment, the best answer will be an assessment. Do not be distracted by an intervention that sounds appropriate.

▶ If the question asks you for an intervention, do not answer with an assessment.

avoid	initial	most
best	first	significant
except	contributing to	likely
not	appropriate	of the following
		most consistent with

FIGURE 1–1.
EXAMPLES OF KEY WORDS AND PHRASES

▶ When two answer choices sound very good, the best one is usually the least expensive, least invasive way to achieve the goal. For example, if your answer choices include a physical exam maneuver or imaging, the physical exam maneuver is probably the better choice provided it will give the information needed.

▶ If the answers include two options that are the opposite of each other, one of the two is probably the correct answer.

▶ When numeric answers cover a wide range, a number in the middle is more likely to be correct.

▶ Watch out for distracters that are correct but do not answer the question, combine true and false information, or contain a word or phrase that is similar to the correct answer.

▶ Err on the side of caution.

Only One Answer Can Be Correct

▶ When more than one suggested answer is correct, you must identify the one that best answers the question asked.

▶ If you cannot choose between two answers, you have a 50% chance of getting it right if you guess.

Avoid Changing Answers

▶ Change an answer only if you have a compelling reason, such as you remembered something additional, or you understand the question better after rereading it.

▶ People change to a wrong answer more often than to a right answer.

Time Yourself to Complete the Whole Exam

▶ Do not spend a large amount of time on one question.

▶ If you cannot answer a question quickly, mark it and continue the exam.

▶ If time is left at the end, return to the difficult questions.

▶ Make educated guesses by eliminating the obviously wrong answers and choosing a likely answer even if you are not certain.

▶ Trust your instinct.

▶ Answer every question. There is no penalty for a wrong answer.

▶ Occasionally a question will remind you of something that helps you with a question earlier in the test. Look back at that question to see if what you are remembering affects how you would answer that question.

ABOUT THE CERTIFICATION EXAMS

The American Nurses Credentialing Center Computerized Exam

The ANCC examination is given only as a computer exam, and each exam is different.

The order of the questions is scrambled for every test, so even if two people are taking the same exam, the questions will be in a different order. The exam consists of 175 multiple-choice questions.

▶ 150 of the 175 questions are part of the test and how you answer will count toward your score; 25 are included to refine questions and will not be scored. You will not know which ones count, so treat all questions the same.

▶ You will need to know how to use a mouse, scroll by either clicking arrows on the scroll bar or using the up and down arrow keys, and perform other basic computer tasks.

▶ The exam does not require computer expertise.

▶ However, if you are not comfortable with using a computer, you should practice using a mouse and computer beforehand so you do not waste time on the mechanics of using the computer.

Know what to expect during the test.

▶ Each ANCC test question is independent of the other questions.

▷ For each case study, there is only one question. This means that a correct answer on any question does not depend on the correct answer to any other question.

▷ Each question has four possible answers. There are no questions asking for combinations of correct answers (such as "a and c") or multiple-multiples.

▶ You can skip a question and go back to it at the end of the exam.

▶ You cannot mark key words in the question or right or wrong answers. If you want to do this, use the scratch paper.

▶ You will get your results immediately, and a grade report will be provided upon leaving the testing site.

INTERNET RESOURCES

▶ ANCC website: www.nursecredentialing.org

▶ ANA bookstore: www.nursesbooks.org. Catalog of ANA nursing scope and standards publications and other titles that may be listed on your test content outline

▶ National Guideline Clearinghouse: www.ngc.gov

PSYCHIATRIC–MENTAL HEALTH NURSE PRACTITIONER ROLE, SCOPE OF PRACTICE, AND REGULATORY PROCESS

Starting in the 1950s with the seminal work of two psychiatric nurses, June Mellow (1968) and Hildegard Peplau (1952), psychiatric nursing has been a well-established, well-recognized sub-specialty of nursing. The emergence of the psychiatric–mental health nurse practitioner (PMHNP) role reflects the growth of the advanced practice role, the acceptance of a brain-based etiology of psychiatric disorders, and an awareness of the need to provide holistic nursing care that does not artificially separate mind and body (Stuart, 2013).

The PMHNP role is built on fundamental, core advanced practice knowledge common to all nurse practitioners. This base of knowledge is expanded to include the very specific knowledge of the subspecialty of psychiatry. This chapter reviews the role of the PMHNP, the scope of practice, and the regulatory process.

Advanced practice nurses specializing in psychiatry are educationally prepared at the master's or doctoral level, possess in-depth knowledge and skills in the specialty area, and provide primary psychiatric care to individuals or families at risk for or currently experiencing a psychiatric disorder.

NURSE PRACTITIONER ADVANCED PRACTICE CORE CONTENT

All nurse practitioners upon graduation are expected to meet a set of core competencies (National Organization of Nurse Practitioner Faculties [NONPF], 2014). Specialty competencies, such as the *Psychiatric–Mental Health Nurse Practitioner Competencies*, are then built upon these core competencies (NONPF, 2013).

Nurse Practitioner Core Competencies
▶ Scientific Foundations
▶ Leadership
▶ Quality

▶ Practice Inquiry

▶ Technology and Information Literacy

▶ Policy

▶ Health Delivery System

▶ Ethics

▶ Independent Practice

NURSE PRACTITIONER ADVANCED PRACTICE SPECIALIZED CONTENT

The specialty competencies are specifically designed for entry-level psychiatric–mental health nurse practitioners. These specialty competencies are to be used with the Nurse Practitioner (NP) Core Competencies. The specialty competencies address the life-span PMHNP focus, including families and populations. As changes occur within the healthcare system, these competencies will also change (NONPF, 2013).

Leadership Competencies

▶ Participates in community and population-focused programs that evaluate programs and promote mental health and prevent or reduce risk of mental health problems

▶ Advocates for complex client and family medicolegal rights and issues

▶ Collaborates with interprofessional colleagues about advocacy, policy to reduce health disparities and improve outcomes for populations

Quality Competencies

▶ Evaluates the appropriate uses of seclusion and restraints in the care process

Policy Competencies

▶ Employs opportunities to influence health policy to reduce the impact of stigma on services for prevention and treatment of mental health problems and psychiatric disorders

Independent Practice Competencies

▶ Develops age-appropriate treatment plans

▶ Includes differential diagnosis

▶ Assesses impact of acute and chronic medical problems on psychiatric treatment

▶ Conducts individual and group psychotherapy

▶ Applies supportive psychodynamic, cognitive, behavioral, and other evidence-based psychotherapies to brief and long-term practice

▶ Applies recovery-oriented principles

▶ Demonstrates best practices of family care approaches

▶ Plans care to minimize the development of complications and promote function

▶ Treats acute and chronic psychiatric disorders and problems

▶ Safely prescribes pharmacologic agents

▶ Ensures client safety through the appropriate prescription of pharmacologic and nonpharmacologic interventions

▶ Explains the risks and benefits of treatment to client and family

▶ Identifies the role of PMHNP in risk mitigation strategies in areas of opiate use and substance abuse

▶ Seeks consultation

▶ Uses self-reflection to improve care

▶ Provides consultation to healthcare providers and others to enhance quality and cost

▶ Guides the client in evaluating the appropriate use of complementary and alternative treatment

▶ Uses individualized outcome measure to evaluate psychiatric care

▶ Manages psychiatric emergencies

▶ Refers clients appropriately

▶ Facilitates the transition of clients across levels of care

▶ Uses outcomes to evaluate care

▶ Attends to the client–NP relationship as a vehicle for change

▶ Maintains a therapeutic relationship over time with individuals and groups

▶ Therapeutically concludes the client–NP relationship

▶ Demonstrates ability to address sexual and physical abuse, substance abuse, sexuality, and spiritual conflicts

▶ Applies therapeutic relationship strategies based on theory and research

▶ Applies principles of self-efficacy, empowerment, and others to effect change

▶ Identifies and maintains professional boundaries

▶ Teaches clients, families, and groups

▶ Provides psychoeducation

▶ Modifies the treatment approach based on client readiness

▶ Considers motivation and readiness to improve self-care

▶ Demonstrates knowledge of appropriate use of seclusion and restraint

▶ Documents appropriate use of seclusion and restraint

HISTORY OF THE NP ROLE

The NP role was introduced in 1965 by Loretta C. Ford, EdD, and Henry K. Silver, MD, at the University of Colorado (Mirr Jansen & Zwygart-Stauffacher, 2006). They identified new roles in which experienced registered nurses (RNs) with advanced education and skills were performing clinical duties traditionally reserved for physicians. Universities were slow to implement NP programs at the master's level. However, RNs embraced the new role and rushed into continuing education programs of varying length, quality, and focus to accomplish the necessary educational preparation for this new role.

In 2008 the License, Accreditation, Certification, and Education (LACE) consensus model was finalized and adopted by many nursing organizations. The consensus model identified four Advanced Practice Registered Nurse roles: Certified Registered Nurse Anesthetist (CRNA), Certified Nurse Midwife (CNM), Clinical Nurse Specialist (CNS), and Certified Nurse Practitioner (CNP). As part of the LACE model, Psychiatric–Mental Health was identified as a population focus. The American Psychiatric Nurses Association (APNA) and International Society of Psychiatric Nurses (ISPN) recommendation was for psychiatric–mental health nurse practitioners (PMHNPs) to be prepared across the life span (APNA, 2011). As of 2015 APRNs in psychiatric–mental health nursing have one certification examination, PMHNP–Life Span, with the American Nurses Credentialing Center (ANCC, 2015). All previous psychiatric–mental health advanced practice certification examinations have been retired as of December 2015 (ANCC, 2015).

Proven competence brought an acceptance of the NP role in the healthcare system, with acceptance and recognition of the title and role by consumers and other health professionals. NP programs are accredited by one of two organizations to achieve standardization and control over quality: the Commission on Collegiate Nursing Education (CCNE, 2016) and the Accreditation Commission for Education in Nursing (ACEN, 2016). NPs are recognized providers under many third-party insurance coverage plans (e.g., Medicare, Medicaid, CHAMPUS, federal programs funding school-based clinics, U.S. military, Veterans Administration).

Growth of the NP Role

▶ Facilitating factors for growth

  ▷ Consumer demand for services

  ▷ Acceptance of the advanced practice nursing role

  ▷ Emergence of the PMHNP role

  ▷ Decreasing stigmatization

  ▷ Emphasis on integrated healthcare services

▶ Constraining factors for growth

  ▷ Growing competition in job market in general for NPs

  ▷ Reimbursement struggles with Medicare and private insurance companies

  ▷ Overlapping scope of practice with other NPs

  ▷ Increased concerns over reimbursement fraud and abuse (e.g., issues of coding and billing for services)

  ▷ Scope of practice and need for formal supervisory or collaborative relationships with physicians

Regulatory and Statutory Dimensions of the NP Role

▶ State legislative statutes

  ▷ Grant *legal authority* for NP practice

  ▷ The *Nurse Practice Act* of every state

    ▶ Provides title protection (who may be called a nurse practitioner)

    ▶ Defines advanced practice

▶ Prevailing state laws that define scope of practice (what NPs may do)

▶ Places restrictions on practice

▶ Sets NP credentialing requirements (e.g., educational requirements, certification)

▶ States grounds for disciplinary action:

   ▷ Practicing without valid license

   ▷ Falsification of records

   ▷ Medicare fraud

   ▷ Failure to use appropriate nursing judgment

   ▷ Failure to follow accepted nursing standards

   ▷ Failure to complete accurate nursing documentation

▶ May specifically require that an NP develop a collaborative agreement with a physician

   ▷ *Collaborative agreement:* Also known as a protocol that describes what types of drugs might be prescribed and defines some form of oversight for NP practice

▶ Statutory law

   ▷ Rules and regulations differ for each state

   ▷ May further define scope of practice and practice requirements

   ▷ May provide restrictions in practice unique to specific state

▶ Licensure

   ▷ A process by which an agency of state government grants permission to persons to engage in the practice of that profession

   ▷ Also prohibits all others from legally doing protected practice

▶ Credentialing

   ▷ Process used to protect the public by ensuring a minimum level of professional competence

▶ Certification

   ▷ A credential that provides title protection

   ▷ Determines scope of practice (i.e., whom NPs can see and what NPs can treat)

   ▷ The process by which a professional organization or association certifies that a person licensed to practice as a professional has met certain predetermined standards specified by that profession for specialty practice

   ▷ Assures the public that a person has mastery of a specified body of knowledge

   ▷ Assures that the person has acquired the skills necessary to function in a particular specialty

▷ The American Nurses Credentialing Center (ANCC), which is a subsidiary of the American Nurses Association, is the only certifying body for advanced practice psychiatric nursing.

▶ Certification offered as a Psychiatric–Mental Health Nurse Practitioner–Life Span (ANCC, 2015)

▶ Scope of practice

▷ Defines NP roles and actions

▷ Identifies competencies assumed to be held by all NPs who function in a particular role

▷ Varies broadly from state to state

▷ Advanced practice PMHNP standards are identified in *Psychiatric-Mental Health Nursing: Scope and Standards of Practice* (ANA, 2014).

▶ Standards of practice

▷ Authoritative statements regarding the quality and type of practice that should be provided

▷ Provide a way to judge the nature of care provided

▷ Reflect the expectation for the care that should be provided to clients with various illnesses

▷ Reflect professional agreement focused on the minimum levels of acceptable performance

▷ Can be used to legally describe the standard of care that must be met by a provider

▷ May be precise protocols that must be followed or more general guidelines that recommend actions

PROFESSIONAL ROLE RESPONSIBILITIES

▶ Confidentiality

▷ The client's right to assume that information given to the healthcare provider will not be disclosed

▷ Protected under federal statute through the Medical Record Confidentiality Act of 1995 (S. 1360)

▷ Pertains to verbal and written client information

▷ Requires that the provider discuss confidentiality issues with clients, establish consent, and clarify any questions about disclosure of information

▷ Requires that provider obtain a signed medical authorization and consent form to release medical records and information when requested by the client or another healthcare provider

▶ HIPAA

▷ The first national comprehensive privacy protection act

▷ Guarantees clients four fundamental rights:

1. To be educated about HIPAA privacy protection,

2. To have access to their own medical records,

3. To request amendment of their health information to which they object, and

4. To require their permission for disclosure of their personal information.

▶ The Health Information Technology for Economic and Clinical Health Act (HITECH) of 2009 (Health Resources and Services Administration [HRSA], 2013)

▷ Incentive payments for sharing specific electronic health record (EHR) data

▷ Meaningful use incentives

▷ Electronic health records can improve both individual and population-based health outcomes (Friedman, Parrish, & Ross, 2013).

▷ Electronic health records can improve quality, safety, efficiency, effectiveness, and outcomes (U.S. DHHS, Office for Civil Rights, 2013).

    ▶ E-prescribing

    ▶ Computerized physician order sets

    ▶ Tracking care and avoiding duplication of services

▶ Telehealth

▷ The use of telephone or videoconferencing tools to deliver mental health care to clients who reside in rural areas or who may otherwise not be able to access care

▷ Must follow the same standards as care delivered in person

▷ Must be practiced in accordance with international, federal, and state regulatory agency standards

▷ Must include provisions for emergency care of the client

▷ The PMHNP must assure that HIPAA regulations regarding confidentiality and maintenance of the health record are followed.

▶ Exceptions to guaranteed confidentiality

▷ When appropriate persons or organizations determine that the need for information outweighs the principle of confidentiality

▷ If a client reveals an intent to harm self or others

▷ Information given to attorneys involved in litigation

▷ Releasing records to insurance companies

▷ Answering court orders, subpoenas, or summonses

▷ Meeting state requirements for mandatory reporting of diseases or conditions

▷ *Tarasoff* principle (Tarasoff v. Regents at the University of California, 1976): Duty to warn potential victim of imminent danger of homicidal clients

▷ In cases of child or elder abuse

▶ Informed consent

▷ The communication process between the provider and the client that results in the client's acceptance or rejection of the proposed treatment

▷ An explanation of relevant information that enables the client to make an appropriate and informed decision

▷ The right of all competent adults or emancipated minors

▶ *Emancipated minors:* Persons younger than 18 years old who are married, parents, or self-sufficiently living away from the family domicile

▷ Elements of informed consent

▶ Nature and purpose of proposed treatment or procedure

▶ Risks or discomforts and benefits of treatment

▶ Risks and benefits of not undergoing treatment

▶ Alternative procedures or treatments

▶ Diagnosis and prognosis

▷ Provider must document in the medical record that informed consent has been obtained from the client.

▷ PMHNP is responsible for ensuring that the client is cognitively capable of giving informed consent.

▶ Ethics

▷ Important aspect of the NP role that deals with moral duties, obligations, and responsibilities

▷ What is right versus what is wrong

▷ Ethical principles that provide foundation and direction for complex decisions:

▶ *Justice:* Doing what is fair; fairness in all aspects of care

▶ *Beneficence:* Promoting well-being and doing good

▶ *Nonmaleficence:* Doing no harm

▶ *Fidelity:* Being true and loyal

▶ *Autonomy:* Doing for self

▶ *Veracity:* Telling the truth

▶ *Respect:* Treating everyone with equal respect

▷ In 2015 the American Nurses Association (ANA) published the *Code of Ethics for Nurses with Interpretive Statements* (ANA, 2015). Its nine provisions are:

1. The nurse practices with compassion and respect for the inherent dignity, worth, and unique attributes of everyone.

2. The nurse's primary commitment is to the client, whether an individual, family, group, community, or population.

3. The nurse promotes, advocates for, and protects the rights, health, and safety of the client.

4. The nurse has the authority, accountability, and responsibility for nursing practice, makes decisions, and takes action consistent with the obligation to promote health and provide optimal care.

5. The nurse owes the same duties to self as to others, including the responsibility to promote health and safety, preserve wholeness of character and integrity, maintain competence, and continue personal and professional growth.

6. The nurse, through individual and collective effort, establishes, maintains, and improves the ethical environment of the work setting and conditions of employment that are conducive to safe, quality health care.

7. The nurse, in all roles and settings, advances the profession through research and scholarly inquiry, professional standards development, and the generation of both nursing and health policy.

8. The nurse collaborates with other health professionals and the public to protect human rights, promote health diplomacy, and reduce health disparities.

9. The profession of nursing, collectively through its professional organizations, must articulate nursing values, maintain the integrity of the profession, and integrate principles of social justice into nursing and health policy.

▷ Important ethical principles in psychiatry

▶ Clients must be involved in decision-making to the full extent of their capacity (mutual decision-making).

▶ Clients have a right to treatment in the least restrictive setting.

▶ Clients have a right to refuse treatment unless a legal process resulting in a mandatory court order for treatment has been obtained.

▷ Ethical dilemma

▶ Occurs in a situation in which there are two or more justifiable alternatives

▶ Occurs when the choice is made to promote good

▶ Which option sacrifices the fewest high-priority values (a harm reduction approach)?

▷ Theoretical approaches to ethical decision-making

▶ *Deontological Theory:* An action is judged as good or bad based on the act itself regardless of the consequences.

▶ *Teleological Theory:* An action is judged as good or bad based on the consequence or outcome.

▶ *Virtue Ethics:* Actions are chosen based on the moral virtues (e.g., honesty, courage, compassion, wisdom, gratitude, self-respect) or the character of the person making the decision.

Ethics of Disclosure by Providers

▶ Clients have a right to know what is happening during the course of their treatment.

▶ Providers have an ethical responsibility to disclose medical errors, accidents, injuries, and negative results to clients.

▶ As a result of the disclosure, a client may have legal right to compensation for harm suffered due to medical misadventures (Sadock, Sadock, & Ruiz, 2015).

Risk vs. Benefits of Disclosure of Disability Regarding Employment

▶ The Americans with Disabilities Act (ADA) works to prevent discrimination by employers with 15 or more employees against qualified persons in hiring, firing, advancement, job training, compensation, and workplace conditions (Buppert, 2012).

▶ The ADA is federal legislation granting Americans who have disabilities, including mental illness, the opportunity for employment on an equal basis with the nondisabled.

▶ Employers are required to make reasonable accommodations for qualified applicants or employees with a disability.

Risk of Disclosure

▶ Employers may find ways to avoid hiring persons known to have a disability.

▶ Coworkers may harass or discriminate against persons with psychiatric illnesses.

▶ Assumption that persons with psychiatric illnesses may be less productive

▶ May limit an employee's chance for advancement in career

▶ Feedback for improvement may not be given to employee because others may attribute the employee's behavior to the psychiatric illness.

▶ Labeling oneself as "disabled" may affect one's beliefs or self-image.

Benefits of Disclosure

▶ Able to request reasonable accommodations

▶ Opportunity to have a job coach come to the worksite and communicate directly with employer

▶ Employee can involve an employment service provider, employee assistance program, or other third party in the development of accommodations.

▶ Easier for employee to come to work during an exacerbation of symptoms

▶ May help with the recovery process

▶ Allows coworkers to offer personal support

▶ May empower another employee to disclose

Legal Considerations

▶ Malpractice insurance

▷ Provides financial protection against claims of malpractice

▶ Coverage for negligent professional acts

▶ Coverage for highly technical or professional skills required by health professionals, including NPs

▷ Recommended universally for all NPs

▷ Does not protect NPs from charges of practicing outside their legal scope of practice

▷ Provides NPs their own legal representation to advocate for them even if their agency also carries malpractice liability insurance protection

▷ Four elements of negligence that must be established to prove malpractice:

1. *Duty:* The NP had a duty to exercise reasonable care when undertaking and providing treatment to the client.

2. *Breach of duty:* The NP violated the applicable standard of care in treating the client's condition.

3. *Proximate cause:* There is a causal relationship between the breach in the standard of care and the client's injuries.

4. *Damages:* The client experiences permanent and substantial damages as a result of the breach in the standard of care.

Competency

▶ A legal, not a medical concept

▶ A determination that a client can make reasonable judgments and decisions regarding treatment and other health concerns

▶ A person is considered competent until a court rules the person to be incompetent.

▶ If a person is deemed incompetent, a court-appointed guardian will make health-related decisions for that person.

Commitment

▶ Process of forcing a person to receive involuntarily evaluation or treatment

▶ Process may differ from state to state

▶ Basic criteria include

▷ Person has a diagnosed psychiatric disorder,

▷ Person is harmful to self or others as a consequence of the disorder,

▷ Person is unaware or unwilling to accept the nature and severity of the disorder, and

▷ Treatment is likely to improve functioning.

▶ Involuntary admission

▷ Admission to a hospital or other treatment facility against the person's will

▷ Clients maintain all civil liberties except the ability to come and go as they please

▷ Amount of time clients can be kept against their wishes varies by state

▶ Voluntary admission

▷ Admission to a hospital or other treatment facility that a person desires or agrees to

▷ Client maintains all civil liberties

▷ Client consents to potential confinement within the structure of a hospital setting

ROLES OF THE PMHNP

Scholarly Activities

▶ It is important for NPs to engage in the following scholarly activities:

▷ Publishing

▷ Lecturing or presenting

▷ Preceptorship

▷ Continuing education

Mentoring

▶ A process in which a more experienced NP agrees to guide and support a junior colleague in the role, competencies, and skills

▶ Requires mutual respect and an interactive process of learning

▶ Needs involvement by both the mentor and the mentee in the relationship

Client Advocacy

▶ Stand up for clients' rights and empower them to become their own advocates

▶ Reduce the stigma of mental illness

▶ Help clients receive available services

▶ Promote mental health by participating in one or more of these professional organizations:

▷ American Nurses Association (ANA)

▷ American Psychiatric Nurses Association (APNA)

▷ International Society of Psychiatric Nurses (ISPN)

Health Policy

▶ Advanced practice nurses have a legal and ethical responsibility to be a client advocate.

▷ Participation in local, state, national, and international health policy activities (Buppert, 2012)

▷ Involvement: Testify at a public meeting, lobby, or work with the media to bring awareness to an issue

▷ Phases of policy-making: formulation, implementation, and evaluation (Abood, 2007)

Case Management

▶ A system of controlled oversight and authorization of services and benefits provided to clients

▶ Consists of coordinating care, ensuring quality outcomes, monitoring plan of care, and doing advocacy

▶ Overall goal is to promote quality, cost-effective outcomes

Risk Assessment

▶ Continuous monitoring for high-risk situations

▶ Assessing persons for nonhealthy behaviors

Risk Management

▶ Activities or systems designed to recognize and intervene to reduce the risk of injury to clients

▶ Appropriate interventions implemented to reduce nonhealthy behaviors in clients and high-risk situations

▶ Recognition and intervention to reduce subsequent claims against healthcare providers

Advance Directives

▶ Durable power of attorney for health care. Also known as healthcare proxy

  ▷ Legally binding in all 50 states

  ▷ Designates, in writing, an agent to act on behalf of a person should he or she become unable to make healthcare decisions

  ▷ Not limited to terminal illness; also covers other aspects of illness, such as making financial decisions during a person's illness

  ▷ Should be considered as an aspect of relapse planning for clients with chronic psychiatric disorders

▶ Living will: Document prepared while client is mentally competent to designate preferences for care if client becomes incompetent or terminally ill

  ▷ Not legally binding in all states

CULTURALLY COMPETENT CARE AND SPECIAL POPULATIONS

▶ Treating clients from diverse cultures, viewing each client as a unique person, and noting a potential relationship between clients' cultural experiences and their symptom presentation and perceptions

▶ Assumes that if the NP becomes more sensitive to cultural issues influencing the client's symptoms and treatment, more comprehensive health care can be provided

▶ Culture: The learned beliefs and behaviors or the socially inherited characteristics that are common among all members of a group; may be a racial, social, ethnic, or religious grouping

▶ Culture-bound syndromes: Specific behaviors related to a person's culture and not linked to a psychiatric disorder

  ▷ Be cognizant of inaccurately judging a client's behavior as psychopathology when it is really related to his or her culture.

Cultural Influences and Determinants of Health

▶ *Family:* A group of adults and children who are usually related and whose adults participate in carrying out the essential functions of providing food, clothing, shelter, safety, and education of children

  ▷ Concept broadened beyond the traditional husband–wife–children pattern

  ▷ Family initially teaches the belief patterns, religion, culture, and mores of a society.

▶ *Ethnicity:* Self-identified race, tribe, or nation with which a person or group identifies and which greatly influences beliefs and behavior

▶ *Community:* A group of families, often sharing the same race, tribe, or culture, who have beliefs or behavior not shared by others

▶ *Environment:* Includes both physical and psychosocial factors; the general circumstances of a person's life:

  ▷ Social contacts
  ▷ Housing surroundings
  ▷ Climate
  ▷ Altitude
  ▷ Temperature
  ▷ Air pollution

  ▷ Fluoride in water
  ▷ Water contamination
  ▷ Crime
  ▷ Poverty
  ▷ Transportation

Homelessness

Homelessness is an enormous problem affecting the United States and the world. It can have devastating effects on individuals' and families' emotional and physical health. Drugs, alcohol, violence, and behavioral problems are just a few major issues faced by persons who are homeless. The practitioner must be aware of the challenges faced by this vulnerable population. Possessing appropriate communication skills and knowledge of available resources are invaluable.

▶ Homeless person

  ▷ Someone who does not have stable or consistent nighttime housing or who maintains permanent residence at shelters, hotels, transitional housing, or public places not appropriate for human beings to live in; someone intended to be institutionalized who is in an institution for transitory residence

  ▷ Men, women, and children make up the homeless population. The number of homeless families is on the rise.

    ▶ The majority of homeless families are headed by a single parent, usually a woman.

      ▷ Female-headed households are at high risk for becoming homeless if the head of household has limited education or employment skills, low-paying employment with little or no benefits, and limited access to affordable housing.

      ▷ Teen mothers are at high risk due to lack of education and incomes that older parents possess.

▷ Reasons for homelessness:

▶ Mental illness

▶ Addictive disorders

▶ Poverty

▶ Unemployment

▶ Inadequate public assistance

▶ Domestic violence

▶ Lifestyle choice

▶ Mental illness and addictive disorders in the homeless population:

▷ Approximately 50% of homeless people have co-occurring substance use disorders and serious mental illness, including bipolar disorder, schizophrenia, and depression.

▷ Schizophrenia accounts for 15% to 45% of the U.S. homeless population (Sadock, Sadock, & Ruiz, 2015).

▷ Symptoms are often active and untreated.

▷ Untreated serious mental illness results in symptoms such as paranoia, hallucinations, mania, anxiety, and depression, making it difficult for people to maintain employment, relationships, and other activities of daily living.

▷ Homeless people with co-occurring disorders are at a greater risk for violence, medication noncompliance, and treatment resistance.

Strategies for Reducing Homelessness

▶ *Outreach*: Introducing services to homeless persons with serious mental illness in various settings, building an empathetic, consistent, and caring relationship to provide *treatment*

▶ *Integrated care*: Treatment combining mental health and medical care to improve overall functioning in the community; may also include access to dental care and pharmacy services

▷ *Colocation:* Providing mental health and primary care services at a single site

▶ *Supporting services to persons in housing*: Effective in moving homeless persons with serious mental illness directly to independent housing with support and intensive attention

▶ *Prevention*: Beginning with discharge planning in inpatient settings, provide resources for mental health care, housing, transitioning service, and follow-up

Migrant and Seasonal Farm Workers

▶ *Migrants*: Persons who leave their permanent residences to take agricultural jobs in different locations

▶ *Seasonal*: Workers who travel from their permanent residences seasonally for agricultural employment

▶ Men, women, and children of all cultures

▶ It is estimated that more than 3 million migrant and seasonal farm workers work in the United States (National Center for Farmworker Health, 2009).

▷ Hard to get an accurate census because families and workers move a great deal

▶ Working conditions, problems with the process of acculturation, isolation, discrimination, and impaired access to health care play a role in a high prevalence of mental illness among migrant and seasonal farm workers.

▶ Very high incidence of depression, anxiety, and substance abuse

▶ Physical and emotional abuse of women is harder to address because of frequent changes of location.

▶ Meeting the mental health needs of this vulnerable population can pose a challenge because of the ways specific cultures perceive mental illness. Displaying an empathic, understanding, and culturally sensitive attitude is imperative when promoting care to this population.

Sexual Orientation

Possessing a thorough understanding of sexuality is of great importance when communicating with clients of different sexual orientations. The practitioner must possess an open, supportive, sensitive, empathetic attitude toward the client. Understanding the client's viewpoint and what he or she is seeking will help facilitate an effective psychiatric evaluation. In addition, an awareness of the factors the client may have faced because of his or her sexuality is crucial.

▶ *Sexual identity:* How people identify psychologically on a continuum between female and male and to whom they are sexually or affectionately attracted (Sadock, Sadock, & Ruiz, 2015)

▶ *Gender identity:* A person's identity along a continuum between normative constructs of masculinity and femininity

▷ Influences of gender identity may consist of biological and social factors.

▷ Biological factors may include pre- and postnatal hormone levels and gene expression.

▷ Social factors may include gender messages from family, mass media, and cultural attitudes.

▶ *Gender dysphoria:* The formal diagnosis to describe a marked incongruence between one's experienced and expressed gender and the gender assigned at birth (American Psychiatric Association [APA], 2013)

▶ *Sexual orientation:* The direction of sexual attraction; preferred over "sexual preference" or "lifestyle," which imply choice, whereas "orientation" does not; some prefer "sexual identity" because it allows people to determine their own identities. Sexual orientation does not always relate to gender identity.

▷ *Asexual:* Not attracted to either sex

▷ *Bisexual:* Attracted to both sexes

▷ *Heterosexual:* Attracted to the opposite sex

▷ *Homosexual:* Attracted to the same sex

▷ *Transgender*: Umbrella term describing persons whose gender identity does not conform to gender norms associated with the gender they were assigned at birth; does not imply a particular sexual orientation

▷ *Transsexual*: Persons who identify as the opposite gender from the one they were assigned at birth; some change their bodies hormonally and surgically to conform to their gender identity

▷ *LGBTQ*: Lesbian, gay, bisexual, transgender, and queer or questioning

▷ Many clients seek treatment from a provider of the same orientation

▶ *Sexual behavior*: The manner in which humans experience and express their sexuality; includes attracting partners, sexual interactions, and social interactions (Sadock, Sadock, & Ruiz, 2015)

Forensics and Corrections

It is estimated that 15% to 24% of U.S. prisoners have severe mental illness resulting in the need for mental health care. Unfortunately, lack of synchronized care among criminal justice, mental, and public health systems results in repeat incarcerations (Baillargeon et al., 2010; Kushel, Hahn, Evans, Bangsberg, & Moss, 2005). It is essential to remain neutral, calm, and objective, and be skilled in self-reflective techniques as well as acknowledging one's own emotional response and biases when providing care for imprisoned clients. Lyons (2009) recommends that the practitioner compartmentalize emotional responses and biases temporarily then debrief afterward.

▶ *Forensic*: The application of scientific knowledge to legal problems and legal proceedings, for example, in forensic anthropology, forensic dentistry, forensic medicine (legal medicine), forensic pathology, and forensic science

▶ *Forensic science*: The application of a broad range of sciences to answer questions of interest to the legal system; a high-technology field using electron microscopes, lasers, ultraviolet and infrared light, advanced analytical techniques, and computerized databanks to analyze and research evidence

▶ *Forensic nursing*: The practice of nursing when health and legal systems intersect; the forensic nurse provides direct services to individual clients; consultation services to nursing, medical, and legal agencies; and expert court testimony in areas dealing with trauma or investigations of questioned deaths, adequacy of services delivery, and specialized diagnoses of specific conditions as related to nursing

Forensic Versus Correctional

▶ *Forensic*: Nurse–client relationship based on crime committed and investigational aspect of the interaction

▶ *Correctional*: Nurse–client relationship based on offender's current mental health and medical conditions

▶ *Locations*: Emergency departments, prisons (high-, medium-, and low-security units), courts, and police stations (Lyons, 2009)

Forensic Knowledge Base

▶ Relies on evidence-based practice as well as past clinical experience

▶ Incorporates both criminal justice and mental health systems

- ▶ The forensic PMHNP should possess theoretical and practical knowledge of the criminal justice and mental health systems
  - ▷ Function of the court
  - ▷ Litigation procedures
  - ▷ Workings of the criminal justice system
  - ▷ Relevant case law and health litigation
  - ▷ Understanding of mental health, distorted thinking patterns, and impaired cognition
  - ▷ *Competence:* Safety, security, management, and assessment of risk; management of aggression and violence; therapeutic relationship; offending behavior knowledge; prison culture; documentation; medical knowledge; psychopharmacology; and crisis de-escalation (Lyons, 2009)

Forensic Risk Assessment vs. Risk Assessment

- ▶ *Forensic risk assessment:* Protect the public from persons with known mental disorders having dangerous, violent, and criminal histories
- ▶ *Risk assessment:* Psychiatric evaluation performed in emergency department after arrest and before person is confined to a correctional facility (Lyons, 2009)

CASE STUDY 1

Karen Harris is a newly graduated PMHNP. She worked as a psychiatric nurse for 5 years before going to graduate school. She is considering a job at the local community mental health center. The director of the center has told her that her role would consist of seeing mainly adult clients with serious, chronic, and persistent mental illness.

On occasions when the psychiatrist is "busy," Ms. Harris is told she may be expected to see a few children in addition to adults. The director expects Ms. Harris to provide medication management to well-known clients and occasionally to assist in diagnostic evaluations of new clients or clients in crisis. He also expects that she will "from time to time" meet the emergent medical needs of clients who have limited access to primary care providers, including the routine, ongoing care of nonpsychiatric disorders such as diabetes, hypertension, and chronic pain. Ms. Harris has many issues to consider before deciding to take or not take the position.

1. Would Ms. Harris be legally authorized to treat both children and adults?

2. What regulation, rule, or standard should Ms. Harris consult to determine if she is legally allowed to treat both children and adults?

3. What regulation, rule, or standard should Ms. Harris consult to determine if she is legally allowed to treat both physical and psychiatric disorders?

4. What is the role of professional psychiatric nursing organizations in assisting Ms. Harris to determine the scope of practice that is appropriate for her as a new graduate?

Ms. Harris decides not to take that job and instead has been working for about a year as a PMHNP in a nurse-managed primary mental health clinic. One day she is asked to assess a client who is clearly psychotic, experiencing hallucinations and delusions, and expressing verbal threats against many persons at another clinical practice in town who had "malpracticed" them. The client is adamant that he does not wish any treatment and that he is not ill. To care for this client, Ms. Harris has many issues to consider.

5. Is Ms. Harris able to treat the client if he is not consenting to care?

6. What legal standards must be met if she is to treat this client without his consent?

About 5 weeks later the above-mentioned client returns to the clinic for follow-up care. He is clinically stable, on medication, and showing no active symptoms. He is interested in developing a relapse prevention plan and asks Ms. Harris to assist him in this process. Ms. Harris has many issues to consider.

7. Is the inclusion of a durable power of attorney an appropriate strategy in relapse planning for this client?

8. What quality indicators should be considered in planning the client's care with him?

9. What risk management and liability issues should Ms. Harris consider?

CASE STUDY 2

A PMHNP working in a rural mental health clinic is asked by a women's clinic to evaluate Ms. M., a 35-year-old female. Ms. M. insists she is not depressed, but that she has been feeling understandably distressed because she was fired from her job for excessive absenteeism related to "head, neck, and back pain." Ms. M. has difficulty falling and staying asleep, wakes up feeling tearful, and doesn't want to get out of bed. She has become socially isolative and spends hours sitting in front of the television. She has been taking 50 mg of amitriptyline for the past 6 months. The medication has been prescribed by a physician's assistant at a women's clinic. She was last seen at the women's clinic 4 months ago. After evaluating Ms. M., the PMHNP decides that she meets criteria for major depression. He decides to continue the amitriptyline but increases the dose.

1. How should the PMHNP explain his rationale for increasing the dose of the amitriptyline to the client?

2. Since amitriptyline is a tricyclic antidepressant, is it reasonable for the PMHNP to continue and even adjust the dose of this medication—in other words, is this treatment within the scope of the PMHNP's practice?

ANSWERS TO CASE STUDY DISCUSSION QUESTIONS

Case Study 1

1. The key word here is "legally." Professional standards and scope of practice documents suggest what is reasonable and prudent practice. Professional nursing organizations will provide information on what is seen as acceptable educational preparation for practice. However, the individual legislative regulations of each state determine what constitutes legal practice for each individual PMHNP.

2. The Nurse Practice Act and related legislation of the state in which she practices will delineate the legal boundaries of her practice.

3. Professional standards and scope-of-practice documents suggest what is reasonable and prudent practice. The individual legislative regulations of each state determine what constitutes legal practice for each individual PMHNP.

4. Professional nursing organizations provide information through a Scope and Standards document about what is seen as an acceptable practice role for PMHNPs, but the PMHNP's practice is ultimately guided by the individual state's Nurse Practice Act.

5. Any client, including a psychiatric client, has the right to refuse treatment. Ms. Harris is legally and ethically bound to honor the client's rights.

6. Ms. Harris must meet the legal standard in the state where she practices to treat a client against his or her wishes. This usually entails performing the legal task of committing a client and in most states, ensuring that the following criteria are met:

   ▷ The person has a diagnosed psychiatric disorder

   ▷ The person is unaware or unwilling to accept the nature and severity of disorder

   ▷ As a result of a mental disorder, a person is harmful to self or others

   ▷ As a result of a mental disorder, a person cannot take care of his or her basic needs of food, clothing, and shelter

7. A durable power of attorney allows a person in a state of health to choose another person to act on his or her behalf should he or she become unable to make his or her own healthcare decisions. Chronic mental illness has the potential to render a person unable to make healthcare decisions, and a durable power of attorney document should be part of relapse planning.

8. Standardized client assessment and rating scales, evidence-based standards of care, and measures of quality, including client and family satisfaction, should be considered.

9. Ms. Harris should adhere to standards and scope of practice and identify factors specific to this client that increase liability exposure.

Case Study 2

1. The PMHNP must discuss the treatment plan in the context of the client's psychiatric symptoms. Without trying to convince the client that she has major depression, the PMHNP can discuss how chronic pain may have led to the distress she is

currently experiencing and that the medication may address many of her distressing symptoms. He will also need to address the potential side effects from this tricyclic antidepressant, and the usual course of treatment in terms of dosing and timeline.

2. Yes, if the PMHNP is using the medication to target the client's depressive symptoms and if he believes the benefit-to-risk ratio is reasonable in this instance, it is reasonable for the PMHNP to continue the medication and adjust the dose. The PMHNP must do all the relevant medical tests to prescribe this medication.

REFERENCES AND RESOURCES

Abood, S. (2007). Influencing health care in the legislative arena. *Online Journal of Issues in Nursing, 12*(1), 3.

Accreditation Commission for Education in Nursing. (2016). *Accreditation manual.* Retrieved from http://www.acenursing.org/accreditation-manual/

American Association of Colleges of Nursing. (2013). *CCNE: Commission on Collegiate Nursing Education.* Retrieved from http://www.aacn.nche.edu/ccne-accreditation/why-accreditation

American Nurses Association. (2000). *Medicare and "incidental to" payment: Coverage of nursing services in hospital outpatient clinics and emergency departments.* Washington, DC: Author.

American Nurses Association. (2014). *Psychiatric–mental health nursing: Scope and standards of practice* (2nd ed.). Silver Spring, MD: Author.

American Nurses Association. (2015). *Code of ethics for nurses with interpretive statements.* Silver Spring, MD: Nursebooks.org.

American Nurses Credentialing Center. (2015). Psychiatric–Mental Health Nurse Practitioner Certification eligibility criteria (across the lifespan) (formerly known as Family Psychiatric–Mental Health Nurse Practitioner). Retrieved from http://www.nursecredentialing.org/FamilyPsychNP-Eligibility.aspx

American Psychiatric Association. (2013). *Diagnostic and statistical manual of mental disorders* (5th ed.). Washington, DC: Author.

American Psychiatric Nurses Association. (2011). APNA Board of Directors endorses APNA/ISPN Joint Task Force recommendation on the implementation of the 'Consensus model for APRN regulation: Licensure, accreditation, certification & education.' Retrieved from http://www.apna.org/files/public/LACE.pdf

Baillargeon, J., Penn, J. V., Knight, K., Harzke, A. J., Baillargeon, G., & Becker, E. A. (2010). Risk of reincarceration among prisoners with co-occurring severe mental illness and substance use disorders. *Administrative Policy in Mental Health, 37*(4),

Brownson, R. C., & Petitti, D. (2006). *Applied epidemiology: Theory to practice* (2nd ed.). London, Eng.: Oxford University Press.

Buppert, C. (2012). *Nurse practitioners business practice and legal guide* (4th ed.). Sudbury, MA: Jones & Bartlett Learning.

Burgess, A. W. (1998). *Advanced practice psychiatric nursing.* Stamford, CT: Appleton & Lange.

Commission on Collegiate Nursing Education. (2016). CCNE accreditation. Retrieved from http://www.aacn.nche.edu/ccne-accreditation

Cotroneo, M., Kurlowicz, L. H., Outlaw, F. H., Burgess, A. W., & Evans, L. K. (2001). Psychiatric–mental health nursing at the interface: Revisioning education for the specialty. *Issues in Mental Health Nursing, 22,* 549–569.

Delaney, K., Chisholm, M., Clement, J., & Merwin, E. (1999). Trends in psychiatric mental health education. *Archives of Psychiatric Nursing, 13*(2), 67–73.

Donabedian, A. (1988). The quality of care. How can it be assessed? *JAMA, 260*(12), 1743–1748.

Edmunds, M. W., Horan, N. M., & Mayhew, M. S. (2000). *Adult nurse practitioner review manual.* Washington, DC: American Nurses Association.

Farnam, C., Zipple, A. M., Tyrell, W., & Chittiinanda, P. (1999). Health status risk factors of people with severe and persistent mental illness. *Journal of Psychosocial Nursing, 37,* 16–19.

Fineout-Overholt, E., Melnyk, B. M., & Schultz, A. (2005). Transforming health care from the inside out: Advancing evidence-based practice in the 21st century. *Journal of Professional Nursing, 21*(6), 335–344.

Friedman, D. J., Parrish, G., & Ross, D. A. (2013). Electronic health records and US public health: current realities and future promise. *American Journal of Public Health, 103*(9), 1560–1567.

Friedman, M. (2002). *Family nursing: Research, theory, and practice* (5th ed.). Stamford, CT: Appleton & Lange.

Ford, L. C. (1992). Advancing nursing practice: Future of the nurse practitioner. In L. H. Aiken & C. M. Fagin (Eds.), *Charting nursing's future: Agenda for the 1990s.* Philadelphia, PA: J. B. Lippincott.

Harris, E., & Barraclough, B. (1999). Excess mortality of mental disorder. *British Journal of Psychiatry, 173,* 476–481.

Health Insurance Portability and Accountability Act (HIPAA). Pub. L. 104–1, 110 Stat. 1936 (1996).

Health Resources and Services Administration. (2013). *Health IT adoption toolbox: Meaningful use.* Retrieved from http://www.hrsa.aquilentprojects.com/healthit/toolbox/HealthITAdoptiontoolbox/MeaningfulUse/index.html

Institute for the Future. (2000). *Health and health care 2010: The forecast, the challenge.* San Francisco, CA: Jossey-Bass.

Institute of Medicine. (2001). *Crossing the quality chasm: A new health system for the 21st century.* Washington, DC: National Academies Press.

Institute of Medicine. (2010). *The future of nursing: Leading change, advancing health.* Available from https://iom.nationalacademies.org/Reports/2010/The-Future-of-Nursing-Leading-Change-Advancing-Health.aspx

Johnson, M., Maas, M., & Moorhead, S. (Eds.). (2003). *Nursing outcomes classification* (3rd ed.). St. Louis, MO: Mosby.

Kushel, M. B., Hahn, J. A., Evans, J. L., Bangsberg, D. R., & Moss, A. R. (2005). Revolving doors: imprisonment among the homeless and marginally housed population. *American Journal of Public Health, 95*(10), 1747–1752.

Lyons, T. (2009). Role of the forensic psychiatric nurse. *Journal of Forensic Nursing, 5,* 53–57.

Macnee, C., & McCabe, S. (2000). Micro stressors: The impact of hassles and uplifts. In V. H. Rice (Ed.), *Handbook of stress and coping: Implications for nursing research, theory, and practice* (pp. 125–142). Thousand Oaks, CA: Sage.

Matlow, A. G., Wright, J. G., & Zimmerman, B. (2006). How can the principles of complexity science be applied to improve the coordination of care for complex pediatric patients? *Quality and Safety in Health Care, 15,* 85–88.

McBride, A., & Austin, J. (1996). *Psychiatric–mental health nursing: Integrating the behavioral and biological sciences.* Philadelphia, PA: W. B. Saunders.

McCabe, S. (2000). Bringing psychiatric nursing into the twenty-first century. *Archives of Psychiatric Nursing, 14*(3), 109–116.

McCabe, S. (2002). The nature of psychiatric nursing: The intersection of paradigm, evolution, and history. *Archives of Psychiatric Nursing, 16*(2), 51–60.

McCabe, S., & Macnee, C. L. (2002). Weaving a new safety net of mental health care in rural America: A model of integrated practice. *Issues in Mental Health Nursing, 23,* 263–278.

McCloskey, J. C., & Bulechek, G. M. (Eds.). (2000). *Nursing interventions classification* (3rd ed.). St. Louis, MO: Mosby/Year Book.

Medical Record Confidentiality Act of 1995, S. 1360, 104th Cong. (1995). Retrieved from https://www.gpo.gov/fdsys/pkg/BILLS-104s1360is/content-detail.html

Mellow, J. (1968). Nursing therapy. *American Journal of Nursing, 68,* 2365–2369.

Melnyk, B. M., Fineout-Overholt, E., Stillwell, S. B., & Williamson, K. (2010). The seven steps of evidence-based practice. *American Journal of Nursing, 110*(1), 51–53.

Mirr Jansen, M., & Zwygart-Stauffacher, M. (2006). *Advanced practice nursing: Core concepts for professional role development* (3rd ed.). New York, NY: Springer Publishing.

Nagle, M., & Krainovich-Miller, B. (2001). Shaping the advanced practice psychiatric nursing role: A futuristic model. *Issues in Mental Health Nursing, 22,* 461–482.

National Center for Farmworker Health. (2009). Migrant and seasonal farmworker demographics. Retrieved from http://www.unctv.org/content/sites/default/files/0000011508-fs-Migrant%20 Demographics.pdf

National Organization of Nurse Practitioner Faculties. (2013). *Psychiatric–mental health nurse practitioner competencies.* Washington, DC: National Panel for Nurse Practitioner Faculties.

National Organization of Nurse Practitioner Faculties. (2014). *Nurse practitioner core competencies content.* Washington, DC: National Panel for Nurse Practitioner Faculties.

Nettina, S. M., & Knudtson, M. (2001). *The family nurse practitioner review manual.* Washington, DC: American Nurses Credentialing Center.

North American Nursing Diagnosis Association. (2000). *Nursing diagnosis: Definitions and classifications 1999–2000.* Philadelphia, PA: Author.

Northouse, P. G. (2007). *Leadership theory and practice* (4th ed.). London, Eng.: Sage Publications.

Peplau, H. (1952). *Interpersonal relations in nursing.* New York, NY: GP Putnam's Sons.

Perese, E. F. (2012). *Psychiatric advanced practice nursing: A biopsychosocial foundation for practice.* Philadelphia, PA: F. A. Davis.

Reinhardt, A. C., & Ray, L. N. (2003). Differentiating quality improvement from research. *Applied Nursing Research, 16*(1), 2–8.

Richardson, K. A., Cilliers, P., & Lissack, M. (2001). Complexity science: A "gray" science for the "stuff in between." *Emergence, Complexity and Organization, 3*(2), 6–18.

Richardson, W. S., Wilson, M. C., Nishikawa, J., & Hayward, R. S. (1995). The well-built clinical question: A key to evidence-based decisions. *ACP Journal Club, 123*(3), A12–A13.

Sadock, B., Sadock, V., & Ruiz, P. (2015). *Kaplan and Sadock's synopsis of psychiatry: Behavioral sciences/clinical psychiatry* (11th ed.). Philadelphia, PA: Wolters Kluwer.

Sherwood, G. D., & Horton-Deutsch, S. (2012). *Reflective practice transforming education and improving outcomes.* Indianapolis, IN: Sigma Theta Tau International.

Shea, C. A., Pelletier, L., Poster, E. C., Stuart, G. W., & Verhey, M. P. (1999). *Advanced practice nursing in psychiatric and mental health care.* St. Louis, MO: Mosby.

Stuart, G. W. (2013). *Principles and practice of psychiatric nursing* (10th ed.). St. Louis, MO: Mosby.

Tarasoff v. Regents at the University of California, 17 Cal. 3d 425, 551 P. 2d 334, 131 Cal. Rptr. 14 (Cal. 1976).

U.S. Department of Health and Human Services. (2000). *Mental health: A report of the Surgeon General.* Washington, DC: Substance Abuse and Mental Health Service Administration, National Institute of Mental Health.

U.S. Department of Health and Human Services. (2005). *Healthy people 2010.* Washington, DC: Office of Disease Prevention and Health Promotion.

U.S. Department of Health and Human Services, Office for Civil Rights. (2013). Modifications to the HIPAA privacy, security, enforcement, and breach notification rules under the Health Information Technology for Economic and Clinical Health Act and the Genetic Information Nondiscrimination Act; other modifications to the HIPAA rules. *Federal Register, 78*(17). https://www.gpo.gov/fdsys/pkg/FR-2013-01-25/pdf/2013-01073.pdf

U.S. Department of Health, Education, and Welfare. (1979). *The Belmont report.* Washington, DC: Author.

World Health Organization. (2010). International classification of diseases (10th rev.). Geneva, CH: World Health Organization Assembly.

CHAPTER 3

THEORETICAL BASIS OF CARE

Although the psychiatric–mental health nurse practitioner (PMHNP) role is relatively new, psychiatric–mental health nursing has a long, well-established, and cherished tradition of advanced practice. As with all other specialty areas of nursing, advanced practice psychiatric nursing is theoretically grounded, and a wide array of theories form the basis of the PMHNP role. These theories help identify the foundational, core concepts of advanced-practice psychiatric nursing. The scope of practice for the PMHNP is based on an understanding of foundational core concepts and theories (Alligood, 2014).

This chapter reviews the concepts of biopsychosocial theories that underpin PMHNP practice.

BIOPSYCHOSOCIAL FRAMEWORK OF CARE

Recovery

▶ Recovery is the single most important goal in the transformation of mental health care of the past 2 decades. Four major dimensions of recovery include: health, home, purpose, and community (U.S. Department of Health and Human Services [DHHS], Substance and Mental Health Services Administration, 2015).

▶ PMHNP interventions follow evidence-based practice guidelines, are always client goal–directed, and take into account the client's ethnicity and culture.

▶ PMHNPs help clients to recognize strengths, set attainable goals, and have hope for their future.

▶ A key part of the PMHNP's work is to use empirical evidence in educating their clients, clients' families, and the community about mental health, psychiatric illness, and effective management of illness.

▶ The PMHNP oversees and guides the psychiatric–mental health nurse in designing evidence-based health information and educational programs that are geared to consumer learning needs, ability, and readiness to learn.

▶ PMHNPs care for people with co-occurring medical and psychiatric disorders.

▶ Principles of mental health recovery are integrated into all levels of mental health care (American Psychiatric Nurses Association [APNA], 2012).

CLASSIFICATION OF PSYCHIATRIC DISORDERS: DSM-5

▶ Prior to May of 2013, psychiatric disorders were classified using standard criteria of the *Diagnostic and Statistical Manual of Mental Disorders* (DSM-IV-TR; American Psychiatric Association [APA], 2000).

▶ Unlike previous editions, the DSM-5 does not use multiaxial classifications (APA, 2013).

▶ The DSM-5 classifies mental illnesses on the basis of specific criteria that have been tested for reliability when used by mental health professionals.

▶ Emphasizes dimensional assessments

THERAPEUTIC RELATIONSHIP

▶ Assumes the client and nurse enter into a mutual, interactive, interpersonal relationship specifically to focus on the identified needs of the client

▶ Therapeutic relationships are focused on the client's needs, and are goal-directed, theory-based, and open to supervision.

▶ The following are a few characteristics of a therapeutic relationship:

▷ Genuineness

▷ Acceptance

▷ Nonjudgment

▷ Authenticity

▷ Empathy

▷ Respect

▷ Professional boundaries

▶ The therapeutic relationship has specific and sequential phases (see Table 3–1).

▶ Transference and countertransference are key concepts in the nurse–client relationship.

▷ *Transference*: Displacement of feelings for significant people in the client's past onto the PMHNP in the present relationship

▷ *Countertransference*: The nurse's emotional reaction to the client based on her or his past experiences

▶ Signs indicating the presence of countertransference in the PMHNP include

▷ Intense emotional reactions, positive or negative, on first contact with client;

▷ Recurrent anxiety or uneasiness while dealing with the client;

▷ Uncharacteristic carelessness in interaction and follow-up with client;

▷ Difficulty empathizing;

▷ Resistance to others treating or interacting with the client;

▷ Preoccupation with or dreaming about the client;

TABLE 3–1.
PHASES OF A THERAPEUTIC NURSE–CLIENT RELATIONSHIP

PHASE	NURSING ACTION	COMMON CLIENT BEHAVIOR
Introduction (Orientation)	Creating a trusting environment Establishing professional boundaries Establishing the length of anticipated interaction Providing diagnostic evaluation Setting mutually agreed-upon treatment objectives	Initial hesitancy by the client to participate fully in assessment and treatment planning (approach avoidance)
Working (Identification and Exploitation)	Clarifying client expectations and mutually set goals Implementing treatment plan Monitoring health Undertaking preventative health care Measuring outcomes of care Evaluating outcomes of care Reprioritizing plan and objectives as indicated	Transference—client (countertransference—nurse) Client resistance to care practices Client resistance to change
Termination (Resolution)	Reviewing client's progress toward objectives Establishing long-term plan of care Focusing on self-management strategies Disengaging from relationship Referring client to other services as needed	Client resistance to termination Regression Reemergence of symptoms or problems

Note. Adapted from Keltner, N., Schwecke, L. H., & Bostrom, C. E. (2006). *Psychiatric nursing* (5th ed.). St. Louis, MO: Mosby.

   ▷ Frequently running overtime or cutting time short with client;

   ▷ Depression or other strong emotions during or after interaction with client; and

   ▷ Feedback from others over involvement with client.

▶ The PMHNP is expected to monitor her or his reaction to clients to constantly assess for the presence of countertransference.

▶ If identified, countertransference is usually dealt with through the supervisory process and in talking to coworkers about the issues.

   ▷ Provided in peer–peer or peer–supervisor relationship

   ▷ Examines interpersonal dynamics inherent in the PMHNP's relationship with clients

DEVELOPMENTAL THEORIES

▶ Growth, change, and development are a part of the dynamic, constant life process of being human.

▶ Humans develop uniquely from simple to complex.

▶ The health states of individuals and families can be viewed over a continuum of development.

▶ Developmental stages and the milestones or tasks that accompany them give insight into age-appropriate behaviors, measure levels of comprehension for client teaching, and provide a context within which to evaluate assessment data (see Table 3–2).

TABLE 3–2.
ERIK ERIKSON'S (1902–1994) STAGES OF HUMAN DEVELOPMENT

DEVELOPMENTAL STAGE	AGE	DEVELOPMENTAL TASK	INDICATIONS OF DEVELOPMENTAL MASTERY	INDICATIONS OF DEVELOPMENTAL FAILURE
Infancy	Birth–1 year	Trust vs. mistrust	Ability to form meaningful relationships, hope about the future, trust in others	Poor relationships, lack of future hope, suspicious of others
Early childhood	1–3 years	Autonomy vs. shame and doubt	Self-control, self-esteem, willpower	Poor self-control, low self-esteem, self-doubt, lack of independence
Late childhood	3–6 years	Initiative vs. guilt	Self-directed behavior, goal formation, sense of purpose	Lack of self-initiated behavior, lack of goal orientation
School-age	6–12 years	Industry vs. inferiority	Ability to work; sense of competency and achievement	Sense of inferiority; difficulty with working, learning
Adolescence	12–20 years	Identity vs. role confusion	Personal sense of identity	Identity confusion, poor self-identification in group settings
Early adulthood	20–35 years	Intimacy vs. isolation	Committed relationships, capacity to love	Emotional isolation, egocentrism
Middle adulthood	35–65 years	Generativity vs. self-absorption or stagnation	Ability to give time and talents to others, ability to care for others	Self-absorption, inability to grow and change as a person, inability to care for others
Late adulthood	>65	Integrity vs. despair	Fulfillment and comfort with life, willingness to face death, insight and balanced perspective on life's events	Bitterness, sense of dissatisfaction with life, despair over impending death

Note. Adapted from Sadock, B. J., Sadock, V. A., & Ruiz, P. (2015). *Kaplan and Sadock's synopsis of psychiatry* (11th ed.). Philadelphia, PA: Wolters Kluwer.

▷ Example: The mental status finding of concrete thinking in a 9-year-old client would be normal and expected; however, the same finding in a 29-year-old client is nonnormative and suggestive of psychopathology (see Table 3–3 for typical age of onset for psychiatric disorders).

FOUNDATIONAL THEORIES SUPPORTING PMHNP ROLE

▶ Psychodynamic (Psychoanalytic) Theory (Sigmund Freud, 1856–1939)

▷ Focus is on concepts of intrapsychic conflict among the structures of the mind

▷ Initially designed to explain neurosis and conditions of high anxiety such as phobias and hysteria

▷ Theory later expanded to include normal and abnormal development and personality development

▷ Basic tenets of psychodynamic theory

▶ Psychoanalytical theory assumes that all behavior is purposeful and meaningful. All behavior has meaning.

▶ *Principle of Psychic Determinism*: Even apparently meaningless, random, or accidental behavior is actually motivated by underlying unconscious mental content.

▷ Example: A person forgets where he parked the car because he really does not wish to go wherever it was that he was headed.

▶ Most mental activity is unconscious—urges, feelings, and fantasies that would be unacceptable to the person's values if consciously experienced.

▶ Conscious behaviors and choices are affected by unconscious mental content.

▶ Childhood experiences shape adult personality.

TABLE 3–3.
EXAMPLES OF TYPICAL AGE OF ONSET FOR COMMON PSYCHIATRIC DISORDERS

DISORDER	AGE OF ONSET
Intellectual Disability	Infancy—usually evident at birth
Attention deficit hyperactivity disorder	Early childhood (per DSM-5, by age 12)
Schizophrenia	18 to 25 years for men 25 to 35 years for women
Major depression	Late adolescence to young adulthood
Dementia	Most common after age 85

Note. Adapted from Sadock, B. J., Sadock, V. A., & Ruiz, P. (2015). *Kaplan and Sadock's synopsis of psychiatry* (11th ed.). Philadelphia, PA: Wolters Kluwer.

▶ Instincts, urges, or fantasies function as drives that motivate thoughts, feelings, and behaviors.

   ▷ Two types of normal drives: sexual drives (libido) and aggressive drives

   ▷ Drives affect behavior as an individual attempts to deal with the associated feelings and seeks gratification through release of the tension that the drives produce.

   ▷ Normally, different actions or behaviors are used at different ages to discharge tension from drives and seek gratification.

   ▷ Psychosexual stages of development have been identified to show the age-related behaviors commonly used for discharging drives and obtaining gratification (see Table 3–4).

▷ Three primary psychic structures make up the mind and personality and are responsible for mental functioning:

  1. The Id

   ▷ Contains primary drives or instincts, urges (hunger, sex, or aggression), or fantasies

   ▷ Drives are largely unconscious, sexual, or aggressive in content, and infantile in nature

   ▷ Operates on the pleasure principle; seeks immediate satisfaction

   ▷ Is present at birth and motivates early infantile actions

   ▷ The id says, "I want"

TABLE 3–4.
FREUD'S PSYCHOSEXUAL STAGES OF DEVELOPMENT

STAGE	AGE	PRIMARY MEANS OF DISCHARGING DRIVES AND ACHIEVING GRATIFICATION	PSYCHIATRIC DISORDER LINKED TO FAILURE OF STAGE
Oral stage	0–18 months	Sucking, chewing, feeding, crying	Schizophrenia Substance abuse Paranoia
Anal stage	18 months–3 years	Sphincter control, activities of expulsion and retention	Depressive disorders
Phallic stage	3–6 years	Exhibitionism, masturbation with focus on Oedipal conflict, castration anxiety, and female fear of lost maternal love	Sexual identity disorders
Latency stage	6 years–puberty	Peer relationships, learning, motor-skills development, socialization	Inability to form social relationships
Genital stage	Puberty forward	Integration and synthesis of behaviors from early stages, primary genital-based sexuality	Sexual perversion disorders

Note. Adapted from Sadock, B. J., Sadock, V. A., & Ruiz, P. (2015). *Kaplan and Sadock's synopsis of psychiatry* (11th ed.). Philadelphia, PA: Wolters Kluwer.

2. The Ego

▷ Contains the concept of *external* reality

▷ Rational mind; responsible for logical and abstract thinking

▷ Functions in adaptation

▷ Mediates between the demands of drives and environmental realities

▷ Operates on the reality principle

▷ Begins to develop at birth as infant struggles to deal with environment

▷ Responsible for use of defense mechanisms

▷ The ego says, "I think, I evaluate"

3. The Superego

▷ Is the ego-ideal

▷ Contains sense of conscience or right versus wrong

▷ Also contains aspirations, ideals, and moral values

▷ Regulated by guilt and shame

▷ Begins to fully develop around age six as a child comes into contact with external authority figures such as other parents, schoolteachers, coaches, or religious figures

▷ The superego says "I should or ought"

▷ Psychic structures commonly come into conflict over what to do to achieve gratification.

▷ Although the exact nature of conflict is often unconscious, conflict is experienced consciously as anxiety.

▷ The function of anxiety is to alert the conscious mind to the presence of conflict.

▷ Conflict is normally dealt with through the use of defense mechanisms (see Table 3–5), which

▶ Are a function of the ego,

▶ Are unconsciously called into action,

▶ Are used to reduce anxiety,

▶ Become part of the personality,

▶ Maintain a sense of safety,

▶ Promote self-esteem and a sense of well-being,

▶ May be used episodically or habitually, and

▶ May be used constantly and become fixed, as seen in neurosis.

▶ Cognitive Theory (Jean Piaget, 1896–1980)

▷ Piaget believed that human development evolves through cognition, learning, and comprehending.

TABLE 3–5.
DEFENSE MECHANISMS

DEFENSE MECHANISM	EXPLANATION
Denial	Avoidance of unpleasant realities by unconsciously ignoring their existence
Projection	Unconscious rejection of emotionally unacceptable personal attributes, beliefs, or actions by attributing them to other people, situations, or events
Regression	Return to more comfortable thoughts, behaviors, or feelings used in earlier stages of development in response to current conflict, stress, or threat
Repression	Unconscious exclusion of unwanted, disturbing emotions, thoughts, or impulses from conscious awareness
Reaction formation	Often called overcompensation; unacceptable feelings, thoughts, or behaviors are pushed from conscious awareness by displaying and acting on the opposite feeling, thought, or behavior
Rationalization	Justification of illogical, unreasonable ideas, feelings, or actions by developing an acceptable explanation that satisfies the person
Undoing	Behaviors that attempt to make up for or undo an unacceptable action, feeling, or impulse
Intellectualization	Attempts to master current stressor or conflict by expansion of knowledge, explanation, or understanding
Suppression	Conscious analog of repression; conscious denial of a disturbing situation, feeling, or event
Sublimation	Unconscious process of substitution of socially acceptable, constructive activity for strong unacceptable impulse
Altruism	Meeting the needs of others in order to discharge drives, conflicts, or stressors

Note. Adapted from Shea, C. A., Pelletier, L., Poster, E. C., Stuart, G. W., & Verhey, M. P. (1999). *Advanced practice nursing in psychiatric and mental health care.* St. Louis, MO: Mosby.

▷   He believed that factors such as native endowment and biological and environmental factors set the course for a child's development.

▷   He described four stages of cognitive development:

1. *Sensorimotor* (Birth–2 years): The critical achievement of this stage is object permanence: the ability to understand that objects have an existence independent of the child's involvement with them

2. *Preoperational* (2–7 years): More extensive use of language and symbolism; magical thinking

3. *Concrete Operations* (7–12 years): Child begins to use logic; develops concepts of reversibility and conservation

    ▷   *Reversibility:* The realization that one thing can turn into another and back again (e.g., water and ice)

    ▷   *Conservation:* Ability to recognize that although the shape of an object may change, it will still maintain characteristics that enable it to be recognized as that object (e.g., clay)

4. *Formal Operations* (12 years–adult): Ability to think abstractly; thinking operates in a formal, logical manner

▶ Interpersonal Theory (Harry Stack Sullivan, 1892–1949)

▷ Behavior occurs because of interpersonal dynamics.

▷ Interpersonal relationships and experiences influence one's personality development, which is called the *self-system* (the total components of personality traits).

▷ Understanding behavior requires understanding the relationships in the person's life.

▷ Two drives for behavior: the *drive for satisfaction* (basic human drives such as sleep, sex, hunger) and the *drive for security* (conforming to social norms of a person's reference group).

▷ When the person's need for satisfaction and security is interfered with by the self-system, mental illness occurs.

▷ Humans experience anxiety and behavior is directed toward relieving the anxiety, which then results in *interpersonal security*.

▷ Sullivan also described stages of *interpersonal development* (see Table 3–6).

▶ Hierarchy of Needs Theory (Abraham Maslow, 1908–1970)

▷ Health model rather than illness model

▷ A hierarchical organization of needs

▷ Hypothesizes that certain needs are more important to than others

▷ States that a person will attempt to meet more important needs first before satisfying other needs

▷ Hierarchy of needs:

  ▶ Survival

    ▷ Water

    ▷ Air

    ▷ Food

    ▷ Sleep

TABLE 3–6.
SULLIVAN'S STAGES OF INTERPERSONAL DEVELOPMENT

STAGE	TIME PERIOD	DEVELOPMENTAL TASK
Infancy	Birth–18 months	Oral gratification; anxiety occurs for the first time
Childhood	18 months–6 years	Delayed gratification
Juvenile	6–9 years	Forming of peer relationships
Preadolescence	9–12 years	Same-sex relationships
Early adolescence	12–14 years	Opposite-sex relationships
Late adolescence	14–21 years	Self-identity developed

Note. Adapted from Sadock, B. J., Sadock, V. A., & Ruiz, P. (2015). *Kaplan and Sadock's synopsis of psychiatry* (11th ed.). Philadelphia, PA: Wolters Kluwer.

- ▶ Safety and security needs
  - ▷ Protection from harm: emotional and physical
- ▶ Love and belonging
  - ▷ Affection, intimacy, and companionship
- ▶ Self-esteem
  - ▷ Sense of worth
- ▶ Self-actualization
  - ▷ Achieving one's potential
  - ▷ Being all that one can be
- ▶ Health Belief Model (Marshall Becker, 1940–1993)
  - ▷ Explains that healthy people do not always take advantage of screening or preventative programs because of the following certain variables:
    - ▶ Perception of susceptibility
    - ▶ Seriousness of illness
    - ▶ Perceived benefits of treatment
    - ▶ Perceived barriers to change
    - ▶ Expectations of efficacy
- ▶ Transtheoretical Model of Change
  - ▷ States that change such as in health behaviors occurs in six predictable stages (Prochaska, Norcross, & DiClemente, 1992):
    1. *Precontemplation:* The person has no intention to change.
    2. *Contemplation:* The person is thinking about changing; is aware that there is a problem but not committed to changing.
    3. *Preparation:* The person has made the decision to change; is ready for action.
    4. *Action:* The person is engaging in specific, overt actions to change.
    5. *Maintenance:* The person is engaging in behaviors to prevent relapse.
- ▶ Motivational Interviewing (Miller & Rollnick, 1991)
  - ▷ Focused, goal-directive therapy
  - ▷ Builds on the Transtheoretical Model of Change
  - ▷ Motivation is elicited from the client
  - ▷ Nonconfrontational, nonadversarial
- ▶ Self-Efficacy and Social Learning Theory (Albert Bandura, born 1925)
  - ▷ Behavior is the result of cognitive and environmental factors.
  - ▷ People learn by observing others, relying on role-modeling.
  - ▷ *Self-efficacy* is the perception of one's ability to perform a certain task at a certain level of accomplishment.

▷ Behavioral change and maintenance are functions of outcome expectations and efficacy expectations.

NURSING THEORIES

▶ Theory of Cultural Care (Madeline Leininger, born 1925)

▷ Regardless of the culture, care is the unifying focus and the essence of nursing.

▷ Health and well-being can be predicted through cultural care.

▶ Theory of Self-Care (Dorothy Orem, 1914–2007)

▷ *Self-care*: Activities that maintain life, health, and well-being

▶ Therapeutic Nurse–Client Relationship Theory or Interpersonal Theory (Hildegard Peplau, 1909–1999)

▷ First significant psychiatric nursing theory

▷ Based in part on interpersonal theory (Sullivan, 1953)

▷ Sees nursing as an interpersonal process in which all interventions occur within the context of the nurse–client relationship

▷ The therapeutic nurse–client relationship is central to nursing

▷ Includes phases of the nurse–client relationship (see Table 3–2 above):

▶ Orientation phase

▶ Working phase (identification, exploitation)

▶ Termination phase (resolution)

▷ Promoting adaptive responses is the goal of nursing

▷ Behavior represents the person trying to adapt to internal or environmental forces

▶ Caring Theory (Jean Watson, born 1940)

▷ Caring is an essential component of nursing.

▷ "Carative factors" guide the core of nursing and should be implemented in health care.

▷ Carative factors are those aspects of care that potentiate therapeutic healing and relationships.

CASE STUDY 1

Thomas is a 19-year-old college freshman. During the second week of classes, he presented to his college's student health services clinic seeking help for "shyness." The PMHNP is responsible for assessment and care planning with this client.

As the PMHNP begins working with him, he gives a chief complaint of feeling uncomfortable meeting new people and desiring to return home and drop out of school. The PMHNP has several issues to consider as he or she continues to work with Thomas.

1. Chronologically, what stage of development should Thomas be experiencing?

2. What are the tasks of this stage?

3. How would the PMHNP assess the actual developmental issues that he is experiencing?

4. What factors does the PMHNP need to consider to determine whether he is experiencing normative or nonnormative behaviors?

5. What characteristic does the PMHNP need to display to establish a therapeutic relationship with him?

Thomas reported that he has not been sleeping well, has experienced a decrease in appetite, and just wants to talk to someone about his problems in adjusting to school. In planning the follow-up care for Thomas, the PMHNP has many issues to consider.

6. What would be the goal of continued work with Thomas?

7. If the PMHNP were to start therapy with him, what kind of therapy would he or she consider?

8. According to DSM-5, does Thomas have a mental illness?

CASE STUDY 2

Jason is an 18-year-old, second-semester business major who presents to his university's mental health clinic because "my parents said I have to come here or they will pull me out of school. I don't think I need to be here." Jason is on academic probation. The PMHNP learns that Jason's parents grew alarmed when, while home on holiday, Jason was brought home by police after he and his friend were pulled over and friend was given a DUI. Jason allows that perhaps he "partied too much" during his first semester at school, but insists he "doesn't drink any more than anybody else." Jason reluctantly agrees to see the PMHNP for an evaluation and for 8 weekly psychotherapy sessions "to please my parents."

1. What defense mechanism(s) is Jason using?

2. How should the PMHNP approach working with this client?

ANSWERS TO CASE STUDY DISCUSSION QUESTIONS

Case Study 1

1. Thomas's chronologic age should align with the developmental stage of adolescence.

2. According to Erikson, the developmental task of adolescence is identity versus role confusion.

3. The PMHNP should assess the degree of development of his personal sense of identity.

4. The PMHNP must have an awareness of the normal milestones of development and the behaviors that indicate failure of developmental stages. The client's history and behaviors are then matched to the known norm for comparison.

5. In order to develop a therapeutic relationship with Thomas, the PMHNP must display genuineness, acceptance, nonjudgmental attitude, authenticity, empathy, and respect professional boundaries.

6. The goals of continued work with Thomas are assisting Thomas to establish insight into behaviors and to increase range and maturity of coping behaviors.

7. Options for psychotherapy depend on factors such as a client's goals, motivation, past experiences with counseling, expectations for therapy, and resources.

8. Mental illness causes a disruption in the usual constitutions of mental health. Mental illness assumes an underlying psychopathology and can be defined as a clinically significant behavioral or psychological syndrome or pattern that occurs in a person that is associated with persistent distress or disability or with a significantly increased risk of death, pain, or an important loss of freedom. Thomas appears to be experiencing mental health concerns but based on available data, does not meet the definition of mental illness.

Case Study 2

1. Jason is using denial and rationalization.

2. The PMHNP needs to work with Jason to establish goals using the principles of the Transtheoretical Model of Change and motivational interviewing.

REFERENCES AND RESOURCES

Alligood, M. R. (2014). *Nursing theorists and their work* (8th ed.). St. Louis, MO: Elsevier Mosby.

American Nurses Association, American Psychiatric Nurses Association, & International Society of Psychiatric-Mental Health Nurses. (2014). *Psychiatric–mental health nursing: Scope and standards of practice* (2nd ed.). Silver Spring, MD: Nursesbooks.org.

American Psychiatric Association. (2000). *Diagnostic and statistical manual of mental disorders* (4th ed., text rev.). Arlington, VA: American Psychiatric Publishing.

American Psychiatric Association. (2013). *Diagnostic and statistical manual of mental disorders* (5th ed.). Arlington, VA: American Psychiatric Publishing.

Burgess, A. W. (1998). *Advanced practice psychiatric nursing*. Stamford, CT: Appleton & Lange.

Erikson, E. H. (1963). *Childhood and society.* New York, NY: Basic Books.

Freud, S. (1934). *The ego and the id*. New York, NY: W. W. Norton.

Freud, S. (1936). *The problem of anxiety*. New York, NY: Basic Books.

Haley, J. (1996). *Learning and teaching therapy*. New York, NY: Guilford Press.

Keltner, N., Schwecke, L. H., & Bostrom, C. E. (2006). *Psychiatric nursing* (5th ed.). St. Louis, MO: Mosby.

Kerr, M., & Bowen, M. (1989). *Family evaluation: An approach based on Bowen theory*. New York, NY: W. W. Norton.

Marsh, D. (1998). Serious mental illness and the family: The practitioner's guide. New York, NY: John Wiley.

Miller, W. R., & Rollnick, S. (1991). *Motivational interviewing: Preparing people for change*. New York, NY: Guilford Press.

Minuchin, S., & Fishman, H. (1981). *Family therapy techniques*. Cambridge, MA: Harvard University Press.

Mohr, W. (2000). Partnering with families. *Journal of Psychosocial Nursing, 38*, 15–19.

National Institute of Mental Health. (1990). *Decade of the brain*. Washington, DC: Author.

Peplau, H. (1952). *Interpersonal relations in nursing*. New York, NY: Putnam.

Prochaska, J., & DiClemente, C. (1984). *The transtheoretical approach: Crossing traditional boundaries therapy*. Homewood, IL: Dow Jones Irwin.

Prochaska, J., Norcross, J., & DiClemente, C. (1992). In search of how people change: Applications to addictive behaviors. *American Psychologist, 47*(9), 1102–1112.

Sadock, B., Sadock, V., & Ruiz, P. (2015). *Kaplan and Sadock's synopsis of psychiatry* (11th ed.). New York, NY: Lippincott Williams & Wilkins.

Shea, C. A., Pelletier, L., Poster, E. C., Stuart, G. W., & Verhey, M. P. (1999). *Advanced practice nursing in psychiatric and mental health care*. St. Louis, MO: Mosby.

Sherman, C. (2000). Assessment is good opportunity to change family dynamics. *Clinical Psychiatric News, 3*, 25–29.

Stuart, G. W., & Laraia, M. (2004). *Principles and practice of psychiatric nursing*. St. Louis, MO: Mosby.

Sullivan, H. S. (1953). *Interpersonal theory of psychiatry*. New York, NY: Basic Books.

U.S. Department of Health and Human Services, Substance and Mental Health Services Administration. (2015). *Recovery and recovery support*. Retrieved from http://www.samhsa.gov/recovery

Yalom, I. (2005). *The theory and practice of group psychotherapy* (5th ed.). New York, NY: Basic Books.

CHAPTER 4

PSYCHIATRIC–MENTAL HEALTH NURSE PRACTITIONER PROFESSIONAL ROLE AND HEALTH POLICY: LEADERSHIP, QUALITY IMPROVEMENT AND SAFETY, PRACTICE INQUIRY, AND HEALTH POLICY

LEADERSHIP

Nurses should be leaders and engage with health professionals to transform and redesign health care (Institute of Medicine [IOM], 2010).

- ▶ The nurse practitioner is educated to lead interdisciplinary treatment teams
    - ▷ Acts as full partner in health care
    - ▷ Designs, implements, evaluates, and advocates to redesign the U.S. healthcare system
    - ▷ Translates research into practice
- ▶ Team leadership model
    - ▷ Decision 1: Should the leader monitor the team or take action?
        - ▶ Seek out information to understand the team
        - ▶ Analyze information
        - ▶ Interpret the information and decide how to act
    - ▷ Decision 2: Should the leader intervene to meet the task or relational need?
        - ▶ Performance functions
        - ▶ Task functions
    - ▷ Decision 3: Should the leader intervene internally or externally?

▶ Assess for conflicts between group members—action to maintain group performance

▷ Assess for unclear goals

▷ Assess for proper support (Northouse, 2007, pp. 209–234)

Reflective Practice

▶ Reflection uses a model or framework to systematically "make sense of experience" (Sherwood & Horton-Deutsch, 2012, p. 4).

▶ Process to tell a story about self and others to gain insight into practice

▶ Enhances critical thinking to problem-solve and enhance clinical reasoning and decision-making

▶ Link theory to practice

Conflict Resolution, Negotiation, Mediation, and Professional Civility

▶ *Conflict*: occurs when a person believes his or her needs, interests, or values are incompatible with others'

▶ *Conflict resolution*: directed by a neutral third party who facilitates a "win-win" situation

▶ *Negotiation*: discussion among two or more people with the goal of reaching an agreement

▶ *Mediation*: voluntary and confidential process in which a third party facilitates discussion to reach an agreement

▶ *Arbitration*: process in which a third party reviews evidence from both sides and makes a decision to settle the case

▶ *Professional civility*: behavior that shows respect toward another person

Critical Thinking

▶ Defined as the acquisition of knowledge with an attitude of deliberate inquiry

▶ Making clinical decisions based on evidence-based practice

▷ Decreases the difficulty of choosing from conflicting or multiple recommendations when diagnosing and treating clients

▶ Develops self-awareness though a metacognitive process to gain new insights about self, and in relation to others

Research

▶ Research utilization: Process of synthesizing, disseminating, and using research-generated knowledge to make a change in practices; a subset of the broader evidence-based practice

▶ *Evidence-based practice:* The integration of best research evidence with clinical expertise and client values and needs. PMHNPs need to know the effectiveness of evidence-based interventions and select the intervention to meet the client need (Perese, 2012, p. 29).

▶ Research utilization and evidence-based practice are two models for reducing the gap between research findings and application to practice

  ▷ Research utilization process

    ▶ Critique research

    ▶ Synthesize the findings

    ▶ Apply the findings

    ▶ Measure the outcomes

▶ Develop a clinical question using the PICO method

  P = patient, population of patients, problem

  I = intervention

  C = comparison (another treatment or therapy, placebo)

  O = outcome

▶ Systematically search for relevant research evidence

  ▷ Critique the research evidence

    ▶ Qualitative hierarchy (Fineout-Overholt, Melnyk, & Schultz, 2005)

      ▷ Randomized controlled trials (RCT), meta-analysis, or systematic review

      ▷ Evidence-based guidelines based on systematic review

      ▷ Evidence from RCT without randomization

      ▷ Evidence from systemic review of descriptive and qualitative studies

      ▷ Evidence from expert opinion or committee reports

    ▶ Quantitative hierarchy (Fineout-Overholt, Melnyk, & Schultz, 2005)

      ▷ Evidence from systematic reviews of descriptive and qualitative studies

      ▷ Evidence from a single descriptive or qualitative study

      ▷ Evidence from expert opinion or committee

      ▷ Evidence-based guideline based on systematic review of RCTs

      ▷ Evidence from well-designed controlled trials without randomization

      ▷ Systematic reviews or meta-analysis

      ▷ Evidence from at least one well-designed RCT

  ▷ Make an evidence-based decision regarding implementation

  ▷ Implement the change, depending on the above decision

  ▷ Evaluate the change

▶ Dissemination

  ▷ Present at local, regional, and national conferences

▷ Publish in peer-reviewed journals

▷ Publish in professional newsletters (Melnyk, Fineout-Overholt, Stillwell, & Williamson, 2010)

▶ Concepts in interpreting research findings

▷ *Internal validity*: The independent variable (the treatment) caused a change in the dependent variable (the outcome)

▷ *External validity*: The sample is representative of the population and the results can be generalized

▷ *Descriptive statistics*: Used to describe the basic features of the data in the study; numerical values that summarize, organize, and describe observations; can be generated by either quantitative or qualitative studies

▶ Examples include

▷ *Mean*: Average of scores

▷ *Standard deviation*: Indication of the possible deviations from the mean

▷ *Variance*: How the values are dispersed around the mean; the larger the variance, the larger the dispersion of scores

▷ *Inferential statistics*: Numerical values that enable one to reach conclusions that extend beyond the immediate data alone; generated by quantitative research designs

▶ Examples include

▷ *t test*: Assesses whether the means of two groups are statistically different from each other

▷ *Analysis of variance (ANOVA)*: Tests the differences among three or more groups

▷ *Pearson's r correlation*: Tests the relationship between two variables

▷ *Probability*: Likelihood of an event occurring; lies between 0 and 1; an impossible event has a probability of 0, and a certain event has a probability of 1

▷ *P value*: Also known as level of significance; describes the probability of a particular result occurring by chance alone (if P = .01, there is a 1% probability of obtaining a result by chance alone)

▶ Ethical considerations in research

▷ *Institutional Review Boards* (IRBs) ensure that

▶ Risks to participants are minimized,

▶ Participant selection is equitable,

▶ Adverse events are reported and risks and benefits are reevaluated,

▶ Informed consent is obtained and documented,

▶ Data and safety monitoring plans are implemented when indicated, and

▶ Overall, that the rights and welfare of human research participants are protected, and has the authority to approve, require modifications, or disapprove of any research activities.

▶ All investigators or persons involved in research studies must take and pass a test on protection of human participants

QUALITY IMPROVEMENT

▶ Agency-specific projects that aim to improve systems, decrease cost, and improve productivity

▶ Provides standardized method to identify gaps in practice and systems to evaluate ways to improve structure, function, and resources in care delivery within complex health systems

▶ Institute of Medicine's quality aims (IOM, 2001)

  ▷ Safe

  ▷ Effective

  ▷ Client-centered

  ▷ Timely

  ▷ Efficient

  ▷ Equitable

▶ Examine internal processes

▶ New knowledge is specific to an organization

▶ Donabedian model

  ▷ Structure

  ▷ Process

  ▷ Outcome

▶ Process of quality improvement can be **PDSA** cycle:

  ▷ **P**lan: Plan the change

  ▷ **D**o: Carry out the plan

  ▷ **S**tudy: Examine the results

  ▷ **A**ct: Decide what actions will improve the process

▶ Translation of research into practice using quality improvement efforts and clinical inquiry leads to improved systems and process, which create improved health outcomes

JUST CULTURE OF SAFETY

▶ American Nurses Association Position Statement (ANA, 2010)

  ▷ Supports collaboration efforts among state boards of nursing, professional organizations, patient safety centers, and health systems to develop Just Culture initiatives

  ▷ Holds people accountable for their behaviors and investigates errors

> ▷ Goal of creating open and fair learning environment to design safe systems and manage choices

> ▷ Mindset that affects work environment to proactively look for system breakdowns and identify ways to improve systems

HEALTH DELIVERY SYSTEMS

▶ Health care is complex and fragmented; complexity science provides a framework to understand, design, and structure change.

▶ Focus is on the interaction of the parts and relationships

▶ Nonlinear process

Access to Care

Access to care is a client-centered care model based on the principle that healthcare services should be coordinated and directed by a single physician or other provider. In this model, clients can access services from multiple entry points. Services can be located in the same facility, or an integrated care network of providers in different locations can be accessed when needed.

Quality of Care

The National Committee for Quality Assurance (NCQA) has developed Health Effectiveness Data Information Sets (HEDIS) to measure health outcomes. Currently, eleven HEDIS measures exist for behavioral health:

1. Antidepressant medication management

2. Follow-up care for children prescribed ADHD medication

3. Follow-up after hospitalization for mental illness

4. Diabetes screening for people with schizophrenia and bipolar disorder who are using antipsychotic medications

5. Diabetes monitoring for people with diabetes and schizophrenia

6. Cardiovascular monitoring for people with cardiovascular disease and schizophrenia

7. Adherence to antipsychotic medications for individuals with schizophrenia

8. Use of multiple concurrent antipsychotics in children and adolescents

9. Metabolic monitoring for children and adolescents on antipsychotic medication

10. Use of first-line psychosocial care for children and adolescents on antipsychotic medication

11. Mental health utilization

Organization of Practices

With the Affordable Care Act (ACA; 2010), practices are being reorganized and redesigned to provided integrated care, including medical and psychiatric care. The client-centered medical (health) home has support of the Health Resources and Services Administration (HRSA) and initiatives to provide client-centered, evidenced-based, coordinated, and quality care are moving forward.

Patient-Centered Care Model (PCC)

▶ *Welcoming environment:* Provide a physical space and an initial personal interaction that is welcoming and familiar, not intimidating.

▶ *Respect for clients' values and expressed needs:* Obtain information about the client's care preferences and priorities; inform and involve the client and family or caregivers in decision-making; tailor care to the person; and promote a mutually respectful, consistent client–provider relationship.

▶ *Client empowerment or "activation":* Educate and encourage the client to expand his or her role in decision-making, health-related behaviors, and self-management.

▶ *Sociocultural competence:* Understand and consider culture, economic and educational status, health literacy level, family patterns and situation, and traditions (including alternative and folk remedies); communicate in language and at a level that the client understands.

▶ *Coordination and integration of care:* Assess the client's need for formal and informal services that may affect health or treatment; provide team-based care, care management, and referrals as needed; advocate for the client and family; and ensure smooth transitions between different providers and phases of care.

▶ *Comfort and support:* Emphasize physical comfort, privacy, emotional support, and involvement of family and friends.

▶ *Access and navigation skills:* Provide what the patient can consider a "medical home"; keep waiting times to a minimum; provide convenient service hours; promote access and client flow; help client attain skills to better navigate the healthcare system.

▶ *Community outreach:* Make demonstrable, proactive efforts to understand and reach out to the local community (Silow-Carroll, Alteras, & Stepnick, 2006).

Health Care Home (Substance Abuse and Mental Health Services Administration [SAMHSA], 2015)

▶ Defined in the Affordable Care Act (2010) as an approach to primary care that provides coordinated care to persons with multiple chronic health conditions, including mental health and substance use

▶ Offers team-based care

▶ Builds on community supports

CONFLICT OF INTEREST

A conflict of interest (COI) is a situation in which a person's financial, professional, or personal situation may affect or appear to affect the person's judgment in his or her professional responsibilities, including healthcare decisions, research, and other matters, with the potential for personal or professional gain or advantage—or, conversely, loss or disadvantage—of any kind and the possibility of potential harm to clients.

▶ Disclosure of potential COIs should be done at least annually and whenever new significant financial interests are received.

▶ Disclosure must be reported to employers, boards, professional agencies, and wherever there is potential for a COI.

▶ Action should be carried out to resolve potential or actual COIs and reduce bias.

▶ Healthcare agencies and educational and research institutions have policies to require the disclosure of any potential COI and to define the limits allowed in any relationship with external organizations and companies.

▶ A COI form indicating any financial or other relationship with the products being discussed must be completed prior to any professional presentation. In addition, if any off-label uses of medications or medical devices will be discussed, this information must also be disclosed.

▶ Types of conflict of interest:

▷ Relationships with pharmaceutical, medical supply, or insurance companies

▷ Money, gifts in kind

▷ Referrals

▷ Fee splitting

RIGHTS OF CLIENTS

▶ Confidentiality

▶ Least restrictive treatment

▶ Give consent for treatment and withdraw consent at any time

HEALTH POLICY DEVELOPMENT

Health policy is decisions, actions, and plans to achieve specific healthcare goals (World Health Organization [WHO], 2016).

▶ Four components of health policy:

1. *Process:* formulation, implementation, and evaluation

2. *Policy reform:* changes in programs and practices

3. *Policy environment:* arena the process takes place in (government, media, public)

4. *Policy makers:* key players and stakeholders

▶ Health policies are developed through law and regulations.

▷ *Branches of law:* executive (implement law), legislative (initial formulation), and judicial (interpret law)

CASE STUDY

A PMHNP who is working at a federally qualified health center (FQHC) is asked to implement routine depression screening for all clients who present to the clinic. The PMHNP is excited about the project but has never implemented a system change and is not sure how to proceed. The PMHNP does have access to the quality improvement department and the clinical manager to get guidance.

1. What depression screening measures are in the public domain and have been found to be sensitive to and specific for depression screening?

2. What is the first step the PMHNP should complete to begin her system change process?

3. Who are key players that should be part of the PMHNP's quality improvement team?

4. What model or framework can the PMHNP use to guide her quality improvement project?

5. When conducting a literature review on depression screening in an FQHC, the PMHNP finds two RCT studies and two expert opinion articles. Which type has the highest level of evidence?

ANSWERS TO CASE STUDY DISCUSSION QUESTIONS

1. The screening measures in the public domain, sensitive to and specific for depression screening are: Patient Health Questionnaire–2 (PHQ2) and Patient Health Questionnaire–9 (PHQ9).

2. The first step in beginning a systems change project is to conduct a systemic needs assessment of the organization.

3. The key players that need to be part of the team include all members of the clinic who will be affected by implementation of the depression screening project.

4. The two models that can be used to conduct a quality improvement project include Donabedian model and Plan Do Study Act cycle.

5. The highest level of evidence in the literature when evaluating quantitative research studies is an RCT.

REFERENCES AND RESOURCES

American Nurses Association. (2010). *Just culture position statement.* Retrieved from http://nursingworld.org/psjustculture

Fineout-Overholt, E., Melnyk, B. M., & Schultz, A. (2005). Transforming health care from the inside out: Advancing evidence-based practice in the 21st century. *Journal of Professional Nursing, 21*(6), 335–344.

Institute of Medicine. (2001). *Crossing the quality chasm: A new health system for the 21st century.* Washington, DC: National Academies Press.

Institute of Medicine. (2010). *The future of nursing: Leading change, advancing health.* Available from http://www.nap.edu/catalog/12956/the-future-of-nursing-leading-change-advancing-health

Melnyk, B. M., Fineout-Overholt, E., Stillwell, S. B., & Williamson, K. (2010). The seven steps of evidence-based practice. *American Journal of Nursing, 110*(1), 51–53.

Northouse, P. G. (2007). *Leadership theory and practice* (4th ed.). London, Eng.: Sage Publications.

Patient Protection and Affordable Care Act, Pub. L. No. 111–148 (2010).

Perese, E. F. (2012). *Psychiatric advanced practice nursing: A biopsychosoical foundation for practice.* Philadelphia, PA: F. A. Davis.

Sherwood, G. D., & Horton-Deutsch, S. (2012). *Reflective practice transforming education and improving outcomes.* Indianapolis, IN: Sigma Theta Tau International.

Silow-Carroll, S., Alteras, T., & Stepnick, L. (2006). *Patient-centered care for underserved populations: Definitions and best practices.* Retrieved from http://hsc.unm.edu/community/toolkit/docs8/Overview.pdf

Substance Abuse and Mental Health Services Administration. (2014). *Advancing behavioral health integration with NCQA recognized patient-centered medical homes.* Retrieved from http://www.integration.samhsa.gov/integrated-care-models/Behavioral_Health_Integration_and_the_Patient_Centered_Medical_Home_FINAL.pdf

Substance Abuse and Mental Health Services Administration. (2015). What is a health home? Retrieved from http://www.integration.samhsa.gov/integrated-care-models/Health_Homes_Fact_Sheet_FINAL.pdf

World Health Organization. (2016). Health policy. Retrieved from http://www.who.int/topics/health_policy/en/

CHAPTER 5

NEUROANATOMY, NEUROPHYSIOLOGY, AND BEHAVIOR

A tremendous expansion of knowledge about the brain has occurred in the past 2 decades. As more has been learned about the brain and its complex functioning, assessment and treatment for psychiatric disorders have been altered dramatically. Increasingly, the links among genetics, altered brain anatomy and physiology, and the symptoms of psychiatric disorders have been identified (Sadock, Sadock, & Ruiz, 2015).

This growing knowledge base will continue to alter the treatment of psychiatric disorders. As new knowledge is disseminated, it is helping diminish the stigma long associated with psychiatric illness.

This chapter reviews the basics of neuroanatomy and physiology that provide the scientific rationale for many of the psychiatric–mental health nurse practitioner (PMHNP) care practices, including psychopharmacological interventions described elsewhere in this review book. PMHNPs need a solid grounding in neurobiology. Increasingly, the roles of the PMHNP require the application of this knowledge to clinical practice.

THE NERVOUS SYSTEM

▶ All human thoughts, feelings, and actions are seated in and start with actions of the nervous system.

▶ Necessary for the PMHNP's role functioning is an understanding of the following basic neuroanatomy and physiology:

▷ Neurodeficits that underlie psychiatric disorders

▷ Actions of and client responses to psychopharmacological treatment agents

▶ The nervous system's primary function is to transfer and exchange information.

The Neuron ("Nerve Cells")

▶ The basic cellular unit of the nervous system

▶ The microprocessor of the brain responsible for conducting impulses from one part of the body to another

▶ Components of the neuron:

▷ *Cell body*: Also known as soma; made up of the nucleus and cytoplasm within cell membrane

▷ *Stem* or *axon*: Transmits signals away from the neuron's cell body to connect with other neurons and cells

▷ *Dendrites*: Collect incoming signals from other neurons and send the signal toward the neuron's cell body

Nervous System

▶ Composed of two separate, interconnected divisions:

▷ Central nervous system (CNS)

  ▶ Composed of the spinal cord and the brain

▷ Peripheral nervous system (PNS)

  ▶ Composed of the peripheral nerves that connect the CNS to receptors, muscles, and glands

  ▶ Includes the cranial nerves just outside the brain stem

  ▶ Comprises the somatic nervous system and the autonomic nervous system:

    ▷ *Somatic nervous system*: Conveys information from the CNS to skeletal muscles; responsible for voluntary movement

    ▷ *Autonomic nervous system*: Regulates internal body functions to maintain homeostasis; conveys information from the CNS to smooth muscle, cardiac muscle, and glands; responsible for involuntary movement; divided into the sympathetic nervous system and the parasympathetic nervous system:

      ▶ *Sympathetic nervous system*: The excitatory division; prepares the body for stress (fight or flight); stimulates or increases activity of organs

      ▶ *Parasympathetic nervous system*: Maintains or restores energy; inhibits or decreases activity of organs

NEUROANATOMY AND THE BRAIN

▶ Brain tissue is categorized as either white matter or gray matter.

▷ *White matter* is the myelinated axons of neurons.

▷ *Gray matter* is composed of nerve cell bodies and dendrites; it is the working area of the brain and contains the synapses, the area of neuronal connection.

▶ Outermost surface of the brain: Structured to contain grooves and dips of corrugated wrinkles within the brain tissue that provide anatomical landmarks or reference points

▷ Functions to increase brain's surface area

▶ Increases working area and cell communication area

▷ Grooves and dips named by size and depth

▶ *Sulci*: Small shallow grooves

▶ *Fissures*: Deeper groves extending into the brain

▷ *Gyri* are the raised tissue areas.

▶ Distinct anatomical areas of brain

▷ The brain is subdivided into the cerebrum and the brainstem.

Cerebrum

▶ Largest part of the brain, which is divided into two halves, the right and left cerebral hemispheres

▷ *Left hemisphere:* Dominant in most people; controls most right-sided body functions

▷ *Right hemisphere:* Controls most left-sided body functions

▷ Normal functioning requires effective coordination of two hemispheres.

▷ Both hemispheres connected by a large bundle of white matter, the *corpus callosum*, an area of sensorimotor information exchange between the two hemispheres

▷ Each hemisphere is divided into four major lobes, which work in an interactive and integrated manner, and each with a distinct function:

▶ *Frontal lobe*: Largest and most developed lobe. Functions include:

▷ *Motor function:* Responsible for controlling voluntary motor activity of specific muscles

▷ *Premotor area:* Coordinates movement of multiple muscles

▷ *Association cortex:* Allows for multimodal sensory input to trigger memory and lead to decision-making

▷ *Seat of executive functions:* Working memory, reasoning, planning, prioritizing, sequencing behavior, insight, flexibility, judgment, impulse control, behavioral cueing, intelligence, abstraction

▷ *Language* (Broca's area): Expressive speech

▷ *Personality variables:* The most focal area for personality development

▷ Problems in the frontal lobe can lead to personality changes, emotional, and intellectual changes

▶ *Temporal lobe*; functions include:

▷ Language (Wernicke's area): Receptive speech or language comprehension

▷ Primary auditory area

▷ Memory

▷ Emotion

▷ Integration of vision with sensory information

▷ Problems in the temporal lobe can lead to visual or auditory hallucinations, aphasia, and amnesia

▶ *Occipital lobe*; functions include:

▷ Primary visual cortex

▷ Integration area: Integrates vision with other sensory information

▷ Problems in the occipital lobe can lead to visual field defects, blindness, and visual hallucinations

▶ *Parietal lobe*; functions include:

▷ Primary sensory area

▷ Taste

▷ Reading and writing

▷ Problems in the parietal lobe can lead to sensory–perceptual disturbances and agnosia

▶ Cerebrum includes the cerebral cortex, limbic system, thalamus, hypothalamus, and basal ganglia.

▷ *Cerebral cortex*

▶ Controls wide array of behaviors

▶ Controls the *contralateral* (opposite) side of the body: The right hemisphere controls the left side of the body, and the left hemisphere controls the right side of the body.

▶ Sensory information is relayed from the thalamus and then processed and integrated in the cortex.

▶ Responsible for much of the behavior that makes us human: speech, cognition, judgment, perception, and motor function

▷ *Limbic system*

▶ Essential system for the regulation and modulation of emotions and memory

▶ Composed of the hypothalamus, thalamus, hippocampus, and the amygdala

▷ *Hypothalamus*: Plays key roles in various regulatory functions such as appetite, sensations of hunger and thirst, water balance, circadian rhythms, body temperature, libido, and hormonal regulation

▷ *Thalamus*: Sensory relay station except for smell; modulates flow of sensory information to prevent overwhelming the cortex; regulates emotions, memory, and related affective behaviors

▷ *Hippocampus*: Regulates memory and converts short-term memory into long-term memory

▷ *Amygdala*: Responsible for mediating mood, fear, emotion, and aggression; also responsible for connecting sensory smell information with emotions

▷ *Basal ganglia*: Also known as the corpus striatum

- ▶ Serves as a complex feedback system to modulate and stabilize somatic motor activity (information conveyed from the CNS to skeletal muscles)

- ▶ Plays a role in movement initiation; complex motor functions with association connections

- ▶ Functions in learning and automatic actions such as walking or driving a car

- ▶ Contains extrapyramidal motor system or nerve tract

- ▶ Functions in involuntary motor activities (e.g., muscle tone, posture, coordination of muscle movement and common reflexes)

- ▶ Many psychotropic medications can affect the extrapyramidal motor nerve track, causing involuntary movement side effects

- ▶ Contains both the *caudate* and the *putamen*

- ▶ Problems in the basal ganglia can lead to bradykinesia, hyperkinesias, and dystonia.

Brainstem

- ▶ Made up of cells that produce neurotransmitters

- ▶ Includes the midbrain, pons, medulla, cerebellum, and reticular formation

  - ▷ *Midbrain*: Houses the ventral tegmental area and the substantia nigra (areas of dopamine synthesis)

  - ▷ *Pons*: Houses the locus ceruleus (area of norepinephrine synthesis)

  - ▷ *Medulla*: Together with the pons, contains autonomic control centers that regulate internal body functions

  - ▷ *Cerebellum*: Responsible for maintaining equilibrium; acts as a gross movement control center (e.g., control movement, balance, posture)

    - ▶ Each hemisphere of cerebellum has *ipsilateral* control (same side of body).

    - ▶ Problems with the cerebellum can lead to ataxia (uncoordinated and inaccurate movements).

    - ▶ Romberg test is important for detecting deficiencies in cerebellar functioning.

  - ▷ Reticular formation system: The primitive brain

    - ▶ Receives input from cortex; an integration area for input from postsensory pathways

    - ▶ Innervates thalamus, hypothalamus, and cortex

    - ▶ Regulation functions include:

      - ▷ Involuntary movement

      - ▷ Reflex

      - ▷ Muscle tone

      - ▷ Vital sign control

▷ Blood pressure

▷ Respiratory rate

▷ Critical to consciousness and ability to mentally focus, to be alert and pay attention to environmental stimuli

NEUROPHYSIOLOGY AND THE BRAIN

▶ Two classes of cells are in the nervous system: glia and neurons.

▷ *Glia*: Structures that form the myelin sheath around axons and provide protection and support

▷ *Neurons*: Nerve cells responsible for conducting impulses from one part of the body to another

▶ Components of a neuron include:

▷ *Cell body*: Also known as *soma*; made up of the nucleus and cytoplasm within the cell membrane

▷ *Dendrites*: Receive information to conduct impulse *toward* the cell body

▷ *Axon*: Sends or conducts information *away* from cell body

▶ *Synapse* or *synaptic cleft*—The connection site and area of communication between neurons where neurotransmitters are released

▷ The synapse converts an electrical signal (action potential) from the presynaptic neuron into a chemical signal (neuron transmitter) that is transferred to the postsynaptic neuron.

▷ Neurotransmitters are released at the synaptic cleft as the result of an electrical activity (action potential).

▷ The two phases of an action potential are:

▶ *Depolarization*: The initial phase of the action potential (an excitatory response), when sodium and calcium ions flow into the cell; and

▶ *Repolarization*: The restoration phase (an inhibitory response), when potassium leaves the cell or chloride enters the cell.

▷ Problems in either the structure or chemistry of the synapse interrupt normal flow of impulses and stimuli, which then contribute to symptoms commonly seen in psychiatric disorders.

▶ *Neurotransmitters:* Chemicals synthesized from dietary substrates that communicate information from one cell to another.

▷ The neurotransmitter will be released from the presynaptic neuron, cross the synapse, and then bind to a specific receptor on the postsynaptic neuron.

▷ Specific criteria must be met for a molecule to be classified as a neurotransmitter (see Table 5–1).

▷ Categories of neurotransmitters: Monoamines, amino acids, cholinergics, neuropeptides

TABLE 5–1.
CLASSIFICATION REQUIREMENTS FOR NEUROTRANSMITTERS

Criteria		
	1.	Neurotransmitter must be present in the nerve terminal.
	2.	Stimulation of neuron must cause release of neurotransmitter in sufficient quantities to cause an action to occur at postsynaptic membrane.
	3.	Effects of exogenous transmitter on postsynaptic membrane must be similar to those caused by stimulation of presynaptic neuron.
	4.	A mechanism for inactivation or metabolism of the neurotransmitter must exist in the area of the synapse.
	5.	Exogenous drugs should alter the dose–response curve of the neurotransmitter in a manner similar to the naturally occurring synaptic potential.

Note. Adapted from Sadock, B., Sadock, V., & Ruiz, P. (2015). *Kaplan and Sadock's synopsis of psychiatry* (11th ed.). Philadelphia, PA: Wolters Kluwer

▶ *Monoamines*: "Biogenic amines"—dopamine, norepinephrine, epinephrine, serotonin

  ▷ *Dopamine:* Known as a *catecholamine*; produced in the substantia nigra and the ventral tegmental area; precursor is tyrosine; removed from the synaptic cleft by monoamine oxidase (MAO) enzymatic action

    ▶ Four dopaminergic pathways: Mesocortical, mesolimbic, nigrostriatal, tuberoinfundibular (see Chapter 10)

  ▷ *Norepinephrine*: Also known as a *catecholamine*; produced in the locus ceruleus of the pons; precursor is tyrosine; removed from the synaptic cleft and returned to storage via an active reuptake process; major neurotransmitter implicated in mood, anxiety, and concentration disorders

  ▷ *Epinephrine*: Also known as a *catecholamine*; produced by the adrenal glands; epinephrine system also referred to as the adrenergic system

  ▷ *Serotonin*: Known as an *indole*; produced in the raphe nuclei of the brainstem; precursor is tryptophan; removed from the synaptic cleft and returned to storage via an active reuptake process; major neurotransmitter implicated in mood and anxiety disorders

▶ *Amino acids*: Glutamate, aspartate, γ-aminobutyric acid (GABA), glycine

  ▷ *Glutamate*: Universal excitatory neurotransmitter; major neurotransmitter involved in process of kindling, which is implicated in seizure disorders and possibly bipolar disorder; imbalance implicated in mood disorders and schizophrenia

  ▷ *Aspartate*: Another excitatory neurotransmitter; works with glutamate

  ▷ *GABA*: Universal inhibitory neurotransmitter; site of action of benzodiazepines, alcohol, barbiturates, and other CNS depressants

  ▷ *Glycine*: Another inhibitory neurotransmitter; works with GABA

▶ *Cholinergics*: Acetylcholine

  ▷ *Acetylcholine*: Synthesized by the basal nucleus of Meynert; precursors are acetylcoenzyme A and choline

▶ *Neuropeptides*: Nonopioid type (substance P, somatostatin); opioid type (endorphins, enkephalins, dynorphins)

▷ Modulate pain; decreased amount of neuropeptides is thought to cause substance abuse

▷ See Table 5–2 for identification of neurotransmitters' role in symptom expression in common psychiatric disorders.

▷ Recovery and degradation of neurotransmitters

▶ After the neurotransmitter reaches the postsynaptic neuron, it may then diffuse off its receptor to be destroyed by enzymes or to be transported back to the presynaptic neuron for reuse.

▶ *Enzymatic destruction* occurs either in the cytosol or in the synapse. The neurotransmitter can be destroyed by the enzymes monoamine oxidase (MAO) in the cytosol or catechol-O-methyl transferase (COMT) intracellularly or in the synapse.

TABLE 5–2.
COMMON PSYCHIATRIC DISORDERS AND NEUROTRANSMITTERS IMPLICATED IN THE COMPLEX PATHOPHYSIOLOGY OF COMMON PSYCHIATRIC DISORDERS

NEUROTRANSMITTER	SUSPECTED IMBALANCE	PSYCHIATRIC PRESENTATION
Acetylcholine	Decrease	Alzheimer's disease Impaired memory
	Increase	Parkinsonian symptoms
Dopamine	Increase	Schizophrenia Psychosis
	Decrease	Substance abuse Anhedonia Parkinson's disease
Norepinephrine	Decrease	Depression
	Increase	Anxiety
Serotonin	Decrease	Depression
		Obsessive–compulsive disorder, anxiety disorders
		Schizophrenia
γ-Aminobutyric acid (GABA)	Decrease	Anxiety disorders
Glutamate	Increase	Bipolar affective disorder Psychosis from ischemic neurotoxicity or excessive pruning
	Decrease	Memory and learning difficulty Negative symptoms of schizophrenia
Opioid neuropeptides	Decrease	Substance abuse

Note. Adapted from Thibodeau, G., & Patton, K. (2015). *Anatomy and physiology* (9th ed.). St. Louis, MO: Mosby.

▶   *Reuptake pumps* can remove the neurotransmitter from acting in the synapse. The neurotransmitter will be reloaded into the presynaptic neuron and will be recycled.

▷   Function of neurotransmitters: see Table 5–3

TABLE 5–3.
COMPARISON OF COMMON CNS NEUROTRANSMITTERS

NEURO-TRANSMITTER	RECEPTORS	GENERAL FUNCTION	SYMPTOMS OF DEFICIT	SYMPTOMS OF EXCESS
Dopamine	D_1-like D_2-like	Thinking Decision-making Reward-seeking behavior Fine muscle action Integrated cognition	*Mild:* Poor impulse control Poor spatiality Lack of abstractive thought *Severe:* Parkinson's disease Endocrine alterations Movement disorders	*Mild:* Improved creativity Improved ability for abstract thinking Improved executive functioning Improved spatiality *Severe:* Disorganized thinking Loose association Tics Stereotypic behavior
Norepinephrine	α1 α2	Alertness Focused attention Orientation Primes "fight or flight" Learning Memory	Dullness Low energy Depressive affect	Anxiety Hyperalertness Increased startle Paranoia Decreased appetite
Serotonin	5HT1a 5HT1d 5HT2 5HT2a 5HT3 5HT4	Regulation of sleep Pain perception Mood states Temperature Regulation of aggression Libido Precursor for melatonin	Irritability Hostility Depression Sleep dysregulation Loss of appetite Loss of libido	Sedation Increased aggression Hallucinations (rare)

CONTINUED

NEURO-TRANSMITTER	RECEPTORS	GENERAL FUNCTION	SYMPTOMS OF DEFICIT	SYMPTOMS OF EXCESS
Acetylcholine	Nicotinic Muscarinic	Attention Memory Thirst Mood regulation REM sleep Sexual behavior Muscle tone	Lack of inhibition Decreased memory Euphoria Antisocial action Speech decrease Dry mouth, blurred vision, constipation	Over-inhibition Anxiety Depression Somatic complaints Self-consciousness Drooling Extrapyramidal movements
GABA	GABAa GABAb	Reduces arousal Reduces aggression Reduces anxiety Reduces excitation	Irritability Hostility Tension and worry Anxiety Seizure activity	Reduced cellular excitability Sedation Impaired memory
Glutamate	AMPA MNDA	Memory Sustained automatic functions	Poor memory Low energy Distractible	Kindling Seizures Anxiety or panic
Peptides: Opioid type	μ (mu) κ (kappa) ε (epsilon) δ (delta) σ (sigma)	Modulate emotions Reward-center function Consolidation of memory Modulate reactions to stress	Hypersensitivity to pain and stress Decreased pleasure sensation Dysphoria	Insensitivity to pain Catatonic-like movement disturbance Auditory hallucinations Decreased memory

Note. Adapted from Sadock, B., Sadock, V., & Ruiz, P. (2015). *Kaplan and Sadock's synopsis of psychiatry* (11th ed.). Philadelphia, PA: Wolters Kluwer.

NEUROIMAGING ASSESSMENT AND DIAGNOSTIC PROCEDURES

▶ Techniques that permit observation of the brain can be divided into three categories: structural imaging, functional imaging, and combined structural and functional imaging.

    ▷ *Structural imaging*: Provides evidence of size and shape of anatomical structures

        ▶ Common structural imaging tests include:

            ▷ *Computed tomography (CT)*: Provides a three-dimensional view of the brain structures; differentiates structures based on density; provides suggestive evidence of brain-based problems but no specific testing for psychiatric disorders

                ▶ *Advantages*: Widely available, relatively inexpensive

                ▶ *Disadvantages*: Lack of sensitivity, cannot differentiate white matter from gray matter; cannot view structures close to the bone tissue; underestimation of brain atrophy; inability to image sagittal and coronal views

▷ *Magnetic resonance imaging (MRI)*: Provides a series of two-dimensional images that represent the brain

▶ *Advantages*: Can view brain structures close to the skull and can separate white matter from gray matter; readily available; resolution of brain tissue superior to CT scanning

▶ *Disadvantages*: Expensive; many contraindications to its use (e.g., clients with pacemakers or any metallic implants such as orthopedic screws or plates, or on ventilators); clients with claustrophobia often are unable to complete study because of design of machinery (an enclosed tubelike structure with a confining environment)

▷ *Functional imaging*: Technique that measures function of areas of the brain and bases the resulting assessment on blood flow; may use radioactive pharmaceuticals to cross the blood-brain barrier; mainly used for research

▶ Common functional imaging tests include

▷ *EEG and evoked potentials testing*: Least expensive tests that convey information on electrical functioning of the CNS

▷ *Magnetoencephalography (MEG)*: Similar to the EEG but detects different electrical activities; often used in a complementary fashion with EEG testing

▷ *Single photon emission computed tomography (SPECT)*: Provides information on the cerebral blood flow; limited availability; expensive but less than positron emission tomography

▷ *Positron emission tomography (PET)*: Provides images of the brain when positron-emitting radionuclei interact with an electron; expensive procedure that requires extensive resources and support team

▷ *Combined structural and functional imaging*: The newest imaging; attempts to examine structure in conjunction with function; currently mainly used for research

▶ Available tests include

▷ Functional MRI (fMRI)

▷ Three-dimensional, event-related functional MRI (3fEMRI)

▷ Fluorine magnetic spectroscopy

▷ Dopamine D_2 receptor binding

GENOMICS

Family History, Family Tree, or Pedigree

▶ Tool in determining likelihood of genetic disorder in family, inheritance patterns, and risk of recurrence in family members

▶ Surgeon General recommended that families know their family history (U.S. Department of Health and Human Services, n.d.)

▶ Pedigree symbols in drawing a family tree indicate male, female, marriage, divorce, adoption, twins, pregnancy, consanguinity (relatives having children), conditions

▶ Family history starts with current family and moves back to grandparents.

▶ Autosomal-dominant conditions may be present in more than one generation and in up to 50% of offspring when one parent is affected (e.g., Marfan syndrome).

▶ Recessive conditions appear only in one generation, affecting people who have two copies of a faulty gene, one from each (unaffected) parent (e.g., hemochromatosis, cystic fibrosis).

▶ X-linked disorders are caused by faulty genes on an X chromosome (e.g., fragile X syndrome, color blindness).

▶ Risk assessment is based on inheritance patterns and may be by percentage of risk.

Genetic Counseling

▶ Genetic counseling is a communication process used when a client has a genetic risk and often involves offering a test that could provide information about the genetic status of the person and possible implications for the family.

▶ A genetic counselor is someone whose primary role is to offer information and support to people concerned about an illness that may have a genetic basis.

▶ A referral to a genetic counselor may be needed when a client is anticipating a pregnancy and concerned for the health of the fetus.

Genetic Terms

▶ Chromosomes are structures of DNA (deoxyribonucleic acid) in the nucleus of cells; there are normally 46 total (23 pairs) in humans.

▶ DNA is made up of two twisted, paired strands, composed of sugars linked by four nucleotide bases—adenine (A), thymine (T), cytosine (C), and guanine (G)—specifying the amino acids that make proteins. A is always paired with T and G is always paired with C.

▶ *Genes* are a sequence of DNA that cause human characteristics to be passed to the next generation; genes direct the production of proteins.

▶ Messenger RNA (mRNA) codes for an amino acid.

▶ The Human Genome Project mapped the entire nucleotide sequence of the human genome in 2003. The genome is a complete set of DNA.

▶ A *phenotype* is the observable characteristic of a specific trait and is connected to the genetic contributions to that trait (e.g., fast metabolizer of CYP4502D6 medications).

▶ Gene therapy involves replacing a faulty copy of a gene with a healthy copy of the same gene.

▶ Personalized medicine is health care based on genetic variability.

Studies of Population Genetics

▶ Family studies investigate the occurrence of disorders in first-degree relatives (parents, siblings, and offspring) and second-degree relatives (grandparents, cousins, aunts, and uncles).

▶ Twin studies survey the concordance rate (presence) of a disorder in monozygotic (identical) and dizygotic (fraternal) twins.

▶ Adoption studies investigate the risk of a disorder developing in children raised in a different environment from the biological parent with a specific disorder.

▶ Strong genetic contributions have been found for most psychiatric disorders, with a range of 40% to 90% heritability for some disorders (e.g., attention-deficit hyperactivity disorder, bipolar disorder).

▶ Genes are risk factors that make a person vulnerable to developing the illness when combined with certain environmental risk factors that increase susceptibility of developing the disorder.

▶ Environmental risk factors include prenatal insults, stress, infections, poor nutrition, exposure to toxins, catastrophic loss, and physical and sexual abuse.

▶ Most diseases are multifactorial, caused by both environmental and genetic factors; single-gene disorders are rare.

Gene Expression and Disease

▶ Single nucleotide polymorphisms (SNP) detect single base changes in DNA sequence.

▶ Reduced penetrance of a gene decreases chances of disease in person at genetic risk.

▶ Variable expression of a gene for a disorder occurs at the cellular level.

Pharmacogenomics

▶ Genes account for differences in the way enzymes metabolize drugs.

▶ Medications may act differently based on how genes affect metabolism.

▶ Genetic testing or profiling helps identify the presence of gene variants that may help determine dosing of medication (e.g., CYP450 test of CYP4502D6, CYP450 2C19, and methylene tetrahydrofolate reductase [MTHFR] genes—see Chapter 7 for further information on pharmacokinetics).

▶ Testing for presence of HLA-B*1502 allele, an inherited variant of HLA-B gene, is required by the FDA in people of Asian descent prior to prescribing the anticonvulsant carbamazepine due to risk of Stevens-Johnson syndrome and toxic epidermal necrolysis (TEN).

CASE STUDY 1

Ms. Franklin is a 24-year-old sales clerk. She has a strong family history of mental illness and is worried that she may experience some problems in her life because of her family history. She presents to her local primary care provider complaining of the following symptoms:

▶ Hyperalertness

▶ Increased startle response

▶ Concern that people are staring at her and watching what she eats

▶ Decreased appetite

▶ Difficulty falling asleep

Ms. Franklin is trying to determine if these experiences are the beginning of a mental illness. She wants to have a brain scan done to determine the answer. She also is getting married soon and wants to know what the risk is that her future children will experience mental illness, because she believes it runs in her family. In working with Ms. Franklin, the PMHNP must consider many issues.

1. Are the symptoms described by Ms. Franklin consistent with a psychiatric disorder?

2. Do psychiatric disorders run in families, as Ms. Franklin believes?

3. Do the symptoms as described by Ms. Franklin link with any known neuroanatomical or neurophysiologic deficit?

4. Is a brain scan warranted for Ms. Franklin?

5. Can the risk of Ms. Franklin's children developing psychiatric disorders be determined?

CASE STUDY 2

Joel is an 18-year-old college freshman who developed psychotic symptoms necessitating a brief hospitalization at his university's medical center. Joel is given haloperidol (Haldol) 5 mg IM with lorazepam (Ativan) 1 mg IM and diphenhydramine (Benadryl) 50 mg IM upon admission and is started on risperidone (Risperdal). One day after admission, Joel presents to the nurses' station complaining of a painful "stiff neck" and "thick tongue."

1. What is the best description of Joel's presentation?

2. What is the best explanation for Joel's presentation?

3. Which neurotransmitters are involved in Joel's presentation?

4. How should the PMHNP address this scenario?

5. In formulating diagnostic conclusions about Joel, what should the PMHNP consider?

ANSWERS TO CASE STUDY DISCUSSION QUESTIONS

Case Study 1

1. More assessment would be needed to determine whether Ms. Franklin's symptoms are consistent with a psychiatric disorder, but they may be consistent with an anxiety or mood disorder.

2. Most psychiatric illnesses have been shown to have, in part, a genetic link and therefore, do tend to run in families.

3. Ms. Franklin's symptoms are consistent with excessive levels of norepinephrine.

4. No. There is insufficient data to warrant the cost of a brain scan at this time.

5. Yes, the risk of Ms. Franklin's children developing psychiatric disorders can be determined but only if Ms. Franklin meets criteria for an actual psychiatric illness. Once this is determined, the genetic risk to her children can be identified through the use of such things as concordant rate tables.

Case Study 2

1. Joel's presentation is consistent with acute dystonia.

2. Both haloperidol and risperidone are high-potency D2 antagonists. Although Joel received prophylactic diphenhydramine, adding risperidone, particularly with aggressive dosing, increases the risk of extrapyramidal side effects.

3. CNS dopamine (DA) and acetylcholine (ACH) have a reciprocal relationship. As DA receptors are antagonized by antipsychotic medication, acetylcholine levels increase, giving rise to extrapyramidal side effects. This is particularly true of first-generation antipsychotics, but also of high-potency second-generation agents.

4. Administer diphenhydramine or benztropine (Cogentin) IM immediately and hold subsequent doses of risperidone until dystonia completely resolves. Resume risperidone at a lower dose along with an oral anticholinergic medication. Adjust the dose of the antipsychotic as indicated. If Joel continues to experience extrapyramidal side effects, switching to a lower-potency antipsychotic may be necessary.

5. Joel may have experienced a sentinel episode of schizophrenia. Joel's symptoms may also have been substance-induced.

REFERENCES AND RESOURCES

Alexander, E., Chen, K., Pietrini, P., Rapoport, S. I., & Reiman, E. M. (2002). Longitudinal PET evaluation of cerebral metabolic decline in dementia: A potential outcome measure in Alzheimer's disease treatment studies. *American Journal of Psychiatry, 159*, 238–245.

Amen, D. G. (1998). Brain SPECT imaging in psychiatry. *Primary Psychiatry, 5*, 83–87.

Amen, D. G. (2010). Brain SPECT imaging in clinical practice. *American Journal of Psychiatry, 167*(9), 1125–1126.

American Nurses Association, American Psychiatric Nurses Association, & International Society of Psychiatric-Mental Health Nurses. (2014). *Psychiatric–mental health nursing: Scope and standards of practice* (2nd ed.). Silver Spring, MD: Nursesbooks.org.

Bartolomeis, A. (2014). Glutamatergic postsynaptic density protein dysfunctions in synaptic plasticity and dendritic spines morphology: relevance to schizophrenia and other behavioral disorders pathophysiology, and implications for novel therapeutic approaches. *Molecular Neurobiology, 49*(1), 484–511.

Boyd, M. A. (2014). *Psychiatric nursing: Contemporary practice* (5th ed.). Philadelphia, PA: Lippincott, Williams & Wilkins.

Burhan, A. M., Bartha, R., Bocti, C., Borrie, M., Laforce, R., Rosa-Neto, P., & Soucy, J. P. (2013). Role of emerging neuroimaging modalities in patients with cognitive impairment: a review of the Canadian consensus conference on the diagnosis and treatment of dementia 2012. *Alzheimers Research and Therapeutics*, July 8 (Suppl 1):5.

Carlson, N. R. (2012). *Physiology of behavior* (11th ed.). Boston, MA: Allyn & Bacon.

Goff, D., & Coyle, J. (2001). The emerging role of glutamate in the pathophysiology and treatment of schizophrenia. *American Journal of Psychiatry, 158*, 1367–1377.

Gong, Q., Dazzan, P., Scarpazza, C., Kasai, K., Hu, X., Marques, T. R., ... Mechelli, A. (2015). A neuroanatomical signature for schizophrenia across different ethnic groups. *Schizophrenia Bulletin, 41*(6), 1266–1275.

Lee, Y., & Song, G. (2014). Genome-wide pathway analysis in attention-deficit/hyperactivity disorder. *Neurological Science, 35*(8), 1189–1196.

Matrisciano, F., Panaccione, I., Grayson, D. R., Nicoletti, F., & Guidotti, A. (2016). Metabotropic glutamate 2/3 receptors and epigenetic modifications in psychotic disorders: A review. *Current in Neuropharmacology, 14*(1), 41–47.

McLeod, T. M., Lopez-Figueroa, A., & Lopez-Figueroa, M. O. (2001). Nitric oxide, stress, and depression. *Psychopharmacology Bulletin, 35*, 24–41.

Mujica-Parodi, L. R., Corcoran, C., Greenberg, T., Saceim, H. A., & Malaspina, D. (2002). Are cognitive symptoms of schizophrenia mediated by abnormalities in emotional arousal? *CNS Spectrums, 7*(1), 58–69.

Power, B. D., Nguyen, T., Hayhow, B., & Looi, J. (2015). Neuroimaging in psychiatry: An update on neuroimaging in the clinical setting. *Australasian Psychiatry*, December. doi: 10.1177/1039856215618525

Sadock, B. J., Sadock, V. A., & Ruiz, P. (2015). *Kaplan and Sadock's synopsis of psychiatry: Behavioral sciences/clinical psychiatry* (11th ed.). Philadelphia, PA: Wolters Kluwer.

Stahl, S. M. (2013). *Essential psychopharmacology: Neuroscientific basis and practical applications* (14th ed.). New York, NY: Cambridge University Press.

Stuart, G. W. (2013). *Principles and practice of psychiatric nursing* (10th ed.). St Louis, MO: Mosby, Inc.

Thibodeau, G., & Patton, K. (2015). Anatomy and physiology (9th ed.). St. Louis, MO: Mosby.

Underwood, M. D., Kassir, S. A., Bakalian, M. J., Galfalvy, H., Mann, J. J., & Arango, V. (2012). Neuron density and serotonin receptor binding in prefrontal cortex in suicide. International *Journal of Neuropsychopharmacology, 15*(4), 435–437.

U.S. Department of Health and Human Services. (n.d.). Surgeon General's family health history initiative. Retrieved from http://www.hhs.gov/familyhistory

Yuta, A., Inokuchi, R., Nakao, T., & Yamasue, H. (2013). Neural bases of antisocial behavior: A voxel-based meta-analysis. *Social Cognitive and Affective Neuroscience, 9*(8), 1223–1231.

CHAPTER 6

ADVANCED HEALTH AND PHYSICAL HEALTH ASSESSMENT

This chapter reviews the role of *psychiatric–mental health nurse practitioners* (PMHNPs) in physical health and advanced health assessment. In this chapter you will review information on the process of completing a physical exam and differential diagnosis, and the appropriate use of diagnostic and laboratory testing in providing competent nursing care for clients and families experiencing psychiatric disorders. The chapter specifically highlights the PMHNP role in the identification of physical health problems.

PHYSICAL EXAM

- ▶ Reasons to be familiar with the physical exam in psychiatry:
    - ▷ To be able to detect underlying medical problems
    - ▷ To be familiar with a screening neurological exam and to be able to rule out neurological problems that may manifest as symptoms of a psychiatric problem
    - ▷ To be able to differentiate normal and abnormal signs and symptoms
    - ▷ To know when to refer
- ▶ Done by the PMHNP in the context of his or her primary psychiatric care role
- ▶ Goals are identifying presence of psychiatric disorders, identifying general health status, and screening for other nonpsychiatric disorders
- ▶ Focuses on physical assessment required to accomplish differential diagnoses to determine client health needs
- ▶ Specifically focuses on assessing for disorders or conditions that explain client presentation
    - ▷ Psychiatric disorders
    - ▷ Nonpsychiatric disorders
- ▶ Not intended to replace the role of primary healthcare provider for the client
    - ▷ PMHNP should assist client to establish primary care provider if he or she does not already have one.

▶ Avoids highly personal or intrusive procedures (e.g., Pap exam, male genital exam, rectal exam, breast exam) that may make the formation of a therapeutic alliance more difficult, but it is important to be familiar with these exams and be able to differentiate normal from abnormal

▶ Requires the PMHNP to have depth of knowledge regarding the common health disorders that can mimic symptoms of a psychiatric disorder

  ▷ Differential diagnostic considerations

▶ Requires the PMHNP to have depth of knowledge regarding the common psychiatric disorders that can mimic or produce symptoms of other disorders

  ▷ Differential diagnostic considerations

  ▷ Comorbid conditions and clinical management issues

▶ Generally, if client's health issues are determined to be nonpsychiatric, client is referred to primary care providers other than the PMHNP.

▶ Because of the brain-based nature of psychiatric disorders, the PMHNP role requires the ability to perform an in-depth neurological exam.

NEUROLOGICAL EXAM

▶ Reflexes (biceps, triceps, brachioradialis, patellar, Achilles, plantar)

  ▷ Grade reflexes and note symmetry between right and left sides.

  ▷ Check primitive reflexes in infants (head lag, flexion, rooting, grasping, Moro, glabellar, Babinski).

  ▷ A positive Babinski (fanning of toes and dorsiflexion of the great toe) is normal in infants up to age 2 years.

▶ Cranial nerves (*mnemonic italicized in parentheses*)

  ▷ *Olfactory*: 1st (*On*)

    ▶ Test sense of smell and ensure patency of the nasal passages.

    ▶ Have the client close eyes and test each nostril separately while other is occluded, asking the client to identify familiar odors.

  ▷ *Optic*: 2nd (*Old*)

    ▶ Test vision using Snellen chart or other suitable chart depending on the client's acuity and ability to cooperate.

    ▶ Examine the inner aspect of the eyes with the ophthalmoscope.

    ▶ Test peripheral vision using the confrontation test.

  ▷ *Oculomotor*: 3rd (*Olympus'*)

    ▶ This is the motor nerve to the five extrinsic eye muscles. Test together with cranial nerve 4 (trochlear) and cranial nerve 6 (abducens; see below).

    ▶ Test the extraocular movements (EOMs).

    ▶ Check the equality of pupils, their reaction to light, and their ability to accommodate.

    ▶ Test the corneal light reflex (when shining a light at the bridge of the nose, the light should appear symmetrically in both eyes).

▷ *Trochlear:* 4th (*Towering*)

  ▶ Use the same process as cranial nerve 3 (oculomotor) and cranial nerve 6 (abducens).

▷ *Trigeminal:* 5th (Motor division; *Top*)

  ▶ Palpate the masseter muscles with the fingertips while the client clenches his or her teeth.

  ▶ Look for disparity in tension between the two muscles, which can indicate paralysis on the weak side.

  ▶ Look for tremor of the lips, involuntary chewing movements, and spasm of the masticatory muscles.

▷ *Trigeminal:* 5th (Sensory division)

  ▶ Test tactile perception of the facial skin by touching with a wisp of cotton.

  ▶ Test corneal reflex with wisp of cotton.

  ▶ Test superficial pain of the skin and mucosa with pinpricks.

  ▶ Test the sense of touch in the oral mucosa.

▷ *Abducens:* 6th (*A*)

  ▶ Use the same process as for cranial nerves 3 (oculomotor) and 4 (trochlear).

▷ *Facial:* 7th (Motor division; *Finn*)

  ▶ Inspect the face in repose for evidence of flaccid paralysis.

  ▶ Test by asking the client to elevate eyebrows, wrinkle forehead, close eyes, frown, smile, and puff cheeks.

▷ *Facial:* 7th (Sensory division)

  ▶ Test taste for sugar, vinegar, and salt.

▷ *Acoustic:* 8th (*And*)

  ▶ Check hearing with the audiometer or by the whisper test.

  ▶ Check for hearing loss using the Weber and the Rinne tests.

▷ *Glossopharyngeal:* 9th (*German*)

  ▶ Test together with cranial nerve 10 (vagus; see below).

▷ *Vagus:* 10th (*Viewed*)

  ▶ Test for elevation of the uvula by having the client open his or her mouth and say "ah."

  ▶ Test the gag reflex by touching the back of throat with a tongue blade.

▷ *Accessory spinal:* 11th (*Some*)

  ▶ Test the strength of the sternocleidomastoid and trapezius muscles against resistance of your hands.

▷ *Hypoglossal:* 12th (*Hops*)

  ▶ Look for tremors and other involuntary movement when the client protrudes his or her tongue.

▶ Coordination and fine-motor skills

  ▷ *Equilibrium*: Check by administering the Romberg test: have the client stand up straight with feet together, arms by sides, and eyes closed. Only slight swaying would be normal, and the client will be able to sustain this pose for approximately 5 seconds. More than slight swaying suggests cerebellar ataxia or vestibular dysfunction.

  ▷ *Diadochokinesia*: Ability to perform rapid alternating movements (such as patting knees alternating palm and back of hands, touching thumb to each finger); the client should be able to smoothly execute these movements and maintain the rhythm.

  ▷ *Dyssynergia*: Finger-to-nose test, heel-to-knee test

  ▷ *Handwriting*

  ▷ *Gait*: Observe client walking.

▶ Sensory functions

  ▷ *Pain*: Check sensation to pain with pinprick, and compare on each side of body.

  ▷ *Temperature*: Check temperature if sensation to pain is abnormal.

  ▷ *Superficial touch*: Test with wisp of cotton.

  ▷ *Two-point discrimination:* Apply pins to skin simultaneously; ask the client if he or she feels one or two pinpricks.

  ▷ *Stereognosis:* Tests the ability to distinguish forms by placing objects in the client's hands while his or her eyes are closed.

  ▷ *Graphesthesia:* Tests the ability to identify figures, letters, or words by tracing the figure on the skin of the palm of the hand.

▶ Motor functions

  ▷ *Muscle mass:* Measure muscle mass to check for atrophy or hypertrophy.

  ▷ *Muscle tone:* Tension is present when the muscle is resting.

  ▷ *Muscle strength:* Check muscular strength against resistance.

  Be aware of abnormal muscle movements.

▶ Neurological soft signs

  ▷ *Dysdiadochokinesia:* Inability to perform rapid alternating movements; result of a lesion to the posterior lobe of the cerebellum

  ▷ *Astereognosis:* Inability to discriminate between objects based on touch alone; result of a lesion in the parietal lobe

  ▷ *Choreiform movements*

  ▷ *Tics*

  ▷ *Agraphesthesia*: Inability to recognize letters or numbers "drawn" on the client's hand with a pointed object

  ▷ *Facial grimacing*

  ▷ *Impaired fine-motor skills*

  ▷ *Abnormal blinking*

  ▷ *Abnormal motor tone*

Be alert for extrapyramidal symptoms (as in Parkinsonism, dystonia, akathisia) in the client taking antipsychotics.

▶ Vital signs

▷ Measure height, weight, blood pressure (on children ages two or older), pulse, respirations, temperature, and head circumference (during the first 2 years).

▷ Use growth charts for infants and children.

▶ Greater than 85th percentile for body mass index (BMI) places a child at increased risk for being overweight.

▷ Use BMI charts

▶ Normal: 20 to 25

▶ Overweight: 26 to 29

▶ Obese: 30 to 35

▷ High BMI is a risk factor for diabetes, heart disease, stroke, hypertension, osteoarthritis, and some forms of cancer.

Be alert for high BMI if the client also is being prescribed psychotropic meds with a propensity for weight gain, especially atypical antipsychotics.

▷ If a client is presenting with elevated temperature and also is taking psychotropic meds such as carbamazepine (Tegretol) or clozapine (Clozaril), be alert for agranulocytosis.

▶ Head, skin, nails

▷ Note the color and integrity of the skin and whether lesions are present.

▷ Note if the skin is well-hydrated, dry, or scaly.

▷ Assess skin turgor.

▷ Palpate the skin's temperature.

▷ Note any unusual moles or other lesions.

▷ Look at hair texture and distribution.

▷ Determine the quality of the nails, noting splitting, clubbing, or onychomycosis.

▷ Check capillary refill.

▷ Examine head, scalp, sutures, and fontanelles (if infant).

▷ Check cranial nerve 7 (facial nerve) for symmetry (have client smile, frown, wrinkle forehead, puff cheeks).

Be alert for Stevens-Johnson syndrome (life-threatening rash), especially if the client is taking carbamazepine or lamotrigine (Lamictal).

▷ Cancerous moles can be detected by using the acronym **ABCDE**—**a**symmetry, **b**order irregularity, **c**olor variation, **d**iameter greater than 6 millimeters, and **e**levation.

▶ Eyes

▷ Check visual acuity using the Snellen chart (tests cranial nerve 2: optic nerve).

▷ Test peripheral vision using the confrontation test (tests cranial nerve 2: optic nerve).

  ▷   Note the symmetry of eyes and the appearance of orbits, eyelids, and brows.

  ▷   Inspect the sclera.

  ▷   Assess corneal sensation with wisp of cotton (tests cranial nerves 5 and 7).

  ▷   Assess papillary reaction to light and accommodation (tests cranial nerves 3, 4, and 6).

  ▷   Assess the six cardinal fields of gaze (extraocular movements; tests cranial nerves 3, 4, and 6).

  ▷   Assess corneal light reflex. Light reflections should appear symmetrically in both pupils (tests cranial nerves 3, 4, and 6).

  ▷   Examine the inner aspect of the eyes with the ophthalmoscope (tests cranial nerve 2).

Be aware that many psychotropics can cause blurry vision (an anticholinergic side effect).

  ▷   Quetiapine (Seroquel) may cause cataracts.

▶   Ears

  ▷   Check for configuration, position, and alignment of auricles.

  ▷   Test auditory acuity (cranial nerve 8) with the whisper test or audiometer.

  ▷   Inspect external auditory canals with otoscope for redness, swelling, or excess cerumen.

  ▷   Tympanic membrane should be translucent pearly gray without retractions or bulges.

▶   Nose and sinuses

  ▷   Note the appearance of the external nose and whether it is smooth, intact, symmetric, midline, has discharge, or is flaring.

  ▷   Assess nasal patency.

  ▷   Assess sense of smell.

  ▷   Inspect internal nasal cavity for patency and septal deviation.

  ▷   Palpate maxillary and frontal sinuses.

▶   Neck

  ▷   Palpate the lymph nodes (preauricular, postauricular, tonsillar, submandibular, submental, anterior cervical) for swelling or masses.

  ▷   Palpate thyroid (usually not palpable except in very thin people).

  ▷   Palpate and auscultate carotid pulse and note any bruits.

▶   Back

  ▷   Inspect skin and respiratory pattern on posterior chest.

  ▷   Palpate cervical, thoracic, lumbar, and sacral spine.

  ▷   Palpate thoracic expansion.

  ▷   Percuss posterior chest for tympany.

  ▷   Auscultate posterior chest for vesicular or bronchovesicular sounds and note any adventitious breath sounds.

▶ Thorax and lungs

▷ Assess respiratory rate and depth, regularity, and ease of respirations.

▷ Note anterior–posterior (AP) diameter, which should be less than the transverse diameter.

▷ Percuss anterior chest for resonance and note the quality and symmetry of percussion notes.

▷ Auscultate anterior chest for lung sounds; normal breath sounds include vesicular over peripheral lung, bronchovesicular over first and second intercostal spaces at the sternal border, and bronchial over the trachea.

▶ Breasts

▷ Inspect breasts in different positions: with client arms relaxed and by side, with arms elevated above head, and with hands on hips. Look for dimpling, retractions, and orange-peel appearance.

▷ Palpate breasts for lumps, including Tail of Spence.

▷ Palpate axillary and epitrochlear lymph nodes.

▷ Palpate supraclavicular lymph nodes (also known as sentinel or Virchow nodes).

Be aware that typical antipsychotics as well as atypical antipsychotics may cause galactorrhea.

▶ Heart

▷ Inspect, palpate, and auscultate the carotid pulse.

▷ Palpate peripheral pulses and check for symmetry (carotid, brachial, radial, femoral, popliteal, pedal, and posterior tibial).

▷ Assess heart rate, rhythm, amplitude, and contour.

▷ Assess anatomic location of the apical pulse.

▷ Palpate precordium for pulsations, thrills, heaves, and lifts.

▷ Auscultate heart sounds with bell and diaphragm and note characteristics of the first and second heart sounds.

▷ Assess for jugular venous distention (JVD).

Be alert for possible electrocardiogram (ECG) changes if the client is taking tricyclic anti-depressants or antipsychotics.

Be aware that lithium and anorexia nervosa can cause peripheral edema.

▶ Abdomen

▷ Inspect the contour of the abdomen and check for scars, abdominal aortic pulsations, and the umbilical cord in the newborn.

▷ Auscultate for bowel sounds and the abdominal aorta for bruits.

▷ Percuss the abdomen, and note areas of tympany and dullness. It is normal to hear tympany over the small and large intestines and dullness over organs and a distended bladder.

▷ Percuss the size of liver and spleen.

▷ Palpate the abdomen for masses and tenderness. Also palpate the liver and spleen, which are not normally palpable (sometimes the liver can be palpable in thin clients).

▶ Musculoskeletal

▷ Assess client's posture for alignment of extremities and spine and for symmetry of body parts.

▷ Test muscle strength of upper and lower extremities.

▷ Note symmetry of muscle mass, tone, and strength.

▷ Assess active range of motion in neck and upper and lower extremities, and note any presence of pain with movement.

▷ Palpate muscles and joints to elicit pain, deformities, crepitus, and passive range of motion.

▷ Check for hip dysplasia in infants.

▷ Check for scoliosis in children and adolescents.

▶ Common indicators of physical child abuse

▷ History of unexplained multiple fractures

▷ Burns, hand or bite marks

▷ Injuries at various stages of healing

▷ Evidence of neglect

▷ Bruising on padded parts of body

Diagnostic and Laboratory Testing

▶ Assessment of diagnostic and laboratory testing is an essential element of the PMHNP role. It is important for the PMHNP to know when to order such tests, how to interpret the findings, and how to appropriately alter care based on the findings.

▶ Reasons to assess diagnostic and laboratory testing in psychiatry:

▷ To assist in the establishment of a diagnosis; as knowledge of underlying pathophysiology grows, diagnostic and laboratory testing use will grow as well

▷ Used to rule out other disorders such as medical causes of psychiatric symptoms; helpful in differential diagnostic assessment

▷ Used to determine whether a client's symptoms are better explained by a nonpsychiatric disorder or by factors such as drug use or abuse

▷ For routine ongoing monitoring such as general health screening, monitoring drug levels of certain psychiatric meds, and assessment and monitoring for complications of psychiatric disorders or adverse effects of drugs

▶ Thyroid function tests

▷ Function of thyroid gland is to take iodine from the circulating blood, combine it with the amino acid tyrosine, and convert it to the thyroid hormones T3 and T4.

▷ The thyroid gland also stores T3 and T4 until they are released into the bloodstream under the influence of thyroid-stimulating hormone (TSH) released from the pituitary gland.

▷ Only a small amount of T3 and T4 are bound to protein.

▷ The free portion of the thyroid hormones is the true determinant of thyroid status.

▶ Free thyroxine T4 (FT4; normal values 0.8 to 2.8 ng/dl)

▷ FT4 composes a small portion of the total thyroxine, is available to the tissues, and is the metabolically active form of this hormone.

▷ FT4 test is commonly done to determine thyroid status, to rule out hypo- and hyperthyroidism, and to evaluate thyroid therapy.

▶ Diseases that have increased thyroid levels include:

▷ Graves' disease

▷ Thyrotoxicosis due to T4

▷ Hashimoto's thyroiditis

▷ Acute thyroiditis

▶ Diseases that have decreased thyroid levels include:

▷ Primary hypothyroidism

▷ Secondary hypothyroidism (pituitary insufficiency)

▷ Tertiary hypothyroidism (hypothalamic failure)

▷ Thyrotoxicosis due to T3

▷ Renal failure

▷ Cushing's syndrome

▷ Cirrhosis

▶ Interfering factors:

▷ Values can be increased during treatment with heparin, aspirin, and propranolol.

▷ Values can be decreased during treatment with furosemide (Lasix) or methadone.

▶ Thyroid-stimulating hormone (normal values 2–10 mU/l)

▷ Stimulation of the thyroid gland by TSH causes release and distribution of stored thyroid hormones.

▶ When T4 and T3 are high, TSH secretion decreases.

▶ When T4 and T3 are low, TSH secretion increases.

▶ In primary hypothyroidism, TSH levels rise because of low levels of thyroid hormone.

▶ If the pituitary gland fails, TSH is not secreted and blood levels of TSH fall.

▷ TSH testing is commonly performed to establish the diagnosis of primary hypothyroidism.

- ▶ Diseases that have increased thyroid levels include:
  - ▷ Primary hypothyroidism
  - ▷ Thyroiditis
- ▶ Diseases that have decreased thyroid levels include:
  - ▷ Hyperthyroidism
  - ▷ Secondary and tertiary hypothyroidism
- ▶ Interfering factors:
  - ▷ Values can be decreased during treatment with T3, acetylsalicylic acid, corticosteroids, and heparin.
  - ▷ Values can be increased during drug therapy with lithium.

▶ Systemic effects of hypothyroidism (decreased T4, increased TSH)

- ▷ Mimics symptoms of unipolar mood disorders
  - ▶ Confusion
  - ▶ Decreased libido
  - ▶ Impotence
  - ▶ Decreased appetite
  - ▶ Memory loss
  - ▶ Lethargy
  - ▶ Constipation
  - ▶ Headaches
  - ▶ Slow or clumsy movements
  - ▶ Syncope
  - ▶ Weight gain
  - ▶ Fluid retention
  - ▶ Muscle aching and stiffness
  - ▶ Slowed reflexes
  - ▶ Somatic discomfort including aching and joint stiffness
  - ▶ Slowed speech and thinking
  - ▶ Sensory disturbances, including hearing
  - ▶ Cerebellar ataxia
  - ▶ Loss of amplitude in ECG

▶ Systemic effects of hyperthyroidism (increased T4, decreased TSH)

- ▷ May mimic symptoms of bipolar affective disorders
  - ▶ Motor restlessness
  - ▶ Emotional lability
  - ▶ Short attention span
  - ▶ Compulsive movement
  - ▶ Fatigue
  - ▶ Tremor
  - ▶ Insomnia
  - ▶ Impotence
  - ▶ Weight loss
  - ▶ Increase in appetite
  - ▶ Abdominal pain
  - ▶ Excessive sweating
  - ▶ Flushing
  - ▶ Elevated upper eyelid leading to decreased blinking, staring, fine tremor of eyelid
  - ▶ Tachycardia
  - ▶ Dysrhythmias

▶ Electrolytes

▷ Carried out as a part of routine screening in acute and critical illness or where there is a known or suspected disorder associated with fluid, electrolyte, or acid-base balance.

▶ Calcium (Ca; normal values 8.8–10.5 mg/dl)

▷ Abnormal values:

▶ <7.0 mg/dl associated with tetany

▶ >11.0 mg/dl associated with hyperparathyroidism

▶ >13.5 mg/dl associated with hypercalcemic coma and metastatic cancer.

▷ Most Ca (99%) is located in bone and the remainder is in the plasma and body cells.

▷ Of the Ca in the plasma, 50% is bound to plasma proteins and 40% is in the free or ionized form. The remaining fraction circulates in the blood.

▷ Ca is the major cation for the structure of bones and teeth.

▷ Functions:

▶ Enzymatic cofactor for blood clotting

▶ Required for hormone secretion

▶ Required for function of cell receptors

▶ Required for plasma membrane stability and permeability

▶ Required for transmission of nerve impulses and the contraction of muscles

▷ Ca balance is mediated by interactions among three hormones: parathyroid hormone, vitamin D, and calcitonin.

▷ Acting together, these substances determine the amount of dietary Ca absorbed and the renal reabsorption and excretion of Ca by the kidney.

▶ Increased levels of Ca can cause:

▷ Acidosis

▷ Hyperparathyroidism

▷ Cancers (for example, of bone, leukemia, myeloma)

▷ Drugs (such as thiazide diuretics, hormones, vitamin D, Ca)

▷ Vitamin D intoxication

▷ Addison's disease

▷ Hyperthyroidism

▶ Decreased levels of Ca can cause:

▷ Alkalosis

▷ Hypoparathyroidism

▷ Renal failure

▷ Pancreatitis

▷ Inadequate dietary intake of calcium, vitamin D

▷ Drugs, including barbiturates, anticonvulsants, acetazolamide, adrenocorticosteroids

▶ Interfering factors:
  ▷ Values are higher in children because of growth and active bone formation.
  ▷ Values can be increased by excessive ingestion of milk or during treatment with lithium, thiazide diuretics, alkaline antacids, or vitamin D.
  ▷ Values can be decreased during treatment with anticonvulsants, aspirin, calcitonin, corticosteroids, heparin, laxatives, diuretics, albuterol, and oral contraceptives.

▶ Systemic effects of hypocalcemia (Ca <8.5 mg/dl):
  ▷ Increase in neuromuscular excitability
  ▷ Confusion
  ▷ Paresthesias around the mouth and in the digits
  ▷ Muscle spasms in the hands and feet
  ▷ Hyperreflexia
  ▷ Convulsions
  ▷ Tetany
  ▷ Continuous severe muscle spasm
  ▷ ECG changes: prolonged QT interval
  ▷ Intestinal cramping
  ▷ Hyperactive bowel sounds

▶ Systemic effects of hypercalcemia (Ca >12.0 mg/dl):
  ▷ Fatigue
  ▷ Weakness
  ▷ Lethargy
  ▷ Anorexia
  ▷ Nausea
  ▷ Constipation
  ▷ Behavioral changes
  ▷ Impaired renal function
  ▷ ECG changes: shortened QT interval, depressed T-waves
  ▷ Bradycardia
  ▷ Heart block

▶ Sodium (Na; normal values 135–148 mEq/l)
  ▷ Na accounts for 90% of the extracellular fluid cations and is the most powerful cation in the extracellular fluid.
  ▷ Na regulates osmolality (interstitial and intravascular fluid volume).
  ▷ Na works with potassium and calcium to maintain neuromuscular irritability for conduction of nerve impulses.
  ▷ Na regulates acid-base balance.
  ▷ Na participates in cellular chemical reactions and membrane transport.
  ▷ Na regulates renal retention and excretion of water.

▷ Na maintains systemic blood pressure.

▶ Increased levels of Na can cause:

▷ Hypovolemia

▷ Dehydration

▷ Diabetes insipidus

▷ Excessive salt ingestion

▷ Gastroenteritis

▷ Drugs such as adrenocorticosteroids, methyldopa, hydralazine, or cough medication

▶ Decreased levels of Na can cause:

▷ Addison's disease

▷ Renal disorder

▷ GI fluid loss from vomiting, diarrhea, nasogastric suction, ileus

▷ Diuresis

▷ Drugs such as lithium, vasopressin, or diuretics

▷ Systemic effects of hyponatremia (Na <135 mEq/l):

▶ Lethargy

▶ Headache

▶ Confusion

▶ Apprehension

▶ Seizures

▶ Coma

▶ Hypotension

▶ Tachycardia

▶ Decreased urine output

▶ Weight gain

▶ Edema

▶ Ascites

▶ Jugular vein distention

▷ Systemic effects of hypernatremia (Na >147 mEq/l):

▶ Convulsions

▶ Pulmonary edema

▶ Thirst

▶ Fever

▶ Dry mucous membranes

▶ Hypotension

▶ Tachycardia

▶ Low jugular venous pressure

▶ Restlessness

▶ Magnesium (Mg; normal values 1.3–2.1 mEq/l)

▷ Mg is a major intracellular cation; 40% to 60% is stored in bone and muscle, with 30% in cells.

▷ A small amount is in the serum, where one-third is bound to plasma proteins and the rest is in ionized form.

▷ Regulation of Mg metabolism is primarily by the kidney.

▷ Low serum levels cause renal conservation of Mg.

▷ Mg is a cofactor in intracellular enzymatic reactions.

▷ Mg is a cause of neuromuscular excitability.

► Increased levels:

▷ Addison's disease

▷ Adrenalectomy

▷ Renal failure

▷ Diabetic ketoacidosis

▷ Dehydration

▷ Hypothyroidism

▷ Hyperthyroidism

► Decreased levels:

▷ Hyperaldosteronism

▷ Hypokalemia

▷ Diabetic ketoacidosis

▷ Malnutrition

▷ Alcoholism

▷ Acute pancreatitis

▷ GI loss from vomiting, diarrhea, nasogastric suction, and fistula

▷ Malabsorption syndrome

▷ Pregnancy-induced hypertension

► Interfering factors:

▷ Hemolysis of a sample leads to falsely elevated levels.

▷ Numerous drugs can alter levels.

▷ Values can be increased by drugs such as antacids, laxatives containing Mg, salicylates, and lithium.

▷ Values can be decreased by drugs such as thiazide diuretics, calcium gluconate, insulin, amphotericin B, neomycin, aldosterone, and ethanol.

▷ Systemic effects of hypomagnesemia (Mg <1.5 mEq/l):

► Depression

► Confusion

► Irritability

► Increased reflexes

► Muscle weakness

► Ataxia

► Nystagmus

► Tetany

► Convulsions

▷ Systemic effects of hypermagnesemia (Mg >2.5 mEq/L):

► Nausea and vomiting

► Muscle weakness

► Hypotension

► Bradycardia

► Respiratory depression

► Depressed skeletal muscle contraction and nerve function

► Chloride (normal values 98–106 mEq/L)

▷ Chloride is the major anion in the extracellular fluid.

▷ It provides electroneutrality in relation to sodium (see above).

▷ Transport of chloride is passive and follows the active transport of sodium so that increases or decreases in chloride are proportional to changes in sodium.

- ▶ Increased levels:
  - ▷ Acidosis
  - ▷ Hyperkalemia, hypernatremia
  - ▷ Dehydration
  - ▷ Renal failure
  - ▷ Cushing's syndrome
  - ▷ Hyperventilation
  - ▷ Anemia

- ▶ Decreased levels:
  - ▷ Alkalosis
  - ▷ Hypokalemia
  - ▷ Hyponatremia
  - ▷ GI loss from vomiting, diarrhea, nasogastric suction, and fistula
  - ▷ Diuresis
  - ▷ Overhydration
  - ▷ Addison's disease
  - ▷ Burns

- ▶ Interfering factors:
  - ▷ Elevated serum triglyceride levels and myeloma proteins may lead to falsely decreased levels.
  - ▷ Values can be increased by potassium chloride, acetazolamide, methyldopa, diazoxide, and guanethidine.
- ▷ Values can be decreased by ethacrynic acid, furosemide, thiazide diuretics, and bicarbonate.
- ▷ No specific symptoms are associated with chloride increase or decrease.
- ▶ Potassium (K+; normal values 3.5–5.1 mEq/l)
  - ▷ K+ is the major intracellular electrolyte.
  - ▷ Total body K+ is about 4,000 mEq, with most of it located in the cells.
  - ▷ Intracellular concentration of K+ is 150 to 160 mEq/l; extracellular concentration is 3.5 to 4.5 mEq/l.
  - ▷ As the predominant intracellular ion, K+ regulates intracellular fluid osmolality and provides the balance for intracellular electrical neutrality.
  - ▷ K+ is required for glycogen deposition in liver and skeletal muscle cells.
  - ▷ K+ maintains resting membrane potential and assists in transmission and conduction of nerve impulses, maintenance of normal cardiac rhythms, and skeletal and smooth muscle contraction.
  - ▷ K+ balance is regulated by the kidney, aldosterone levels, insulin secretion, and changes in pH.
    - ▶ Increased levels:
      - ▷ Acidosis
      - ▷ Insulin deficiency
      - ▷ Addison's disease
      - ▷ Acute renal failure
      - ▷ Hypoaldosteronism
      - ▷ Infection
      - ▷ Dehydration

▶ Decreased levels:
  ▷ Alkalosis
  ▷ Excessive insulin
  ▷ GI loss
  ▷ Laxative abuse
  ▷ Burns
  ▷ Trauma
  ▷ Surgery
  ▷ Cushing's syndrome
  ▷ Hyperaldosteronism
  ▷ Thyrotoxicosis
  ▷ Anorexia nervosa
  ▷ Diet deficient in meat and vegetables

▶ Interfering factors:
  ▷ False elevations can occur with vigorous pumping of the hand during venipuncture, hemolysis of the sample, or high platelet counts during clotting.
  ▷ False decreases are seen in anticoagulated samples left at room temperature.
  ▷ Values can be decreased by drugs such as furosemide, ethacrynic acid, thiazide diuretics, insulin, aspirin, prednisone, cortisone, gentamycin, lithium, and laxatives.
  ▷ Values can be increased by drugs such as amphotericin B, tetracycline, heparin, epinephrine, potassium-sparing diuretics, and isoniazid.
  ▷ Chronic marijuana use can elevate K+ level.

▷ Systemic effects of hyperkalemia (K+ >5.5 mEq/l):
  ▶ Muscle weakness
  ▶ Paralysis
  ▶ Tingling of lips and fingers
  ▶ Restlessness
  ▶ Intestinal cramping
  ▶ Diarrhea
  ▶ ECG changes: narrow and taller T-waves
    ▷ Mild hyperkalemia: shortened QT interval
    ▷ Severe hyperkalemia: depressed ST segment, prolonged PR interval, widened QRS complex leading to cardiac arrest

▷ Systemic effects of hypokalemia (K+ <3.5 mEq/l):
  ▶ Impaired carbohydrate metabolism
  ▶ Impaired renal function
  ▶ Polyuria
  ▶ Polydipsia
  ▶ Skeletal muscle weakness
  ▶ Smooth muscle atony

- ▶ Cardiac dysrhythmias
- ▶ Paralysis and respiratory arrest

▶ Liver function tests

▷ Used to monitor liver disease or damage caused by hepatotoxic drugs, as confirmed by elevated levels

▶ Alanine aminotransferase (ALT; normal values 5–35 U/l)

▷ Formerly known as glutamic-pyruvic transaminase (SGPT), ALT is an enzyme produced by the liver that acts as a catalyst in the transamination reaction necessary for amino acid production.

▷ ALT is found in liver cells in high concentrations and in moderate amounts in body fluids, heart, kidneys, and skeletal muscles.

▷ When liver damage occurs, serum levels of ALT rise to as much as 50 times normal.

- ▶ Pronounced elevated levels (>300 U/l):
    - ▷ Liver disease or damage, such as hepatic cancer, hepatitis, or infectious mononucleosis
- ▶ Moderately elevated levels (100–300 U/l):
    - ▷ Biliary tract obstruction
    - ▷ Recent cerebrovascular accident
    - ▷ Muscle injury from intramuscular injections, trauma, infection, and seizures
    - ▷ Muscular dystrophy
    - ▷ Acute pancreatitis
    - ▷ Intestinal injury
    - ▷ Myocardial infarction
    - ▷ Congestive heart failure
    - ▷ Renal failure
    - ▷ Severe burns
- ▶ Interfering factors:
    - ▷ Uremia and hemodialysis can cause falsely decreased levels.
    - ▷ Values can be increased with acetaminophen, allopurinol, aspirin, ampicillin, carbamazepine, cephalosporins, codeine, digitalis, indomethacin, heparin, isoniazid, methotrexate, methyldopa, oral contraceptives, phenothiazines, propranolol, tetracycline, and verapamil.

▶ Aspartate aminotransferase (AST; normal values 5–40 U/l)

▷ Previously known as serum glutamate oxaloacetate transaminase (SGOT), AST measures the level of the enzyme that catalyzes the reversible transfer of an amino group between the amino acid, aspartate, and alphaketoglutamic acid.

▷ AST exists in large amounts in both liver and myocardial cells and in smaller but significant amounts in skeletal muscles, kidneys, the pancreas, and the brain.

▷ Serum AST rises when there is cellular damage to the tissues in which the enzyme is found.

- ▶ Pronounced elevation (>5× normal):
  - ▷ Acute hepatocellular damage
  - ▷ Myocardial infarction
  - ▷ Shock
  - ▷ Acute pancreatitis
  - ▷ Infectious mononucleosis

- ▶ Moderate elevation (3–5× normal):
  - ▷ Biliary tract obstruction
  - ▷ Cardiac arrhythmias
  - ▷ Congestive heart failure
  - ▷ Liver tumors
  - ▷ Chronic hepatitis
  - ▷ Muscular dystrophy
  - ▷ Dermatomyositis

- ▶ Slight elevation (2–3× normal):
  - ▷ Pericarditis
  - ▷ Cirrhosis, fatty liver
  - ▷ Pulmonary infarction
  - ▷ Delirium tremens
  - ▷ Cerebrovascular accident
  - ▷ Hemolytic anemia

- ▶ Interfering factors:
  - ▷ Numerous drugs may elevate levels, including antihypertensives, cholinergic agents, anticoagulants, digitalis, erythromycin, isoniazid, methyldopa, oral contraceptives, opiates, salicylates, hepatotoxic medications, and verapamil.
  - ▷ Exercise can cause increased levels.

▶ Gamma glutamyl transpeptidase (GGT; normal values 10–38 IU/l)

▷ GGT is an isoenzyme of alkaline phosphatase and assists with the transfer of amino acids and peptides across cellular membranes.

▷ Hepatobiliary tissues and renal tubular and pancreatic epithelium contain large amounts of GGT.

▷ Other sources of GGT include the prostate gland, brain, and heart.

▷ GGT is used to evaluate and monitor a client with known or suspected alcohol abuse, because levels rise even after ingestion of small amounts of alcohol.

▷ Also used to evaluate elevated alkaline phosphatase of uncertain etiology.

▷ Pronounced early increases in GGT are found in in hepatic disease.

    ▷   Modest elevation in GGT occurs in cirrhosis and in pancreatic or renal disease.

        ▶   Elevated GGT:

           ▷   Hepatobiliary tract disorders

           ▷   Hepatocellular carcinoma

           ▷   Hepatocellular degeneration such as cirrhosis

           ▷   Hepatitis

           ▷   Pancreatic or renal cell damage or neoplasm

           ▷   Congestive heart failure

           ▷   Acute myocardial infarction (after 4–10 days)

           ▷   Hyperlipoproteinemia

           ▷   Diabetes mellitus with hypertension

           ▷   Seizure disorder

           ▷   Significant alcohol ingestion

        ▶   Interfering factors:

           ▷   Alcohol, barbiturates, and phenytoin can elevate GGT levels.

           ▷   Late pregnancy, oral contraceptives, and clofibrate can lower GGT levels.

DISEASE PREVENTION ACTIVITIES

Immunization

Immunizations are critical to preventing disease, according to the U.S. Centers for Disease Control and Prevention (CDC). Immunizations protect individual children and adults from developing potentially serious diseases while also protecting the community by reducing the spread of infectious disease.

   ▶   Schedules for children and adults are available on the CDC website at www.cdc.gov/vaccines/schedules/index.html.

   ▶   Seasonal influenza vaccination (as live attenuated influenza vaccine or as inactivated type).

   ▶   All persons age 6 months or older should receive annual influenza vaccination.

      ▷   Children 6 months to 8 years of age require two doses of influenza vaccine (4 weeks apart) during their first season of vaccinations.

      ▷   LAIV should not be used in persons younger than 2 years of age or older than 49 years of age.

      ▷   Persons with egg allergy should always receive the vaccination from a health care provider familiar with potential reaction and should be observed for at least 30 minutes post injection for signs of reaction.

      ▷   Immunocompromised persons should not receive live vaccination.

      ▷   Use live vaccine or inactivated vaccine for healthy nonpregnant adults younger than 50 years of age with no high-risk medical conditions. All others should receive the inactivated vaccine only (Grohskopf et al., 2015).

▶ HPV vaccination for girls is recommended at age 11 or 12 years with catch-up vaccination at ages 13 through 26 years to prevent genital human papillomavirus infection, which can cause cervical cancer and genital warts.

  ▷ HPV4 may be administered to males age 9 through 26 years to prevent genital warts.

▶ Measles, mumps, rubella (MMR; live vaccine)

  ▷ Not for pregnant women; people with cancer, weakened immune systems, or HIV or AIDS with T-cell counts below 200; or people currently being treated with high-dose steroids or who have received a blood transfusion within the previous 2 weeks

▶ Diphtheria, tetanus, acellular pertussis

  ▷ Td (tetanus, diphtheria) vaccine should be given every 10 years beginning at age 11 years, with Tdap (tetanus, diphtheria, acellular pertussis) substituted once for Td but no less than 5 years after the last DTaP dose was given. DTaP should not be given to anyone 7 years of age or older.

▶ Shingles (also known as *herpes zoster*) vaccine (CDC, 2015b)

  ▷ Recommended for anyone age 60 or older who has had chickenpox.

  ▷ Do not give shingles vaccine to persons with weakened immune systems or HIV or AIDS with T-cell counts below 200, or to persons being treated with high-dose steroids.

  ▷ Shingles is an inflammatory condition in which a virus produces painful vesicular eruptions along the distribution of the nerves from one or more dorsal root ganglia.

▶ Varicella (chickenpox) vaccine

  ▷ Not for pregnant women; persons with weakened immune systems, HIV or AIDS with T-cell counts below 200, or cancer; or for people being treated with high-dose steroids or who received a blood transfusion within the previous 2 weeks

Anticipatory Guidance

Anticipatory guidance is a framework for implementation of prevention strategies.

▶ Based on the premise that information can be provided to people to help them cope more effectively with events that occur along the life span. Within the framework of anticipatory guidance, the practitioner seeks to determine the specific informational needs of the client in a systematic, standard way.

▶ *Pediatrics:* Soliciting information from parents about their concerns in parenting and providing information specific to their concerns. Teaching parents about health hazards and strategies to prevent harm, such as car seat safety, water safety, wearing helmets, and so forth.

▶ *Bright Futures* (www.brightfutures.org/) is a national health promotion initiative (launched by the Health Resources and Services Administration in partnership with other agencies) dedicated to the principle that every child deserves to be healthy and that optimal health involves trusting relationships among the health professional, the child, the family, and the community as partners in health practice. Expansion of the model includes screening, care management, and education about mental health problems and disorders in developmental context.

▶ In specific healthcare situations, anticipatory guidance can be used to assist people in meeting healthcare challenges across the life span. Some examples include

▷ Coping with terminal illness or death and dying (anticipatory grief)

▷ Coping with disease progression, such as with Alzheimer's dementia, in a loved one

▷ Coping with change and limitations resulting from spinal cord injuries

▷ Can be implemented in each "well check" to identify information needs pertinent to the client's current life situation. Some examples:

   ▶ Responsible alcohol use for the adolescent going off to college

   ▶ Domestic violence

   ▶ Life after the loss of a loved one (through divorce or death)

   ▶ Planning for retirement

GENDER-BASED MEDICAL TESTING AND SCREENING RECOMMENDATIONS FOR THE GENERAL PUBLIC

Tanner Stages Assessment

Defines physical measurements of development in children, adolescents, and adults. The development of primary and secondary sex characteristics (breasts, genitalia, and pubic hair) are assessed by stages to describe the onset and progression of puberty in both males and females. Because of natural variability, males and females pass through the stages at different rates based on timing of puberty.

Girls: Breast Development

Stage 1: Prepubertal

Stage 2: Breast bud stage with elevation of breast and papilla; enlargement of areola

Stage 3: Further enlargement of breast and areola; no separation of their contour

Stage 4: Areola and papilla from a secondary mound above level of breast

Stage 5: Mature stage: projection of papilla only, related to recession of areola (Jarvis, 2011)

Boys: Development of External Genitalia

Stage 1: Prepubertal

Stage 2: Enlargement of scrotum and testes; scrotum skin reddens and changes in texture

Stage 3: Enlargement of penis (length at first); further growth of testes

Stage 4: Increase in size of penis with growth in breadth and development of glans; testes and scrotum larger, scrotum skin darker

Stage 5: Adult genitalia (Jarvis, 2011)

Boys and Girls: Pubic Hair

Stage 1: Prepubertal (can see vellus hair similar to abdominal wall)

Stage 2: Sparse growth of long, slightly pigmented hair, straight or curled, at base of penis or along labia

Stage 3: Darker, coarser, and curlier hair, spreading sparsely over junctions of pubes

Stage 4: Adult-type hair, but covering smaller area than in adult, no spread to medial surface of thighs

Stage 5: Adult type and quantity, with horizontal distribution (Jarvis, 2011)

Women

Ages 18 through 39

▶ Monthly: Skin and oral self-exams

▶ Yearly: Blood pressure; blood tests and urinalysis; physical exam; Pap smear (beginning at age 21 or within 3 years of sexual activity, whichever comes first), pelvic exam, sexually transmitted infection (STI) detection

▶ All persons age 13 to 64 should be tested at least once for HIV (CDC, 2016)

Ages 40 through 49

▶ Monthly: Skin and oral self-exams

▶ Yearly: Blood pressure; blood tests and urinalysis; physical exam; Pap smear (every 2 or 3 years after three consecutive negative smears), pelvic exam, STI detection; electrocardiogram (ECG) every 4 years

Ages 50+

▶ Monthly: Skin and oral self-exams

▶ Yearly: Blood pressure; blood tests (complete blood count, metabolic panel, thyroid-stimulating hormone) and urinalysis; physical exam; Pap smear (65 and older not recommended if person had proper recent normal Pap smear and is not at high risk for cervical cancer), pelvic exam, STI detection; mammography every 2 years; routine bone density screening starting at age 65 and older (beginning at 60 if increased risk for osteoporotic fractures)

▶ Every 4 years: Electrocardiogram (ECG)

▶ Every 5 years through age 75: flexible sigmoidoscopy or double-contrast barium enema or CT colonography (if any of these tests are positive, a colonoscopy should be done), or colonoscopy every 10 years

▶ Consult provider: Hearing, vision

Additional Colorectal Cancer Screening for High-Risk Women

The American Cancer Society recommends that some people be screened using a different schedule because of their personal or family history.

Men

Ages 18 through 39

▶ Monthly: Self-exams (testicles, skin, and oral)

▶ Yearly: Blood pressure; blood tests (complete blood count, metabolic panel, thyroid-stimulating hormone) and urinalysis; physical exam

▶ Screening at least once a year for syphilis, chlamydia, and gonorrhea for all sexually active gay, bisexual, and men who have sex with men up to age 64 (CDC, 2016)

▶ All persons age 13 to 64 should be tested at least once for HIV (CDC, 2016)

Ages 40 through 49

▶ Monthly: Testicles, skin, and oral self-exams

▶ Yearly: Blood pressure; blood tests (complete blood count, metabolic panel, thyroid-stimulating hormone) and urinalysis; physical exam; ECG every 4 years

Ages 50+

▶ Monthly: Testicles, skin, and oral self-exams

▶ Yearly: Blood pressure; blood tests (complete blood count, metabolic panel, thyroid-stimulating hormone) and urinalysis; physical exam; electrocardiogram (ECG) every 3 years

▶ Every 5 years through age 75: Flexible sigmoidoscopy or double-contrast barium enema or CT colonography (if any of these tests are positive, a colonoscopy should be done), or colonoscopy every 10 years

▶ Consult provider: Testosterone blood test; hearing and vision screening

HEALTH BEHAVIOR GUIDELINES

Exercise

Exercise benefits both physical and mental health. Inactivity has a direct link to obesity, a major health problem in this country. In results of recent studies, exercise has demonstrated effects comparable to antidepressant therapy in the treatment of depression.

▶ Key factor in staying healthy: strengthens bones, heart, and lungs, tones muscles, improves vitality, relieves depression, and helps to improve sleep. It is particularly beneficial to persons with comorbid medical conditions such as diabetes, obesity, and hypertension.

▶ Mind–body connection: improves cognition and enhances mood

▶ Neurobiological explanation: promotes increased concentrations of serotonin, norepinephrine, and endorphins

▶ Integrative psychiatry includes strategies to improve lifestyle practices (diet, exercise, smoking cessation, decrease or cease drug and alcohol use) and reduce stress to prevent illness.

▶ Client teaching regarding exercise:

▷ Check with provider before starting an exercise program.

▷ Begin exercising gradually. Don't expect results overnight. If you are consistent, you will see improvement within 3 months.

▷ Work hard enough to sweat, but not so hard that you cannot carry on a conversation.

▷ Plan an exercise routine that lasts at least 30 minutes, and perform the workout at least 3 to 5 days a week. Warming up before exercise helps avoid injury.

▷ Include both aerobic and strengthening activities in exercise program.

▷ Exercise programs need to be modified for children, pregnant women, the elderly, clients who are obese or disabled, and heart attack survivors as well as modified for high altitudes and extreme hot or cold conditions.

▷ Monitor the intensity of exercise by measuring heart rate. The target heart rate during physical activity should be 60% to 90% of the maximum heart rate. Use the following formula to calculate target heart rate:

▶ 220 (beats per minute) minus age = maximum heart rate

▶ Maximum heart rate multiplied by the intensity level = target heart rate

▶ Physical activity at 60% to 70% of the maximum heart rate is considered moderate-intensity exercise.

▷ CDC recommends 60 minutes (1 hour) or more of physical activity each day for children and adolescents.

▷ CDC recommends 150 minutes of moderate-intensity aerobic activity (such as brisk walking) every week and muscle-strengthening activities 2 or more days a week for adults, including healthy older adults (CDC, 2015a).

Self-Awareness

▶ Requires reflection on one's personal beliefs, thoughts, emotions, motives, biases, and limitations and being aware of how they influence behavior toward others

▶ A trusted person who can give open, honest feedback to self-examination is helpful.

▶ Personal experiences influence communication patterns and responses to clients.

▶ Social biases, feelings, and beliefs projected onto the client may affect the nurse–client relationship.

▶ Being nonjudgmental and objective cultivates trust in the relationship.

▶ Clinical supervision by colleague provides ongoing feedback for therapeutic development of the helper, including supporting change as needed.

▶ If personal values and beliefs make it difficult to be therapeutic with a particular client, refer the client to another provider.

Self-Disclosure

▶ Revealing personal information to the client changes the focus away from the client.

▶ When asked personal questions, self-disclosure can be limited by redirecting, giving a vague answer, or reminding the client that you will not share your personal information.

▶ Self-disclosure may be therapeutic only when it is purposeful and has an identified therapeutic outcome, such as role modeling.

Health Promotion and Disease Prevention Education

▶ Preventative care and screening practices are essential aspects of the PMHNP role.

▶ Screening for physical health problems in the psychiatric client

▶ Usually guided by Healthy People 2020 (U.S. Department of Health and Human Services, 2016), which identifies national health objectives, including behavioral health

▶ Mental health promotion and education includes:

▷ Teaching about interventions and ways to cope with specific stressors

▷ Validating "normalcy" of feelings; ensuring clients that they are not "crazy"

▷ Helping clients recognize and identify their feelings or behaviors

▷ Helping clients identify resources in the community

PUBLIC HEALTH PRINCIPLES

▶ *Primary prevention:* Aimed at decreasing the incidence (number of new cases) of mental disorders

▷ Helping people avoid stressors or cope with them more adaptively

▶ *Example*: Stress management classes for graduate students, smoking prevention classes, Drug Abuse Resistance Education (DARE) Keepin' It REAL elementary and middle school curriculum (DARE, 2015)

▶ *Secondary prevention:* Aimed at decreasing the prevalence (number of existing cases) of mental disorders

▷ Early case finding

▷ Screening

▷ Prompt and effective treatment

▶ *Example:* Telephone hotlines, crisis intervention, disaster responses

▶ *Tertiary prevention:* Aimed at decreasing the disability and severity of a mental disorder

▷ Rehabilitative services

▷ Avoidance or postponement of complications

▶ *Example:* Day treatment programs; case management for physical, housing, or vocational needs; social skills training

Risk Factors

▶ Predisposing characteristics that make it more likely that a person will develop a disorder

▶ *Biological risk factors:* History of mental illness in family, poor nutritional status, poor general health

▶ *Psychological risk factors:* Poor self-concept, external locus of control, poor ego defenses

▶ *Social risk factors:* Stressful occupation, low socioeconomic status, poor level of social integration

Preventative Factors

▶ Factors that prevent or protect the person from the disorder

▶ Coping mechanisms or resources that facilitate a healthy response to stress

▶ *Biological preventative factors:* No history of mental illness in the family, healthy nutritional status, good general health

▶ *Psychological preventative factors:* Good self-esteem or self-concept, internal locus of control, healthy ego defenses

▶ *Social preventative factors:* Low-stress occupation, higher socioeconomic status, higher level of education

CASE STUDY 1

Mr. J. is a 79-year-old married man, being treated by the PMHNP for major depression. Mr. J. was started on citalopram 10 mg 4 weeks ago and has now been taking 20 mg p.o. q.a.m. for the past 3 weeks.

Pertinent medical history includes hypertension, which is well controlled by benazepril and hydro-chlorothiazide (Lotensin HCT). He also takes finasteride (Proscar) for benign prostatic hyperplasia.

1. How should the PMHNP think about what may be going on with Mr. J.?

2. How should the PMHNP intervene?

Mr. J. arrives at his follow-up appointment, accompanied by his spouse. He tells you his primary care provider checked his sodium level, which was low, and Mr. J. was instructed to stop the citalopram. He is not on any antidepressant treatment and reports he has been feeling progressively more tired, his stomach has been upset, and he feels "a little foggy." These symptoms began "about a week ago."

3. How would this presentation change the PMHNP's treatment plan?

4. What is the appropriate intervention for Mr. J.?

CASE STUDY 2

Ms. Smith, a 27-year-old single woman who works in a retail store, has been referred by her primary care provider to the PMHNP for evaluation and treatment of "mood swings." Ms. Smith tells the PMHNP that she has been feeling "pretty good" for the past week after coming through a 3-week period of depression. Her PCP discontinued her fluoxetine 20 mg several days ago. She is mildly euphoric, but there is also evidence of irritability. Her speech is pressured and she is hyperverbal, but she is easily redirected. She reports she has been sleeping "about 4 to 5 hours a night," and describes her energy as "pretty good!" There is no evidence of psychosis. Her insight and judgment are intact, and she tells the NP "I think I'm a little high. I'm worried it's going to get me in trouble at work."

Past psychiatric history is significant for depressive episodes beginning in early teens, during which she experienced suicidal ideation. She has been treated with many selective serotonin reuptake inhibitors (SSRIs) over the years, all prescribed by her primary care provider and in each case, she noticed rapid improvement of her mood and discontinued the drug after several months. She denies a history of hypomania until the past year.

Medical history is noncontributory.

Family history is significant for bipolar I disorder in dad and possibly paternal grandmother. Mother has a long history of untreated "depression and anxiety."

The PMHNP and Ms. Smith discuss treatment options and decide to start lithium carbonate.

1. What client teaching should be included in preparation for beginning lithium?

2. What tests should be ordered before beginning this drug?

3. If Ms. Smith were an older adult, what additional test should be ordered before treating her with lithium?

Three months after beginning lithium, Ms. Smith presents with lethargy, constipation, and bradycardia.

4. What should the PMHNP consider as etiology?

5. What labs tests should be ordered?

6. What adjustment should be made to the client's medication?

ANSWERS TO CASE STUDY DISCUSSION QUESTIONS

Case Study 1

1. All SSRIs and some other antidepressants have been implicated in hyponatremia. Owing to diminished renal functioning and frequent polypharmacy, hyponatremia is more common in the elderly. In addition to citalopram, Mr. J. is taking hydrochlorothiazide, which may also cause hyponatremia.

2. The signs and symptoms of hyponatremia vary, depending on how quickly sodium levels drop. Slow decrease in sodium may lead to a subtle presentation such as feeling tired, and slightly "foggy." Clients experiencing a more precipitous drop will present with dramatic changes in level of consciousness and severe headache owing to cerebral edema. The PMHNP should assess for signs and symptoms of hyponatremia and order a sodium level.

3. An assessment should be made if the client has had trials on another SSRI. Assessment of his depression needs to be completed and use of a depression scale, such as the PHQ-9 or GDS, are indicated.

4. If the client has not had another trial on a SSRI it is indicated to place Mr. J. on a SSRI and follow his response.

Case Study 2

1. The client should be taught about the potential risks and benefits of taking lithium. Women of childbearing age should be educated about the risk of birth defects, including Ebstein's anomaly. Consideration of lithium dose and maintenance blood levels should be included in discussing the relative risk. The client should be taught about the signs and symptoms of lithium toxicity.

2. Baseline labs consisting of a metabolic panel, TSH, and complete blood count (CBC) should be done. Women of childbearing age should have a pregnancy test.

3. Clients over the age of 65 or those who have a history of heart disease should have a baseline ECG.

4. Lethargy and constipation may be due to hypothyroidism or hypercalcemia, both of which may be caused by lithium.

5. The client should have TSH, free T4, and electrolytes drawn.

6. The lithium should be tapered off and an alternative medication used for mood stabilization.

REFERENCES AND RESOURCES

American Nurses Association, American Psychiatric Nurses Association, & International Society of Psychiatric-Mental Health Nurses. (2014). *Psychiatric–mental health nursing: Scope and standards of practice* (2nd ed.). Silver Spring, MD: Nursesbooks.org

American Psychiatric Association. (2000). *Practice guidelines for the treatment of patients with major depressive disorder.* Washington, DC: Author.

American Psychiatric Association. (2006). *Practice guideline for psychiatric evaluation of adults.* Washington, DC: Author.

American Psychiatric Association. (2013). *Diagnostic and statistical manual of mental disorders* (5th ed.). Washington, DC: Author.

American Psychiatric Association, Work Group on Eating Disorders. (2000). Practice guideline for the treatment of patients with eating disorders. *American Journal of Psychiatry, 157*(Suppl. 1), 1–39.

Anandarajah, G., & Hight, E. (2001). Spirituality and medical practice: Using the hope questions as a practical tool for spiritual assessment. *American Family Physician, 63*(1), 81–88.

Bakerman, S. (2002). *ABCs of interpretive laboratory data* (4th ed.). Greenville, NC: Interpretive Laboratory Data.

Bickley, L. S. (2007). *Bates' guide to physical examination and history taking* (9th ed.). Philadelphia, PA: Lippincott.

Center for Disease Control. (2015a). Physical activity basics. Retrieved from http://www.cdc.gov/ physicalactivity/basics/

Center for Disease Control. (2015b). Shingles (herpes zoster) vaccination. Retrieved from http:// www.cdc.gov/vaccines/vpd-vac/shingles/

Center for Disease Control. (2016). STD & HIV screening recommendations. Retrieved from http://www.cdc.gov/std/prevention/screeningreccs.htm

Clinical Evidence Organization. (2000). *Clinical evidence international sourcebook.* London, Eng.: BMJ Publishing Group.

DARE. (2015). D.A.R.E.'s keepin' it REAL elementary and middle school curriculums adhere to lessons from prevention research principles. Retrieved from http://www.dare.org/d-a-r-e-s-keepin-it-real-elementary-and-middle-school-curriculums-adhere-to-lessons-from-prevention-research-principles/

Davidson, J. R. (2000). Trauma: The impact of post-traumatic stress disorder. *Journal of Psychopharmacology, 14*(Suppl. 1), S5–S12.

Faulkner, G. (2000). *Behavioral outcomes and guidelines sourcebook.* New York, NY: Faulkner & Gray.

Grohskopf, L. A., Sokolow, L. Z., Olsen, S. J., Bresee, J. S., Broder, K. R., & Karron, R. A. (2015). Prevention and control of influenza with vaccines: Recommendations of the advisory committee on immunization practices, United States, 2015–16 influenza season. *Morbidity and Mortality Weekly Report, 64*(30). Retrieved from http://www.cdc.gov/mmwr/preview/mmwrhtml/mm6430a3.htm

Jarvis, C. (2011). *Physical health examination and health assessment* (6th ed.). St Louis: Elsevier.

Margolin, G., & Gordis, E. B. (2000). The effects of family and community violence on children. *Annual Review of Psychology, 51*, 445–479.

National Institute of Mental Health. (2006). Statistics. Retrieved from http://www.nimh.nih.gov/ health/statistics/index.shtml

National Institutes of Health. (2013). Cultural respect. Retrieved from www.nih.gov/clearcommunication/culturalcompetency.htm

O'Reilly, D. J. (2000). Thyroid function tests: Time for reassessment. *British Medical Journal, 320*, 1332–1334.

Sadock, B. J., Sadock, V. A., & Ruiz, P. (2015). *Kaplan and Sadock's synopsis of psychiatry: Behavioral sciences/clinical psychiatry* (11th ed.). New York, NY: Wolters Kluwer.

Schatsburg, A., Cole, J., & DeBattista, C. (2007). *Manual of clinical psychopharmacology* (6th ed.). Washington, DC: American Psychiatric Association.

Strub, R. (2000). *The mental status examination in neurology.* Philadelphia, PA: Oxford University Press.

Stuart, G. W., & Laraia, M. T. (2004). *Principles and practice of psychiatric nursing* (8th ed.). St. Louis, MO: Mosby.

U.S. Department of Health and Human Services. (2016). Healthy People 2020. Retrieved from http://www.healthypeople.gov/

CHAPTER 7

PHARMACOLOGICAL PRINCIPLES

Psychopharmacology, one of the most active and developing areas of psychiatric research, is the use of psychotropic medication to treat psychiatric disorders. *Psychiatric–mental health nurse practitioners* (PMHNPs) must have a thorough understanding of the science and art of prescribing—of the pharmacokinetic and pharmacodynamic actions of a given drug, as well as the client's motivation to take the drug. The basic pharmacological principles are discussed in this chapter.

CONCEPTS IN PHARMACOLOGICAL MANAGEMENT

▶ *Pharmacology:* Study of what drugs do and how they do it

▶ *Pharmacokinetics:* Study of what the body does to drugs; includes absorption, distribution, metabolism, and excretion

▶ *Pharmacodynamics:* Study of what drugs do to the body; target sites for drug actions include receptors, ion channels, enzymes, and carrier proteins

Pharmacokinetics

▶ *Absorption:* Method and rate at which drugs leave the site of administration

▷ With oral medications, absorption normally occurs in the small intestine and then in the liver.

▶ *Distribution:* Occurs after the drug leaves the systemic circulation and enters the interstitium and cells

▷ Drugs are redistributed in organs according to their fat and protein content.

▷ Most psychotropic medications are lipophilic and highly protein-bound. Only the unbound (free) portion of the drug is active. Therefore, people with low protein (albumin) levels, such as in malnutrition, wasting, or aging, can potentially experience toxicity (see below) from an increased amount of free drug. People with high fat-to-lean body mass ratio (as in older adults) will have erratic amounts of active drug in their system.

▶ *Metabolism:* Process by which the drug becomes chemically altered in the body

▶ *First-pass metabolism:* Process by which the drug is metabolized by cytochrome P450 (P450) enzymes in the intestines and liver prior to going to the systemic circulation

▶ *Elimination:* Process by which the drug is removed from the body

▶ *Half-life (T ½):* Time needed to clear 50% of the drug from the plasma

▷ The half-life also determines the dosing interval and the length of time to reach a steady state.

▶ *Steady state:* Point at which the amount of drug eliminated between doses is approximately equal to the dose administered.

▷ Drugs usually are administered once every half-life to achieve a steady state.

▷ It takes approximately five half-lives to achieve a steady state and five half-lives to completely eliminate a drug.

▶ Alterations in pharmacokinetics

▷ Hepatic cytochrome P450 enzyme interactions can induce or inhibit the metabolism of certain drugs, thus changing their desired concentration levels (see Table 7–1).

▷ Approximately 10% of Caucasians are poor metabolizers of the P450 2D6 enzyme.

▷ Approximately 20% of Asians may have reduced activity of the P450 2C19 enzyme.

▷ First-pass metabolism activity of P450 enzymes 2C9, 2C19, 2D6, and 3A4 in young children may exceed rates of adolescents and adults and give rise to underexposure to certain medications Conversely, the ontogeny of the 1A2 pathway is delayed, possibly leading to toxic effects from drugs that are substrates of this pathway (e.g., some antipsychotics).

▷ Enzyme inducers can decrease the serum level of other drugs that are substrates of that enzyme, thus possibly causing subtherapeutic drug levels.

TABLE 7–1.
CYTOCHROME P450 INHIBITORS AND INDUCERS

INHIBITORS	INDUCERS
Buproprion	Carbamazepine
Clomipramine	Hypericum (St. John's Wort)
Cimetidine	Phenytoin
Clarithromycin	Phenobarbital
Fluoroquinolones	Tobacco
Grapefruit and grapefruit juice	
Ketoconazole	
Nefazodone	
SSRIs	

▷ Enzyme inhibitors can increase the serum level of other drugs that are substrates of that enzyme, thus possibly causing toxic levels.

▷ Liver disease will affect liver enzyme activity and first-pass metabolism, possibly resulting in toxic plasma drug levels.

▷ Kidney disease or drugs that reduce renal clearance, such as nonsteroidal anti-inflammatory drugs (NSAIDs), may increase serum concentration of drugs that are excreted by the kidneys (such as lithium). Older adults are more sensitive to psychotropics because of their decreased intracellular water, protein binding, low muscle mass, decreased metabolism, and increased body fat concentration.

  ▶ Most psychotropics are lipophilic and highly protein-bound. Thus, because older adults have more body fat and less protein, they are more likely to develop toxicity due to accumulation and erratic blood levels of drug.

Pharmacodynamics

▶ Target sites for drug actions include receptors. Several types of pharmacodynamics involve receptors:

  ▷ *Agonist effect:* Drug binds to receptors and activates a biological response

  ▷ *Inverse agonist effect:* Drug causes the opposite effect of agonist; binds to same receptor

  ▷ *Partial agonist effect:* Drug does not fully activate the receptors

  ▷ *Antagonist effect:* Drug binds to the receptor but does not activate a biological response

▶ Another site for drug actions is ion channels, which exist for many ions such as sodium, potassium, chloride, and calcium and can be open at some times and closed at other times. Neurotransmitters or drugs may be excitatory or inhibitory depending on the type of ion channel they gate.

  ▷ *Excitatory response:* Depolarization; involves the opening of sodium and calcium channels so these ions go into the cell

  ▷ *Inhibitory response:* Repolarization; involves the opening of chloride channels so chloride goes into the cell, potassium leaves, or both

▶ Another site for drug actions are enzymes, which are important for drug metabolism and play an important role in the chemical alteration of the drug. Some drugs (e.g., monoamine oxidase inhibitors [MAOIs]) inhibit the action of a particular enzyme, thus increasing the availability of the neurotransmitter.

▶ Another site for drug actions is carrier proteins or reuptake pumps, which transport neurotransmitters out of the synapse and back into the presynaptic neuron to be recycled or reused. Some drugs, such as selective serotonin reuptake inhibitors (SSRIs), will inhibit reuptake pumps, thus increasing the synaptic availability of the neurotransmitter.

Other Terminology

▶ *Potency:* Relative dose required to achieve certain effects

▶ *Therapeutic index:* Relative measure of the toxicity or safety of a drug; ratio of the median toxic dose to the median effective dose

▷ Drugs with a high therapeutic index (e.g., divalproex, 50–125 mcg/ml) have a high margin of safety; that is, the therapeutic dose and the toxic dose are far apart.

▷ Drugs with a low therapeutic index (e.g., lithium, 0.5–1.2 mEQ/L) have a low margin of safety; that is, the therapeutic dose and the toxic dose are close *together.*

▶ *Tolerance:* The process of becoming less responsive to a particular drug over time

▶ *Tachyphylaxis:* An acute decrease in the therapeutic response

PMHNP PHARMACOLOGICAL MANAGEMENT ROLE

▶ Pharmacological management process:

▷ Make a diagnosis and identify the target symptoms.

▷ Consider the phase of illness (such as acute, relapse, recurrence).

▷ Assess prior personal and family history of response to certain medications.

▷ Assess the client's motivation for and any misgivings about treatment.

▷ Identify potential interactions between the currently prescribed medications.

▷ Identify cultural implications of certain drugs.

▷ Discuss the risks and benefits of the treatment.

▷ Document informed consent and the client's understanding of target symptoms, benefits, risks, and alternatives to treatment.

▷ Monitor response and side effects.

▶ Follow-up and role of the PMHNP

▷ Use of standards of care:

▶ Assist in determining length of treatment.

▶ Do relapse planning.

▷ It is helpful and advised to use standardized clinical rating scales to establish the client's baseline and to monitor progress or decompensation over time. Screening tests also will aid in making a diagnosis and ruling out other disorders. (See corresponding chapters for a list of relevant screening tools.)

▷ It is important to recognize the large body of evidence-based data supporting the combined use of pharmacological and nonpharmacological treatments as offering psychiatric clients the best possibility for significant clinical improvement.

▷ Nonadherence is a common problem with all chronic illness, including psychiatric disorders, and should be a continuous focus of concern for the PMHNP.

▷ Common medications used in the clinical management of psychiatric disorders and usually prescribed by the PMHNP are identified in Table 7–2. See corresponding chapters for specific information on each medication.

▷ A Drug Enforcement Administration (DEA) number is required for prescription of controlled substances.

    ▶ Schedule of controlled substances

        ▷ Schedule I

            ▶ Nonmedicinal substances

TABLE 7–2.
MEDICATIONS COMMONLY USED IN THE CLINICAL MANAGEMENT OF PSYCHIATRIC DISORDERS

MEDICATIONS USED TO TREAT SCHIZOPHRENIA AND OTHER PSYCHOTIC DISORDERS	
Typical Antipsychotics	Haloperidol (Haldol), haloperidol decanoate (Haldol Decanoate)
	Loxapine (Loxitane)
	Thioridazine (Mellaril)
	Thiothixene (Navane)
	Fluphenazine (Prolixin), fluphenazine decanoate (Prolixin Decanoate)
	Mesoridazine (Serentil)
	Trifluoperazine (Stelazine)
	Chlorpromazine (Thorazine)
	Perphenazine (Trilafon)
Second-Generation Antipsychotics	Clozapine (Clozaril)
	Ziprasidone (Geodon)
	Risperidone (Risperdal)
	Quetiapine (Seroquel)
	Olanzapine (Zyprexa)
	Aripiprazole (Abilify)
	Paliperidone (Invega)
	Iloperidone (Fanapt)
	Asenapine (Saphris)
	Lurasidone (Latuda)
MEDICATIONS USED TO TREAT MOOD DISORDERS AND BIPOLAR AFFECTIVE DISORDERS	
Mood Stabilizers	Valproic acid (Depakene)
	Divalproex sodium (Depakote)
	Lithium carbonate (Eskalith, Lithobid, Lithonate, Lithotabs)
	Lamotrigine (Lamictal)
	Carbamazepine (Tegretol)
	Carbamazepine ER (Equetro)
	Oxcarbazepine (Trileptal; off-label)

CONTINUED

MEDICATIONS USED TO TREAT MOOD DISORDERS, UNIPOLAR AFFECTIVE DISORDERS, AND DEPRESSIVE DISORDERS

Tricyclics (TCAs)	Clomipramine (Anafranil)
	Amoxapine (Asendin)
	Amitriptyline (Elavil)
	Desipramine (Norpramin)
	Nortriptyline (Pamelor)
	Doxepin (Sinequan)
	Trimipramine (Surmontil)
	Imipramine (Tofranil)
	Protriptyline (Vivactil)
Serotonin Selective Reuptake Inhibitors (SSRIs)	Citalopram (Celexa)
	Fluvoxamine (Luvox)
	Paroxetine (Paxil)
	Paroxetine mesylate (Pexeva)
	Fluoxetine (Prozac)
	Sertraline (Zoloft)
	Escitalopram (Lexapro)
Monoamine Oxidase Inhibitors (MAOIs)	Phenelzine (Nardil)
	Tranylcypromine sulfate (Parnate)
	Selegiline transdermal (EMSAM)
SNRIs and Other Agents	Trazodone (Desyrel)
	Venlafaxine (Effexor)
	Desvenlafaxine (Pristiq)
	Mirtazapine (Remeron)
	Nefazodone (Serzone)
	Bupropion (Wellbutrin, Forfivo, Aplenzin)
	Duloxetine (Cymbalta)
	Vilazodone (Viibryd)
	Vortioxetine (Brintellix)
	Levomilnacipran (Fetzima)

MEDICATIONS USED TO TREAT ANXIETY DISORDERS

Benzodiazepines (BNZs)	Lorazepam (Ativan)
	Clonazepam (Klonopin)
	Chlordiazepoxide (Librium)
	Oxazepam (Serax)
	Clorazepate (Tranxene)
	Alprazolam (Xanax)
Anxiolytics	Buspirone (BuSpar)
Other Agents	Propranolol (Inderal)
	Atenolol (Tenormin)

MEDICATIONS USED TO TREAT ATTENTION DEFICIT DISORDER AND ATTENTION DEFICIT HYPERACTIVITY DISORDER	
Stimulants	Amphetamine/dextroamphetamine (Adderall)
	Dexmethylphenidate (Focalin)
	Dextroamphetamine (Dexedrine)
	Methylphenidate (Ritalin)
	Methylphenidate (Concerta)
	Lisdexamfetamine dimesylate (Vyvanse)
Other Agents	Guanfacine (Intuniv)
	Clonidine (Kapvay)
	Atomoxetine (Strattera)
	Antidepressants such as desipramine (Norpramin), venlafaxine (Effexor), and bupropion (Wellbutrin) are also used in the clinical management of ADHD.

- ▶ High abuse potential
- ▶ Used for research purposes only
- ▶ Not legally available by prescription
- ▶ Examples include heroin and marijuana
- ▷ Schedule II
  - ▶ Medicinal drugs in current use
  - ▶ High potential for abuse and dependency
  - ▶ Written prescription only
  - ▶ No telephone orders allowed
  - ▶ No refills allowed on prescription
  - ▶ Examples include morphine sulfate, codeine, fentanyl, methadone, hydromorphone (Dilaudid), oxycodone (OxyContin, Percocet), hydrocodone (Vicodin and others), amphetamine salts, methylphenidate
- ▷ Schedule III
  - ▶ Medicinal drugs with less abuse potential than Schedule II drugs
  - ▶ Still greater potential for abuse than Schedule IV drugs
  - ▶ Telephone orders if followed by written prescription
  - ▶ Prescription must be renewed every 6 months
  - ▶ Refills limited to five
  - ▶ Examples include appetite suppressants, butalbital, testosterone, buprenorphine/naloxone
- ▷ Schedule IV
  - ▶ Medicinal drugs with less abuse potential than Schedule III drugs

▶ Examples include dextropropoxyphene (Darvon), pentazocine (Talwin), benzodiazepines (such as alprazolam [Xanax], chlordiazepoxide [Librium], clonazepam [Klonopin], diazepam [Valium], clorazepate [Tranxene], and lorazepam [Ativan]), modafinil (Provigil), phenobarbital, zolpidem (Ambien), eszopiclone (Lunesta), temazepam (Restoril), armodafinil (Nuvigil)

▷ Schedule V

▶ Medicinal drugs with the lowest abuse potential

▶ Handled in manner similar to noncontrolled drugs

▶ Examples include buprenorphine (Buprenex), cheratussin (Robitussin) with codeine, promethazine (Phenergan) with codeine, diphenoxylate/atropine (Lomotil)

Other Pharmacological Considerations

▶ It is vital to be aware of the teratogenic nature of many psychotropic agents. It is important to discuss the risks versus the benefits of medications during pregnancy.

▷ Possible risks of psychotropic medications during pregnancy include:

▶ Problems with appetite

▶ Transient agitation or sedation

▶ Premature labor

▶ Drug discontinuation symptoms

▶ Teratogenic effects of certain psychotropics

▷ Possible risks of not taking psychotropic medications during pregnancy include

▶ Recurrence of symptoms

▶ Adverse effects on mother–infant bonding

▶ Poor maternal self-care

▶ Federal Drug Administration (FDA) pregnancy ratings for medications

▷ **A:** Controlled studies show no risk

▷ **B:** No evidence of risk in humans

▷ **C:** Risk cannot be ruled out

▷ **D:** Positive evidence of risk

▷ **X:** Absolutely contraindicated in pregnancy

▶ Teratogenic risks of common psychiatric medications

▷ Benzodiazepines: Floppy baby syndrome, cleft palate

▷ Carbamazepine (Tegretol): Neural tube defects

▷ Lithium (Eskalith): Epstein anomaly

▷ Divalproex sodium (Depakote): Neural tube defects, specifically spina bifida, atrial septal defect, cleft palate, and possible long-term developmental deficits

▶ Some common medications can induce depression or mania (see Table 7–3).

▶ Remember that some medications can *possibly* cause a false urinary drug screen result (see Table 7–4).

TABLE 7–3.
MEDICATIONS THAT INDUCE DEPRESSION OR MANIA

MEDICATIONS THAT INDUCE DEPRESSION	MEDICATIONS THAT INDUCE MANIA
• Beta blockers	• Steroids
• Steroids	• Disulfiram (Antabuse)
• Interferon	• Isoniazid (INH)
• Isotretinoin (Accutane)	• Antidepressants in persons with bipolar disorder
• Some retroviral drugs	
• Antineoplastic drugs	
• Benzodiazepines	
• Progesterone	

TABLE 7–4.
MEDICATIONS THAT CAN CAUSE DRUG SCREEN FALSE POSITIVE RESULTS

FALSE POSITIVE FOR	DRUG RESPONSIBLE
Amphetamines	• Stimulants (i.e., amphetamine/dextroamphetamine [Adderall], methylphenidate [Ritalin])
	• Bupropion (Wellbutrin)
	• Fluoxetine (Prozac)
	• Trazodone
	• Ranitidine
	• Nefazodone (Serzone)
	• Nasal decongestants
	• Pseudoephedrine
Alcohol	• Valium
Benzodiazepines	• Sertraline (Zoloft)
Cocaine	• Amoxicillin
	• Most antibiotics
	• NSAIDs
Heroin or morphine	• Quinolones
	• Rifampin
	• Codeine
	• Poppy seeds
Methadone or PCP	• Over-the-counter cough medicine (such as Nyquil) Dextromethorphan

CASE STUDY 1

Ms. J., a 74-year-old client whom the PHMNP has been seeing for depression, presented at her appointment with complaints of tremors, diaphoresis, headache, and nausea over the past week. She is currently being prescribed amitriptyline (50 mg q.h.s.), which was increased at her last visit, and sertraline (100 mg q.d.). She denies depression but admits to increased confusion and memory problems.

1. What is the biggest pharmacological concern with the combination of medication the client is being prescribed?

2. What would be the PHMNP's plan of action?

3. What pharmacokinetics should the PHMNP keep in mind when treating older adults?

CASE STUDY 2

Ms. M. is a 30-year-old married Chinese woman who is in the midst of a first major depressive episode. Ms. M. is employed as a grade school teacher but is currently on summer break. Despite participating in 6 months of cognitive behavioral therapy with an experienced therapist, her symptoms have not improved. Ms. M describes feeling sad and cries easily. She feels anxious and has trouble shutting her thoughts off, particularly when trying to fall asleep at night. She feels tired upon awakening, despite getting 7 to 8 hours of sleep, and she has trouble getting out of bed. Her energy remains low throughout the day. She notes a worsening in her motivation as well. Her weight and appetite are unchanged. She denies suicidal ideation. After careful evaluation, the PMHNP suggests a trial of fluoxetine and prescribes 20 mg p.o. q.a.m. with food.

Ms. M. calls the PMHNP before her scheduled follow-up appointment, requesting to come in sooner because she feels "worse." She describes more difficulty falling asleep, feels "revved up" much of the time, and is having mild nausea and headaches.

1. What are possible reasons for Ms. M. feeling "worse"?

2. What should the PMHNP suggest as the next intervention for Ms. M.?

CASE STUDY 3

Ms. S. is a 22-year-old woman who presents to the PMHNP with signs and symptoms of major depression. Ms. S. has a strong family history of major depression and both her mother and older sister have been treated with an antidepressant. Ms. S. herself has never been treated for depression before, and she says she is nervous about taking medication because she "gets side effects from everything."

1. How should the PMHNP respond to Ms. S.'s concerns about taking medication?

2. How should the PMHNP begin to think about medication management for Ms. S.?

Ms. S. is started on sertraline 50 mg. She calls within a few days of starting the drug and says that she is experiencing an upset stomach, headache, difficulty sleeping, and an overall feeling of being "edgy."

3.   What is the most likely reason for Ms. S.'s reported side effects?

4.   What is the most reasonable intervention by the PMHNP?

5.   Other than potential side effects, what information should the PMHNP include in client teaching when starting a person on a new medication?

ANSWERS TO CASE STUDY DISCUSSION QUESTIONS

Case Study 1

1. The SSRI is potentially increasing the concentration of the TCA to toxic levels.

2. Check the blood level of amitriptyline and decrease the dose; consider tapering Ms. J. off the TCA.

3. Higher body fat content, decreased gastric acid secretion, and decreased hepatic and renal functioning all predispose an older adult to the potential toxic effects of medications. Anticholinergic effects and orthostasis are particularly common and problematic.

Case Study 2

1. Fluoxetine may cause uncomfortable activation in some clients. In addition, Ms. M. appears to be having multiple side effects. Fluoxetine is metabolized primarily by cytochrome P450 2D6. People who are deficient in 2D6 are considered "slow metabolizers," and may need significantly lower doses of medications that are substrates of 2D6. Finally, all clients started on antidepressants must be monitored closely for a switch from depression to hypomania or mixed mania. While Ms. M.'s increase in insomnia and feeling "revved up" and "worse" are likely side effects from fluoxetine, this could signal beginning symptoms of a shift into a bipolar spectrum mood state.

2. Unless agitation is prominent, the first prudent intervention would be to lower the dose of the fluoxetine. If this is not helpful in diminishing side effects, prescribing a low dose of lorazepam or other benzodiazepine used as a "bridge" medication until the SSRI is effective may be prudent. If neither of these interventions proves helpful, the medication should be changed.

Case Study 3

1. The PMHNP should ask Ms. S. to tell her more about being anxious about taking medicine, and ask about the medications her immediate family members are taking, whether or not the family members have had problems with side effects, and finally, whether any medication has been particularly helpful to her family members.

2. A genetic polymorphism screening test to determine gene variants may be reasonable. Because mood and anxiety disorders have a genetic component, beginning with a medication that has been beneficial in the treatment of similar symptoms in a first-degree relative is a reasonable starting point of treatment.

3. The sertraline was started at too high a dose.

4. Lower the dose to 25 mg. Make sure Ms. S. is taking the medication with food. If not already doing so, switch the time of dosing to after breakfast.

5. During client teaching, the PMHNP should cover the usual course of treatment: typical time until benefit, typical therapeutic dosing, and expected length of treatment. The PMHNP should also emphasize that most side effects are transient and can usually be managed, such as by adjusting the dose.

REFERENCES AND RESOURCES

American Psychiatric Association. (2000). *Practice guidelines for the treatment of patients with major depressive disorder.* Washington, DC: Author.

Antai-Otong, D. (Ed). (2008). *Psychiatric nursing: Biological and behavioral concepts* (2nd ed.). New York, NY: Delmar.

Beck, A. T., Ward, C. H., Mendelson, M., Mock, J., & Erbauh, J. (1961). An inventory for measuring depression. *Archives of General Psychiatry, 4,* 561–571.

Berlin, C. M., Jr. (2015). *Overview of drug treatment in children.* Retrieved from http://www.merckmanuals.com/professional/pediatrics/principles_of_drug_treatment_in_children/overview_of_drug_treatment_in_children.html

Boyd, M. A. (2002). *Psychiatric nursing: Contemporary practice* (2nd ed.). Philadelphia, PA: Lippincott.

De Wildt, S. N., Tibboel, D., & Leeder, J. S. (2014). Drug metabolism for the paediatrician. *Archive of Disease in Childhood, 99*(12), 1137-1142.

Dipiro, J. T., Talbert, R. L., & Yee, G. C. (Eds.). (2002). *Pharmacotherapy: A pathophysiological approach* (5th ed.). New York: McGraw-Hill.

Fuller, M., & Sajatovic, M. (2005). *Lexi-Comp's psychotropic drug information handbook (mental health).* Cleveland, OH: Lexi-Comp.

Hirschfeld, R., & Holzer, C. (2003). Validity of the mood disorder questionnaire: A general population study. *American Journal of Psychiatry, 160,* 178–180.

Kay, S. R., & Fiszbein, A. (1987). The positive and negative syndrome scale for schizophrenia. *Schizophrenia Bulletin, 13,* 261–275.

Kroenke, K., Spitzer, R. L., & Williams, J. B. (2001). The PHQ-9: Validity of a brief depression severity measure. *Journal of General Internal Medicine, 16*(9), 606–613.

Overall, J. E., & Gorham, C. R. (1962). The brief psychiatric rating scale. *Psychological Reports, 10,* 790–812.

Rapuri, S., Ramaswamy, S., Madaan, V., Rasimas, J., & Krahn, L. (2006). "WEED" out false positive urine drug screens. *Current Psychiatry, 5*(8), 107–110.

Sadock, B. J., Sadock, V. A., & Ruiz, P. (2015). *Kaplan and Sadock's synopsis of psychiatry: Behavioral sciences/clinical psychiatry* (11th ed.). Philadelphia, PA: Wolters Kluwer.

Schatsburg, A., Cole, J., & DeBattista, C. (2015). *Manual of clinical psychopharmacology* (8th ed.). Washington, DC: American Psychiatric Association Press.

Stahl, S. (2013). *Stahl's essential psychopharmacology: Neuroscientific basis and practical applications* (4th ed.). New York, NY: Cambridge University Press.

CHAPTER 8

NONPHARMACOLOGICAL TREATMENT

This chapter discusses nonpharmacological interventions such as individual psychotherapies, group therapy, family therapies, and complementary and alternative therapies. Because medications alone do not treat a person's environmental or interpersonal stressors and his or her responses to these stressors, an integrated approach is the most beneficial in treating mental illnesses. Although some people seek counseling for self-discovery, the most common issues for individual therapy are:

▶ Losses

▶ Interpersonal conflicts

▶ Symptomatic presentations such as panic, phobias, and negativity

▶ Unfulfilled expectations at life transitions

▶ Characterological issues such as narcissism or aggressiveness

Confidentiality may be broken when there is increased potential for self-harm or harm to others; abuse of a child, older adult, or person with disabilities; when the therapist determines that the person needs hospitalization; and when clients request that their information be released to a third party.

INDIVIDUAL THERAPY

▶ Psychoanalytic Therapy

　▷ Originated by Sigmund Freud (1856–1939), who believed that behavior is determined by unconscious motivations and instinctual drives (see also Chapter 3)

　▷ Promotes change by the development of greater insight and awareness of maladaptive defenses

　▷ Attends to past developmental and psychodynamic factors, which shape present behaviors

▶ Cognitive Therapy

　▷ Originated by Aaron Beck (born 1921)

  ▷ Purports that external events do not cause anxiety or maladaptive responses

  ▷ States that a person's expectations, perceptions, and interpretations of events cause anxiety

  ▷ Allows clients to view reality more clearly through an examination of their central distorted cognitions

  ▷ Goal is to change clients' irrational beliefs, faulty conceptions, and negative cognitive distortions

▶ Behavioral Therapy

  ▷ Originated by Arnold Lazarus (born 1932)

  ▷ Focuses on changing maladaptive behaviors by participating in active behavioral techniques such as exposure, relaxation, problem-solving, and role-playing

▶ Dialectical Behavioral Therapy

  ▷ Originated by Marsha Linehan (born 1943)

  ▷ Commonly used with people with borderline personality disorder

  ▷ Focuses on emotional regulation, tolerance for distress, self-management skills, interpersonal effectiveness, and mindfulness, with an emphasis on treating therapy-interfering behaviors

  ▷ Goals

    ▶ Decrease suicidal behaviors

    ▶ Decrease therapy-interfering behaviors

    ▶ Decrease emotional reactivity

    ▶ Decrease self-invalidation

    ▶ Decrease crisis-generating behaviors

    ▶ Decrease passivity

    ▶ Increase realistic decision-making

    ▶ Increase accurate communication of emotions and competencies

▶ Existential Therapy

  ▷ Originated by Viktor Frankl (1905–1997)

  ▷ A philosophical approach in which reflection on life and self-confrontation is encouraged

  ▷ Emphasizes accepting freedom and making responsible choices

  ▷ States that a basic dimension of humans includes finding meaning and purpose in life—"Why am I here? What is my purpose?"

  ▷ Goals are to live authentically and to focus on the present and on personal responsibility

▶ Humanistic Therapy

  ▷ Originated by Carl Rogers (1902–1987)

  ▷ Also known as *person-centered therapy*

▷ Concepts include self-directed growth and self-actualization; people are born with the capacity to direct themselves toward self-actualization

▷ Each person has the potential to actualize and find meaning.

▶ Interpersonal Therapy

▷ Originated by Gerald L. Klerman (1928–1992) and Myrna M. Weissman (born 1940)

▷ Evidence-based therapy with focus on interpersonal issues that are creating distress

▷ Time-limited, active, focused on the present and on interpersonal distress

▷ Developed to treat aspects of depression and is effective for adults and adolescents

▷ Has been applied to treat interpersonal distress related to other disorders, including bipolar, substance use, and eating disorders

▶ Eye Movement Desensitization and Reprocessing (EMDR)

▷ Originated by Francine Shapiro (born 1948)

▷ A form of behavioral and exposure therapy

▷ Involves the use of bilateral stimulation—moving the eyes back and forth, alternating tapping on hand or knee, or sounds in ears

▷ Most commonly used in post-traumatic stress disorder

▷ Goal is to achieve adaptive resolution

▷ *Desensitization phase:* The client visualizes the trauma, verbalizes the negative thoughts or maladaptive beliefs, and remains attentive to physical sensations. This process occurs for a limited time while the client maintains rhythmic eye movements. He or she is then instructed to block out negative thoughts; to breathe deeply; and then to verbalize what he or she is thinking, feeling, or imagining.

▷ *Installation phase:* The client installs and increases the strength of the positive thought that he or she has declared as a replacement of the original negative thought.

▷ *Body scan:* The client visualizes the trauma along with the positive thought and then scans his or her body mentally to identify any tension within.

GROUP THERAPY

▶ Benefits

▷ Increases insight about oneself

▷ Increases social skills

▷ Is cost-effective

▷ Develops sense of community

▶ Irvin Yalom (born 1931) was the first person to put a theoretical perspective on group work and identified 10 therapeutic factors that differentiate group therapy from individual therapy.

1. *Instillation of hope:* Participants develop hope for creating a different life. Members are at different levels of growth; thus, they gain hope from others that change is possible.

2. *Universality:* Participants discover that others have similar problems, thoughts, or feelings and that they are not alone.

3. *Altruism:* This results from sharing oneself with another and helping another.

4. *Increased development of socialization skills:* New social skills are learned, and maladaptive social behaviors are corrected. The group can provide a "natural laboratory."

5. *Imitative behaviors:* Participants are able to increase their skills by imitating the behaviors of others.

6. *Interpersonal learning:* Interacting with others increases adaptive interpersonal relationships.

7. *Group cohesiveness:* Participants develop an attraction to the group and other members as well as a sense of belonging.

8. *Catharsis:* Participants experience catharsis as they openly express their feelings, which were previously suppressed.

9. *Existential factors:* Groups enable participants to deal with the meaning of their own existence.

10. *Corrective refocusing:* Participants reexperience family conflicts in the group, which allows them to recognize and change behaviors that may be problematic.

▶ Group phases (Tuckman, 1965)

▷ *Pregroup phase:* The leader considers the direction and framework of the group.

  ▶ Purpose

  ▶ Goals

  ▶ Membership criteria

  ▶ Membership size

  ▶ Pregroup interview

  ▶ Informed consent

▷ *Forming phase:* Members are concerned about self-disclosure and being rejected. Goals and expectations are identified, and boundaries are established. The development of trust and rapport is very important.

▷ *Storming phase:* Members are resistant and may begin to use testing behaviors. Issues related to inclusion, control, and affection begin to surface. Leaders' tasks are to allow expression of both positive and negative feelings, assist the group in understanding the underlying conflict, and examine nonproductive behaviors.

    ▷ *Norming phase:* Resistance to the group is overcome by members. A strong attraction to the group and others emerges. Open and spontaneous communication occurs, and the group norms are established.

    ▷ *Performing phase:* The group's work becomes more focused. Creative problem-solving and solutions begin to emerge. Experiential learning takes place. Group energy is directed toward completion of goals.

    ▷ *Adjourning phase:* Preparation is made to end the group. (Remember that the work of termination begins during the first stage of the group.) Both members and leaders express their feelings about each other and termination. A discussion and overview of what has been learned, as well as what issues still need to be worked on, takes place.

▶ Reminiscence Therapy

    ▷ Characterized by a progressive return of memories of past experiences

    ▷ Used with older adults

    ▷ Enables participants to search for meaning in their lives and strive for some resolution of past interpersonal and intrapsychic conflicts

FAMILY THERAPIES

▶ Family system concepts

    ▷ A *system* is any unit structured on feedback—such as the family.

    ▷ The process by which all family members operate together is referred to as the *family system.*

    ▷ Family systems theory is based on the idea that one could not understand any family member (part) without understanding how all family members operate together (system).

    ▷ The family system operates based on a set of rules that may be overt or covert.

    ▷ *Boundaries:* Barriers that protect and enhance the functional integrity of families, individuals, and subsystems. System boundaries can be physical or psychological.

    ▷ *Types of boundaries*

        ▶ *Clearly defined boundaries:* Maintain person's separateness while emphasizing belongingness

        ▶ *Rigid or inflexible boundaries:* May lead to distant relationships and to disengagement

        ▶ *Diffuse boundaries:* Blurred and indistinct boundaries; lead to enmeshment

    ▷ *Circular causality:* An ongoing feedback loop; a series of actions and reactions that maintain a problem. Individuals and emotional problems are best understood within the context of relationships and through assessing interactions within an entire family.

    ▷ *Family homeostasis:* Tendency of families to resist change and to maintain a steady state

▷ *Morphogenesis:* A family's tendency to adapt to change when changes are necessary

▷ *Morphostasis:* A family's tendency to remain stable in the midst of change

▶ Family Systems Therapy

▷ Originated by Murray Bowen (1913–1990), who believed that a person's problematic behavior may serve a function or purpose for the family or be a symptom of dysfunctional patterns

▷ Focus is on chronic anxiety within families

▷ Treatment goals are to increase the family's awareness of each member's function within the family and to increase levels of *self-differentiation* (the level at which one's sense of self-worth is not dependent on external relationships, circumstances, or occurrences).

▶ *Triangles:* Dyads that form triads to decrease stress; the lower the level of family adaptation, the more likely a triangle will develop

▶ *Nuclear family emotional system:* Level of differentiation of the parents is usually equal to the level of differentiation for the entire family

▶ *Multigenerational transmission process:* Dysfunction present over several generations

▶ *Family projection process:* Parents transmitting their own level of differentiation on the most susceptible child

▶ *Emotional cutoffs:* Attempting to break contact with the family of origin

▶ *Sibling position:* Influences interactions and personality characteristics

▶ Structural Family Therapy

▷ Originated by Salvador Minuchin (1913–1990), who placed emphasis on how, when, and to whom family members relate in order to understand and then change the family's structure

▷ A person's symptoms are rooted in the context of family transaction patterns. The symptom is a function of the health of the whole family and is maintained by structural problems in the system.

▷ The main treatment goal is to produce a structural change in the family organization to more effectively manage problems—changing transactional patterns and family structure.

▶ *Family structure:* An invisible set of functional demands that organize the way members interact with each other, made up of subsystems (e.g., marital, parental, sibling), coalitions (e.g., two members joining forces against a third member), and boundaries

▶ *Structural mapping* (genogram): Mapping relationships using symbols to represent overinvolvement, conflict, coalitions, and so forth

▶ *Hierarchies:* Distribution of power

▶ Experiential Therapy

▷ Originated by Virginia Satir (1916–1988)

▷ Behavior is determined by personal experience and not by external reality.

▷ Focus is on being authentic, on freedom of choice, on human validation, and on experiencing the moment

▷ Treatment goals are to develop authentic, nurturing communication and increased self-worth of each family member; overall goal is growth rather than symptom reduction alone.

▷ It does not focus on particular techniques.

► Strategic Therapy

▷ Originated by Jay Haley (1923–2007)

▷ Symptoms are viewed as metaphors and reflect problems in the hierarchal structure. Symptoms are a way to communicate metaphorically within a family.

▷ Treatment goal is to help family members behave in ways that will not perpetuate the problem behavior.

▷ Interventions are problem-focused. Strategic therapy is more symptom-focused than structural therapy.

▷ Strategic family therapists are concerned mainly with those techniques that change the sequence of interactions that is maintaining the problem.

▷ Techniques are straightforward directives, paradoxical directives, and reframing belief systems.

  ► *Straightforward directives:* Tasks that are designed in expectation of the family member's compliance

  ► *Paradoxical directives:* A negative task that is assigned when family members are resistant to change and the member is expected to be noncompliant (use this technique with caution)

  ► *Reframing belief systems:* Problematic behaviors are relabeled to have more positive meaning (e.g., *jealousy* reframed to *caring*)

► Solution-Focused Therapy

▷ Originated by Steve deShazer (1940–2005), Bill O'Hanlon (born 1952), and Insoo Berg (1934–2007)

▷ Focus is to rework for the present situation solutions that have worked previously

▷ Treatment goal is effective resolution of problems through cognitive problem-solving and use of personal resources and strengths.

▷ Techniques include the use of miracle questions, exception-finding questions, and scaling questions.

  ► *Miracle questions:* "If a miracle were to happen tonight while you were asleep, and tomorrow morning you awoke to find that the problem no longer existed, what would be different?" "How would you know the miracle took place?" "How would others know?"

  ► *Exception-finding questions:* Directing clients to a time in their lives when the problem did not exist, which helps them move toward solutions by assisting them in searching for any exceptions to the pattern. "Was there a time when the problem did not occur?"

▶ *Scaling questions:* "On a scale of 1–10, with 10 being very anxious and depressed, how would you rate how you are feeling now?" This is useful for highlighting small increments of change.

COMPLEMENTARY AND ALTERNATIVE THERAPIES (CATS)

▶ CATs deal with the connection between the mind and the body and are viewed as holistic health care (dealing with the biopsychosocial and spiritual components of the person).

▷ *Complementary therapies:* Used in addition to traditional medical practices

▷ *Alternative therapies:* Used in place of traditional medical practices

▷ *Integrative therapies:* Recent term used to describe the use of traditional complementary therapies

▶ Why people use CATs

▷ Desire for more control over decision-making

▷ Decreased insurance coverage for traditional medical therapies, therefore making the use of CATs cheaper

▷ Preference for natural rather than synthetic medications

▷ Increased costs of prescriptions and services

▷ Failure of conventional medications

▶ Mind–body interventions

▷ Guided imagery

▷ Meditation

▷ Yoga

▷ Biofeedback

▶ Biologically based therapies

▷ Herbal products

▷ Vitamins

▷ Supplements

▷ Aromatherapy

▶ Manipulative and body-based therapies

▷ Acupressure and acupuncture

▷ Massage

▷ Reflexology

▶ Acupressure and Acupuncture

▷ Based on the basic tenet of Chinese medicine that vital energy (*chi*) flows along specific pathways that have many points of access and that manipulating these points, by either hands or needles, corrects imbalances by stimulating or removing blockages to energy flow

- ▷ Thought to produce effects by regulating the nervous system and aiding the activity of endorphins and immune system cells at different sites in the body
- ▷ Also thought to alter brain chemistry by changing the release of neurohormones and neurotransmitters

- ► Biofeedback
  - ▷ A process providing a person with visual or auditory information about the autonomic physiologic functions of his or her body, such as blood pressure, muscle tension, and brain wave activity
  - ▷ The person learns to consciously control these processes, which were previously regarded as involuntary.
  - ▷ Uses
    - ► Stress-related symptoms (e.g., anxiety)
    - ► Pain
    - ► Insomnia
    - ► Neuromuscular problems (e.g., migraines, muscular tension, tension headaches, Raynaud's disease, urinary incontinence)
    - ► Neurobehavioral disorders
    - ► Enhancement of healing
    - ► Athletic and work performance
  - ▷ Desired outcome
    - ► Positive change in baseline measures
    - ► Demonstrated skill at self-regulation
    - ► Improvement in symptoms
    - ► Improved use of skills in daily life
    - ► Reduction of muscle bracing
    - ► Increased sense of self-efficacy

- ► Aromatherapy
  - ▷ Therapeutic use of plants or oils to obtain many therapeutic effects, such as analgesic, psychological, and antimicrobial benefits
  - ▷ In psychiatry, olfactory stimulation used to elicit feelings or memories during psychotherapy

- ► Herbal Products and Supplements
  - ▷ Practice of herbal medicine originated in China and is the oldest system of medicine
  - ▷ Relies on plants to cure illnesses and maintain health
  - ▷ Similar to prescription medications, many plants contain active compounds that produce physiological effects
  - ▷ Food and Drug Administration (FDA) approval is not required; thus no uniform standards ensure quality control or potency

▷ Common supplements and interactions include:

▶ *Omega-3 fatty acids*

▷ Used for attention deficit hyperactivity disorder, dyslexia, cognitive impairment, dementia, cardiovascular disease, asthma, lupus, and rheumatoid arthritis

▷ Interacts with warfarin (Coumadin), increasing anticoagulant effect (people cautioned to stop using before surgery)

▶ *Sam-e*

▷ Used for depression, osteoarthritis, and liver disease

▷ May cause hypomania, hyperactive muscle movements, and possible serotonin syndrome

▶ *Tryptophan*

▷ Used for depression, obesity, insomnia, headaches, and fibromyalgia

▷ Found in high concentrations in turkey

▷ Increased risk of serotonin syndrome with use of selective serotonin reuptake inhibitors (SSRIs), monoamine oxidase inhibitors (MAOIs), and St. John's wort

▶ *Vitamin E*

▷ Used for enhancing the immune system and protecting cells against effects of free radicals

▷ Used for neurological disorders, diabetes, and premenstrual syndrome

▷ Interacts with warfarin, increasing anticoagulant effect; antiplatelet drugs; and statins, increasing additive effect and risk of rhabdomyolysis

▶ *Melatonin*

▷ Used for insomnia, jet lag, shift work, and cancer

▷ Sets timing of circadian rhythms and regulates seasonal responses

▷ Interacts with aspirin, nonsteroidal anti-inflammatory drugs (NSAIDs), beta blockers, corticosteroids, valerian, kava kava, and alcohol

▷ Can inhibit ovulation in large doses

▶ *Fish oil*

▷ Used for bipolar disorder, hypertension, lowering triglycerides, and decreasing blood clotting

▷ Interacts with warfarin, aspirin, NSAIDs, garlic, and ginkgo

▷ May alter glucose regulation

▷ Most herbals are contraindicated during pregnancy and, because they are secreted in breast milk, during lactation.

▷ Common herbals with psychoactive effects include:

▶ *Black cohosh:* Menopausal symptoms, premenstrual syndrome, dysmenorrhea

- ▶ *Belladonna:* Anxiety
- ▶ *Catnip:* Sedation
- ▶ *Chamomile:* Sedation, anxiety
- ▶ *Ginkgo:* Delirium, dementia, sexual dysfunction caused by SSRIs
- ▶ *Ginseng:* Depression, fatigue
- ▶ *Valerian:* Sedation

- ▶ Massage
  - ▷ Believed to increase blood circulation, improve lymph flow, improve musculoskeletal tone, and have a relaxing effect on the mind
- ▶ Meditation
  - ▷ Consciously directing one's attention to alter one's state of consciousness
  - ▷ Produces physiological effects such as decreased heart rate, blood pressure, and respiratory rate; decreased anxiety; and increased alpha brain waves
- ▶ Reflexology
  - ▷ Stimulates the body's natural healing power through massaging the feet, hands, and ears
  - ▷ Alleviates tension by cleaning crystalline deposits under the skin that may interfere with the natural flow of the body's energy
  - ▷ Based on the mapping of body parts on the soles and sides of the feet, hands, and ears
  - ▷ Treats disorders related to the represented body parts by application of pressure
  - ▷ Used for back pain, migraines, infertility, sleep disorders, digestive disorders, and stress-related conditions
- ▶ Macrobiotics
  - ▷ Foods classified as yin (cold and wet) and yang (hot and dry)
  - ▷ Goal is to keep the dietary yin and yang in balance in attempt to live in harmony with nature
- ▶ Yoga
  - ▷ Originated in Indian religious practices
  - ▷ Combines mind and body connection
  - ▷ Uses breathing, physical movements, and meditation

CASE STUDY

You are a psychiatric–mental health nurse practitioner working with Jill, who has depression. In session Jill states, "Nothing good ever happens to me. I'm just a failure and should accept that people at work think I'm inadequate to do my job."

1. What therapeutic approach would be most helpful in working with Jill?

2. Specifically, what cognitive and behavioral techniques would be helpful for Jill?

3. Which scales would be helpful to use in assessing her depression and negative thoughts?

4. If you chose a CBT approach to work with Jill, what is the three-question technique?

5. What types of distortions does Jill have and, as her therapist, how would you begin to address her distortions?

ANSWERS TO CASE STUDY DISCUSSION QUESTIONS

1. The therapy that would be most helpful for Jill is cognitive behavioral therapy.

2. In working with Jill, having her complete a thought record to identify situations that lead to automatic thoughts, emotions, and her responses would be helpful.

3. Scales that would be useful to track Jill's progress in therapy include: PHQ-9, Beck Depression Scale, and Schema questionnaire.

4. The three-question technique when using CBT involves Socratic questioning. For example, asking the following: (1) Evidence for her negative belief; (2) How else can she interpret the situation?; (3) If it is true, what are the implications?

5. The types of distortions Jill has are all-or-nothing thinking and overgeneralization. A technique that would be helpful to address Jill's distortion are using a scale will help her put the distortions on a continuum to help her respond differently to low scale items.

REFERENCES AND RESOURCES

Corey, M., Corey, G., & Corey, C. (2010). *Groups: Process and practice* (8th ed.). Pacific Grove, CA: Brooks/Cole.

Goldenberg, I., & Goldenberg, H. (2013). *Family therapy: An overview* (8th ed.). Boston, MA: Brooks/Cole Cengage Learning.

Sadock, B. J., Sadock, V. A., & Ruiz, P. (2015). *Kaplan and Sadock's synopsis of psychiatry: Behavioral sciences/clinical psychiatry* (11th ed.). New York, NY: Wolters Kluwer.

Scharf, R. (2013). *Theories of psychotherapy and counseling* (5th ed.). Boston, MA: Brooks/Cole Cengage Learning.

Snyder, M., & Lindquist, R. (Eds.). (2010). *Complementary & alternative therapies in nursing* (6th ed.). New York, NY: Springer.

Tusaie, K., & Fitzpatrick, J. (2013). *Advanced practice psychiatric nursing integrating psychotherapy, psychopharmacology, and complementary and alternative approaches.* New York, NY: Springer Publishing Company.

Weisz, J. & Kazdin, A. (2010). *Evidence-based psychotherapies for children and adolescents* (2nd ed.). New York, NY: Guilford Press.

Wheeler, K. (2014). *Psychotherapy for the advanced practice psychiatric nurse* (2nd ed.). New York, NY: Springer Publishing Company.

Yalom, I. (2005). *Theory and practice of group psychotherapy* (5th ed.). New York, NY: Basic Books.

CHAPTER 9

DEPRESSIVE DISORDERS AND BIPOLAR DISORDERS

This chapter reviews the mood disorders and evidence-based practice guidelines that psychiaric–mental health nurse practitioners (PMHNPs) use in treating clients who have these disorders. As a childhood disorder, Disruptive Mood Dysregulation Disorder will be discussed in Chapter 15.

Mood disorders are the most common of all psychiatric illnesses.

It has become increasingly common for mood disorders to be treated in primary care settings, and often clients first present in such settings because of the high degree of somatic symptomatology that accompanies these disorders.

Sadness is a common, normal human emotion. PMHNPs caring for clients who present for evaluation of depression must distinguish between normal levels of sadness and pathological levels that are symptomatic of an underlying brain-based illness called major depression. Major depression requires treatment and generally will not fully abate without therapeutic intervention. Untreated, major depression predisposes people to other serious health problems, so pathological levels of depression should not go untreated.

SADNESS AS A COMMON EMOTIONAL STATE

▶ Sadness, one of the most common human emotions, exists on a continuum ranging from the absence of depression at one end to pathological levels that produce significant symptoms of a psychiatric disorder called major depression at the other.

▶ Cultural differences affect behavioral manifestations of depression.

▶ Mild depression can be a healthy reaction to life stressors that motivates a person to deal with events and emotions

   ▷ Sadness can be pathological if:

      ▶ It is disproportionate to events and sustained over a significant time period;

      ▶ It significantly impairs normal social functioning (e.g., occupational, social, school, relational functioning);

▶ It significantly impairs normal somatic functioning (e.g., loss of appetite, altered sleep, altered self-care activities, altered sexual functioning); or

▶ It is apparently unrelated to any identifiable event or situation in a person's life.

MAJOR DEPRESSIVE DISORDER (MDD)

Description

▶ One of the most common psychiatric disorders; the primary unipolar affective disorder

▶ A complex brain-based illness with a primary characteristic of a persistent disturbance in mood

▶ An excessive or distorted degree of sadness that manifests with behavioral, affective, cognitive, and somatic symptoms

▶ May have a known precipitating event, situation, or concern but often occurs without any precipitating stressor identified

▶ Significantly interferes with daily functioning and goal attainment

▶ Has complex genetic, biochemical, and environmental etiological factors

Etiology

▶ Multiple theories of the etiology of depression fall into two categories: psychological and neurobiological.

▶ Psychodynamic theories

▷ Object Loss Theory (Ronald Fairbairn, D. W. Winnicott, Harry Guntrip; Gilbert, 2006)

▶ This theory assumes that early psychological developmental issues lay the foundation for depressive responses in later life; that the accomplishment of the first stage of development in which the child is able to form relationships is normal; and that, during second stage of development, the child experiences traumatic separation from significant objects of attachment (usually a maternal object).

▶ Loss may be related to maternal death, illness, or emotional lack of availability and is unexpected and overwhelming.

▶ Depth of loss produces constellation of responses dominated by separation anxiety, grief, mourning, and despair.

▶ This critical object loss event predisposes the child to respond in similar ways to any future losses or significant separation.

▷ Aggression-Turned-Inward Theory (Sigmund Freud)

▶ This theory assumes that early psychological developmental issues lay the foundation for depressive responses in later life; that the accomplishment of the first stage of development in which the child is able to form relationships is normal; and that, during second stage of development, the child experiences the loss of the significant mothering person.

▶ The loss can be a real or imagined and is unexpected and overwhelming.

▶ The loss may be related to maternal death, illness, or emotional lack of availability or to the birth of a new sibling and the child's perception of losing undivided, individualized attention from the mother. The child's initial reaction is anger; however, the child feels unsafe to express this anger openly and directly. This may relate to the child's fearing further loss if he or she responds with anger or his or her subjective perception that anger is unacceptable.

▶ The child uses defense mechanisms to deal with conflict created by desire for the love object but co-occurring with anger for the love object.

▶ Instead of anger being expressed outward at the maternal figure, it turns inward because it is more acceptable and safer to be angry at oneself than at the mother.

▶ Anger at oneself is rationalized as the child assumes that loss of the mother was related to something bad that he or she did rather than to the caregiver's actions.

▶ Excessive guilt becomes a manifestation of the process of dealing with aggression experienced with the loss of the mother's attention.

▶ A similar emotional reaction (such as low self-esteem, excessive guilt, inability to cope with anger, self-destructive impulses) occurs as an adult whenever a loss is experienced.

▷ Cognitive Theory (Aaron Beck, 1979)

▶ This theory represents a cognitive diathesis–stress model in which developmental experiences sensitize a person to respond to stressful life events in a depressed manner.

▶ Cognitive theory assumes that people with a tendency to be depressed think about the world differently than nondepressed people and that depressed people are more negative and believe that bad things are going to happen to them because of their own personal shortcomings and inadequacies.

▶ This thinking promotes low self-esteem and beliefs that the person deserves to have bad things happen to him or her and promotes pessimistic perceptions about the world at large and about his or her future, as well as globalizes the negativity to all events, situations, and people in his or her life.

▶ When confronted by stressful events, these people tend to appraise them and the potential consequences in a negative, hopeless manner and therefore are more depressed than people with different cognitive styles.

▷ Learned Helplessness-Hopelessness Theory (Martin Seligman)

▶ This theory is a modified aspect of cognitive theory, which assumes that a person becomes depressed due to perceptions of lack of control over life events and experiences. These perceptions are learned over time, especially as the person perceives others seeing him or her as inadequate.

▶ Perceptions of lack of control lead to the person not adapting or coping.

▶ The person's behavior becomes passive and nonreactive because of self-perceptions of personal characteristics of being helpless, hopeless, and powerless.

▶ Biological theories

▷ Genetic predisposition

▶ There is a clear genetic predisposition to depressive disorders; one assumption is a polygenic single nucleotide polymorphism (SNP) disorder.

▶ Having a depressed parent is the single strongest predictor of depression. Children of depressed parents are three times more likely to experience MDD in their lifetimes than the general population and have a 40% chance of having a depressive episode before age 18 years.

▶ The earlier the age of onset for MDD and the more severe the symptoms, the more likely it is that a person has a strong genetic predisposition for depression.

▷ Endocrine dysfunction

▶ MDD has symptoms that suggest endocrine abnormalities as part of the etiologic picture.

▶ Neurovegetative symptoms commonly seen in MDD (e.g., sleep disturbances, appetite disturbances, libido disturbances, lethargy, anhedonia) are related to functions of the hypothalamus and pituitary and the hormones they secrete.

▶ A high incidence of postpartum mood disturbances is suggestive of endocrine dysfunction.

▶ Dysphoria is often triggered by changes in levels of sex steroids that occur during the menstrual cycle.

▶ Deregulation of the *hypothalamic–pituitary–adrenal axis* (HPA, which controls the physiological response to stress and consists of interconnected feedback pathways between the hypothalamus, pituitary gland, and adrenal glands) is another theory of an endocrine basis for MDD. In this theory, MDD is presumed to be, at least in part, a result of an abnormal stress response related to HPA dysregulation.

▷ In response to stress, the hypothalamus releases corticotropin-releasing hormone (CRH), which then stimulates the pituitary to release adrenocorticotropic hormone (ACTH). This then stimulates the adrenals to release cortisol.

▷ Hyperactivity of the HPA has been shown to be present in people with MDD, as have possible elevated cortisol levels.

▷ Over time, elevated cortisol levels damage the central nervous system (CNS) by altering neurotransmission and electrical signal conduction.

▷ Evidence supports that cortisol over time can cause changes in size and function of brain tissue.

▷ Evidence supports that major depression may be associated with proinflammatory cytokine activation

▶ HPA dysregulation is the rationale and scientific basis for the dexamethasone suppression test (DST), a screening test for depression, which has proved to be too nonspecific and is not commonly used in clinical practice.

▷ Abnormalities of neurotransmitter function

▶ All of the following are possible neurotransmitter function abnormalities causing depression:

▷ Dysregulation of one or more biogenic amine neurotransmitters: dopamine, serotonin, norepinephrine

▷ Low levels of endogenous catecholamines in specific areas of the brain

▷ Serotonin levels were shown to be low in postmortem studies on people who commit suicide and in people with MDD.

▷ Low level of precursor tryptophan

▷ Low levels of serotonin metabolite 5HTIAA

▷ Receptor sensitivity for neurotransmitters set unusually high in specific areas of the brain

▶ A stronger neurotransmitter receptor cascade is required to induce neuronal activity.

▷ Low density of receptor sites in specific areas of the brain

▷ Hypometabolism in specific areas of the brain regulating mood, appetite, and cognition

▷ Complexity of brain functions implies that the etiology of complex disorders such as MDD involves the relative balance of available neurotransmitters and not just a low level of one neurotransmitter.

▷ Structural brain changes

▶ Neuroimaging has shown consistent abnormalities in certain structures of the brain in people with chronic and severe depression.

▷ Hypovolemic hippocampus

▷ Hypovolemic prefrontal cortex–limbic striatal regions

▶ MDD is a common comorbidity in people who have experienced brain damage, including damage from stroke and trauma.

▷ Chronobiological theory

▶ Desynchronization of circadian rhythms produces the symptom constellation collectively called MDD.

▶ Circadian rhythms control biological processes that are frequent problems in depressed persons.

▷ Interrupted sleep–rest cycle

> ▷ REM abnormalities

> ▷ Frequent waking

> ▷ Intensified dreaming

> ▷ Diurnal variations to circadian-related behaviors

> ▷ Decreased arousal and energy levels

> ▷ Decreased activity patterns

> ▷ Increased cortisol secretion

> ▷ Increased emotional reactivity

Incidence and Demographics

▶ MDD is a common illness, with approximately 5% of the U.S. population ages 18 and older in a given year, or 15 million U.S. adults, having the disorder.

▶ MDD is the leading cause of disability in the United States and is the most common psychiatric illness seen in primary care practices; however, only 50% of people with MDD ever receive treatment.

▶ MDD can occur at any age; however, the average age of onset is mid-20s.

▶ During reproductive years, the lifetime risk for MDD varies with gender—25% for women, 12% for men; the risk is equal for the genders before puberty and after menopause.

▶ MDD is a greater source of morbidity for women than any other illness.

▶ MDD is associated with high mortality; 15% of people with MDD will die by suicide. People with MDD have a 4-times-greater risk of premature death than the normal control population.

▶ The disease course is variable and can involve isolated episodes separated by many years, clusters of episodes, or a severe episode with some remission of symptoms but with chronic symptoms persisting over time.

▶ If left untreated, an episode of MDD usually lasts four months or longer.

▶ MDD tends to be a chronic, recurrent illness.

▶ One year after initial diagnosis of MDD, symptoms often persist.

> ▷ 40% of clients have significant enough symptoms to meet full *Diagnostic and Statistical Manual of Mental Disorders* (*DSM-5*; American Psychiatric Association, 2013) criteria for MDD.

> ▷ 20% of clients do not meet full *DSM-5* criteria but still have a significant symptom level that impairs functioning.

> ▷ 40% have no symptoms.

▶ The number of prior episodes predict the likelihood of future episodes (Judd et. al., 2000).

▶ People with first episode of major depression have approximately a 60% risk of a second episode.

▷ People who experience a second episode have approximately a 70% risk of a third episode.

▷ People who experience a third episode have approximately a 90% risk of a fourth episode.

Risk Factors

▶ Genetic loading

  ▷ Family history, especially a first-degree relative

▶ Prior episode of MDD

▶ Female gender

▶ Postpartum period

▶ Medical comorbidity

▶ Single marital status

▶ Significant environmental stressors, especially multiple losses

Prevention and Screening

▶ Provide at-risk family education.

▶ Provide community education to help reduce stigma, to convey signs and symptoms of illness, and to emphasize the treatment potential for control of symptoms.

▶ Provide significant screening efforts to help recognize, intervene, and initiate treatment early.

▶ Provide healthcare provider education to facilitate early recognition and effective treatment.

▶ Significant and protracted prodromal symptom period usually noted before full onset of illness.

Assessment

Conduct baseline screening with a tool such as the Patient Health Questionnaire 9 (PHQ-9) or Edinburgh Postnatal Depression Scale (EPDS) (Siu & U.S. Preventive Task Force, 2016). Or the Beck Depression Inventory (BDI), or Hamilton Depression Rating Scale (HAM-D), and repeat throughout the course of treatment to evaluate initial symptoms and response to treatment.

History

▶ Detailed history of present illness, including time frame, progression, and any associated symptoms

▶ Social history, including present living situation, marital status, occupation, spirituality; education, alcohol, tobacco, and illicit drug use

▶ Medication use, including prescription, over-the-counter, alternative, supplements, and home remedies

▶ Recent medical illness or surgery

▶ Initial and periodic functional history and assessment

▶ Validation of history with family member

   ▷ Initial presentation: often manifests as vague somatic complaints

      ▶ Bodily aches, pains

      ▶ Headaches

      ▶ Muscle pains

      ▶ Lack of energy

      ▶ Gastrointestinal problems

▶ When mood is the presenting complaint, often client word choice may be vague or indirect.

   ▷ The person may describe mood as *depressed, discouraged, sad, "blue," "blah,"* or *"down in the dumps."*

   ▷ Irritable mood is a frequent subjective state validated by a significant person in the client's life.

▶ Characteristic low energy is seen, so assess for individual activity intolerance without other apparent cause.

▶ Anhedonia is almost always present to some degree.

▶ Sleep disturbance is almost always present.

   ▷ Typically problems occur with middle or terminal insomnia.

   ▷ Hypersomnia can be present.

   ▷ Diurnal variations can be present.

▶ A prodromal episode consisting of a high level of subjective anxiety and mild depressive symptoms often develops over days to weeks before onset of a full episode.

▶ Women often report symptoms occurring in fixed pattern around several days before onset of menses, so assess menstrual history.

▶ Psychotic features can be present, so always assess for their presence.

▶ Assess for client's symptoms according to *diagnostic criteria for MDD:*

   ▷ Anhedonia or a depressed mood, or both

   ▷ Depressed mood most of the day, nearly every day, as indicated by subjective reports or observations of others

      ▶ In children, irritable mood

   ▷ Marked anhedonia in all or almost all activities of daily living

   ▷ At least three or more significant symptoms present during the same 2-week period that represent a change in previous functioning

   ▷ Significant, unintentional weight loss or gain of more than 5% of body weight; with increased appetite and usually a concurrent craving for specific foods, such as carbohydrates or sweets

   ▷ Hypersomnia or insomnia nearly every day

▷ Psychomotor agitation or retardation

▷ Fatigue or loss of energy

▷ Self-deprecating comments or thoughts

▷ Feelings of worthlessness or excessive or inappropriate guilt nearly every day

▷ Decreased concentration and memory

▷ Recurrent morbid thoughts or suicidal ideation

▷ Symptoms that begin within 2 months of significant loss such as death of a loved one and do not persist beyond 2 months are generally considered bereavement and not MDD.

Physical Exam Findings

▶ There are no specific physical findings.

▶ People with certain other disorders (such as diabetes, myocardial infarction, carcinomas, stroke) have a statistically significant increased risk for MDD.

▷ Prognosis for treatment of other disorders is poor if MDD is not recognized and effectively treated.

▶ Clients with MDD may have trouble participating in assessments related to the cognitive problems of the disorder.

▷ Impaired ability to report chronological timeline of illness

▷ Poor decision-making

▷ Slowed thought processes

▷ Poor concentration

▶ Clients with MDD often have psychomotor findings.

▷ Agitation

▷ Retardation

Mental Status Exam Findings

▶ Appearance

▷ Unkempt

▷ Tired-looking

▷ Clothing showing little attention or care about how the person looks

▷ Dark-colored, loose-fitting clothing

▷ Significant weight change from baseline

▶ Mood

▷ Sad

▷ "Depressed"

▷ Anxious

▷ Irritable

▶ Affect

▷ Constricted or blunted

▷ Sad, tearful

▷ Anxious

▷ Irritable

▶ Speech

▷ Underproductive

▷ Slowed response times

▷ Monotonal intonation

▶ Thought process

▷ Usually organized but may be disorganized if psychosis present

▷ Slowing

▷ Distractible

▷ Ruminative

▶ Thought content

▷ Morbid preoccupation

▷ Suicidal ideation exists on continuum of severity:

  ▶ Guilt for not being able to overcome the depression or for what they are "putting loved ones through"

  ▶ Thoughts that others would be better off if the person was "gone"

  ▶ Transient recurrent thoughts of suicide

  ▶ Nonspecific thoughts of active action to commit suicide

  ▶ Specific plan for committing suicide

  ▶ Specific plan with timeline for completion

  ▶ Specific plan with acquisition of the means to carry out plan (suicidal motivation differs for different clients)

  ▶ Desire to give up struggle

  ▶ Attempt to end significant emotional pain

  ▶ Lack of any visible options for dealing with stressors, hopeless, helpless

  ▶ Anger and frustration with poor impulse control

▷ Research evidence supports that it is not possible to predict accurately whether or when a person will attempt suicide (see Table 9–1 for review of suicide assessment).

▷ Suicide risk especially high for persons with certain symptoms or history:

  ▶ Presence of psychotic symptoms

  ▶ History of past attempts

  ▶ History of first-degree relative who committed suicide

TABLE 9–1.
ASSESSING FOR SUICIDAL BEHAVIOR

Past history for suicide attempts or completed suicide in client or family
Negativity and morbidity
Suicidal ideation currently
Plan and intent for suicide action
Means and access to commit suicide
Perceived social supports
Lethality of intended suicide action: *High lethality:* Jumping from significant height, gun, hanging *Moderate lethality:* Overdose of toxic agents (such as aspirin, sleeping pills) *Low lethality:* Superficial wrist-cutting, breath-holding
Impulsivity
Substance abuse or dependence
History of psychiatric disorder

> ▶ Concurrent substance abuse or dependency

> ▶ Current serious health problem (see below for clinical management of suicidality)

▶ Orientation

> ▷ Client is usually oriented to person, place, and time unless psychosis is present.

▶ Memory

> ▷ Usually impaired recent and short-term memory

▶ Concentration

> ▷ Usually significantly impaired

▶ Abstraction

> ▷ Abstract ability on proverb testing usually intact

> ▷ If concrete, assess for other psychotic findings

▶ Insight

> ▷ May be intact or impaired

▶ Judgment

> ▷ May be impaired for self-welfare

Diagnostic and Laboratory Findings

▶ No lab findings specific to MDD exist

▶ Complete blood count (CBC), chemistry profile, thyroid function tests, or B_{12} and folate levels to rule out metabolic causes or unidentified conditions; consider referral for sleep study if snoring, apnea, or suspicion of other sleep disorder

▶ Drug toxicity screening, if indicated by history

▶ Depression related to a differential diagnosis

▷ Endocrine disorders

  ▶ Hypothyroidism

  ▶ Diabetes

  ▶ Hyperaldosteronism

  ▶ Cushing's or Addison's disease

▷ Neurological disorders

  ▶ Stroke

  ▶ Epilepsy

  ▶ Dementia

  ▶ Huntington's disease

  ▶ Sleep apnea

  ▶ Wilson's disease

  ▶ Neoplasms

  ▶ Head trauma

  ▶ Multiple sclerosis

  ▶ Parkinson's disease

▷ Cardiac disorders

  ▶ Myocardial infarction

  ▶ Congestive heart failure

  ▶ Hypertension

▷ Infectious and inflammatory states

  ▶ Mononucleosis

  ▶ AIDS

  ▶ Pneumonia: viral and bacterial

  ▶ Systemic lupus erythematous

  ▶ Temporal arteritis

  ▶ Tuberculosis

▷ Nutritional disorders

  ▶ Pernicious anemia

  ▶ Pellagra

▷ Other disorders

  ▶ Fibromyalgia

  ▶ Chronic fatigue syndrome

  ▶ Bereavement or grief reaction

  ▶ Electrolyte imbalance

  ▶ Uremia and other renal conditions

▷ Psychiatric disorders

▶ Anxiety disorders

▶ Eating disorders

▶ Bipolar affective disorder

▶ Substance dependence–related disorders

▷ Medications that can cause altered mood states as side effects

▶ Steroids

▶ Estrogen compounds

▶ Antihypertensive agents

▶ Anti-Parkinson's agents

▶ Antineoplastic agents

▶ Antibacterial and antifungal agents

▶ Analgesics

▶ Isotretinoin (Accutane)

▶ Benzodiazepines

Clinical Management

▶ The top goal in the acute phase of MDD is ensuring client safety.

▶ A general consideration is to rule out or treat any conditions that may contribute to depression and cognitive impairment.

▶ Assess for the acuity level of client presentation.

▷ Reasons for brief hospitalization during acute episodes of MDD:

▶ Ensure client safety

▶ Initiate medication change, when doing so as an outpatient poses undue risk

▶ Restabilize on medication

▶ Monitor suicidality

▶ Ensure client compliance with treatment to reach stabilization.

▷ Clinical management during nonacute episodes occurs most often in community settings.

▶ Obtain baseline labs as indicated before initiation of treatment.

▷ Pharmacological management

▷ Nonpharmacological management (psychotherapy)

Pharmacological Management

▶ Inform client that therapeutic effect may take at least 4 to 6 weeks.

▶ Once started, continue antidepressants for a minimum of 6 to 12 months.

▷ If client has more than two prior episodes of MDD, consider continuing antidepressants indefinitely.

▶ Not all symptoms of MDD will respond to pharmacological interventions.

  ▷ Identify clear, measurable target symptoms and educate the client about these symptoms (see Table 9–2).

▶ Research has found that the most effective intervention is a combination of medication and psychotherapy.

▶ Antidepressant rebound is common when stopping antidepressants abruptly, particularly when drugs with short half-lives are involved.

▶ Antidepressants may induce mania or mixed mania in susceptible persons.

▶ All antidepressants have "black box" warnings regarding suicidality for children, adolescents, and young adults.

▶ Classes of antidepressants

  ▷ Selective serotonin reuptake inhibitors (SSRIs)

    ▶ Act primarily to increase serotonin levels in central nervous system (CNS) by inhibiting their presynaptic reuptake

    ▶ See Table 9–3 for examples

  ▷ Tricyclic antidepressants (TCAs)

    ▶ Elevate serotonin and norepinephrine levels primarily by inhibiting their presynaptic reuptake

    ▶ See Table 9–4 for examples.

  ▷ Monoamine oxidase inhibitors (MAOIs)

    ▶ Elevate serotonin and norepinephrine levels primarily by inhibiting MAO, the enzyme that breaks down monoamine neurotransmitters

    ▶ See Table 9–5 for examples.

  ▷ Serotonin norepinephrine reuptake inhibitors (SNRIs)

    ▶ Inhibit dual reuptake of norepinephrine and serotonin

    ▶ Action very selective on neurotransmitters

TABLE 9–2.
TARGET SYMPTOMS OF ANTIDEPRESSANT TREATMENT

Depressed mood
Sleep–rest disturbances
Anxiety
Irritability
Impaired concentration
Impaired memory
Appetite disturbance
Agitation
Anhedonia
Impaired energy and motivation

TABLE 9–3.
DRUGS FOR MOOD DISORDERS: ANTIDEPRESSANTS—SELECTIVE SEROTONIN REUPTAKE INHIBITORS

AGENT	BRAND NAME	DOSAGE FORMS DAILY DOSAGE	SIDE EFFECTS	COMMENTS
Citalopram	Celexa	Tablet 20–40 mg/day	Sedation Sexual dysfunction Agitation Yawning GI disturbances Weight gain	Pregnancy Category C Lactation Category L2 2011 warning about prolonged QTc interval in doses above 40 mg (20 mg in older adults) and in those susceptible to prolonged QTc
Escitalopram	Lexapro	Tablet 10–20 mg/day	Somnolence Headache Sexual dysfunction GI disturbances	Pregnancy Category C Lactation Category L2
Fluoxetine	Prozac	Capsule, tablet, or liquid 20–80 mg/day	Insomnia Headache GI disturbances Sexual dysfunction	Long half-life Pregnancy Category C Lactation Catagory L2 Discontinuation syndrome unlikely
Fluvoxamine	Luvox	Tablet 100–300 mg/day	Sedation Sexual dysfunction Agitation GI disturbances	Doses above 150 mg should generally be given b.i.d. Pregnancy Category C Lactation Category L2
Paroxetine	Paxil CR, Pexeva	Tablet or liquid 20–60 mg/day	Headache GI disturbances Somnolence Sexual dysfunction	Pregnancy Category D Lactation Category L2 Discontinuation syndrome very common
Sertraline	Zoloft	Tablet 50–200 mg/day	Sexual dysfunction GI disturbances Somnolence Headache	Pregnancy Category C Lactation Category L2
Serotonin partial agonist reuptake inhibitor (SPARI)				
Vilazodone	Viibryd	Tablet 20–40 mg	Diarrhea Nausea Dry mouth (lower risk of sexual side effects)	Pregenancy Category C Lactation Category: Unknown, is excreted in breast milk

▶ Elevate serotonin and norepinephrine levels by inhibiting their presynaptic reuptake

▶ See Table 9–7 for examples.

TABLE 9–4.
TRICYCLIC ANTIDEPRESSANTS

AGENT	BRAND NAME	DOSAGE FORMS DAILY DOSAGE	COMMENTS
Amitriptyline	Elavil	Tablet or IM 50–300 mg/day	Also used for chronic pain (particularly neuropathic), insomnia Pregnancy Category C Lactation Category L2
Clomipramine	Anafranil	Capsule 100–250 mg/day	Approved for obsessive–compulsive disorder; 250 mg/day maximum because of increased seizure risk Pregnancy Category C Lactation Category L2
Desipramine	Norpramin	Tablet or capsule 100–300 mg/day	Also used for attention-deficit hyperactivity disorder (off-label for pediatric clients and for ADHD) Pregnancy Category C Lactation Category L2
Doxepin	Sinequan	Capsule or liquid 100–300 mg/day	Also used for insomnia Pregnancy Category C Lactation Category L5 Avoid
Imipramine	Tofranil	Tablet, capsule, or IM 100–300 mg/day	Also used for enuresis and separation anxiety Pregnancy Category D Lactation Category L2
Nortriptyline	Pamelor	Capsule or liquid 50–150 mg/day	Also used for enuresis and attention deficit hyperactivity disorder Pregnancy Category D Lactation Category L2
Protriptyline	Vivactil	Tablet 15–60 mg/day	Pregnancy Category C Lactation Category: Inadequate data
Trimipramine	Surmontil	Capsule 100–300 mg/day	Pregnancy Category C Lactation Category: Inadequate data

▶ Norepinephrine dopamine reuptake inhibitors (NDRIs)

▷ Inhibit dual reuptake of norepinephrine and dopamine

▷ Action very selective on neurotransmitters

▷ Elevate dopamine and norepinephrine levels by inhibiting their presynaptic reuptake

▷ See Table 9–6 for examples.

▶ Serotonin agonist and reuptake inhibitors (SARIs)

▷ Dual action

▷ Agonist of serotonin 5HT-2 receptors

▷ Action very selective on neurotransmitters

▷ Elevate serotonin levels by inhibiting serotonin reuptake

TABLE 9–5.
MONOAMINE OXIDASE INHIBITORS

DRUG	BRAND NAME	DOSAGE FORMS		COMMENTS
		DAILY DOSAGE		
Isocarboxazid	Marplan	Tablet 20–60 mg/day		Also used for panic disorder, phobic disorders, selective mutism
Phenelzine	Nardil	Tablet 45–90 mg/day		*Caution:* High-tyramine diet; sympathomimetic agents
				Divided dosing: b.i.d. and q.i.d.
Tranylcypromine	Parnate	Tablet 30–60 mg/day		All Pregnancy Category C
				Lactation Category: Inadequate Information
Selegiline	EMSAM	Transdermal patch 6–12 mg		No dietary restrictions with 6 mg dosage; may need higher dose to see antidepressant effect
				Pregnancy Category C
				Lactation Catagory L4 Avoid

TABLE 9–6.
TYRAMINE-FREE DIETARY CONSIDERATIONS

CATEGORY OF FOOD	SPECIFIC FOODS TO AVOID
Cheeses	Aged cheeses, such as blue, brie, Camembert, and Roquefort
Meat	Smoked, aged, and cured meats such as sausages, pastrami, and salami
Fish	Smoked, aged, and cured fish such as pickled herring and salted fish
Beverages	Any aged and fermented beverages such as red wine, aged liquors, whiskey (gin and vodka permissible), beer (bottled and pasteurized permissible)
Other	Bean curd (tofu), soy products, sauerkraut, miso, yeast extract, MSG, ripe bananas, avocado

▷ See Table 9–6 for examples.

▶ The various antidepressants differ markedly in characteristics such as

  ▷ Cost

  ▷ Side-effect profile

  ▷ Safety in overdose

  ▷ Safety in clients with other disorders

  ▷ Drug–drug interactions

  ▷ Cytochrome P450 liver effects

▶ To achieve best control of symptoms, match client's symptom profile to the pharmacodynamic and pharmacokinetic properties of specific antidepressant agents.

SSRIs

▶ First-line treatment for first episode of major depression with mild to moderate symptoms

▶ Serious side effects are rare

▶ Much safer in overdose than TCAs

▶ Also effective for panic disorder, obsessive–compulsive disorder, bulimia, generalized anxiety disorder, social phobia, posttraumatic stress disorder, and premenstrual dysphoric disorder

TCAs

▶ Considered second-line drugs for treating MDD (see Table 9–4).

▶ Affect many neurotransmitters, leading to more side effects and possibly poor adherence.

   ▷ *Anticholinergic:* Dry mouth, blurred vision, constipation, memory problems (from muscarinic receptor blockade)

   ▷ *Antiadrenergic:* Orthostatic hypotension (from alpha 1 receptor blockade)

   ▷ *Antihistaminergic:* Sedation and weight gain (from histamine receptor blockade)

   ▷ Electrocardiogram (EKG) changes and cardiac dysrhythmias possible; avoid in clients known to have susceptibility (personal or family history). Monitor EKG before treatment and annually in older adults.

   ▷ Unsafe in many co-occurring disorders (such as cardiac disease)

   ▷ Known to induce hypomania in susceptible clients

▶ Well-identified serum blood levels guide dosing (particularly nortriptyline) and predict toxicity.

▶ Inexpensive and available in generic forms.

▶ Anticholinergic properties may be highly problematic but may also be useful in those who have significant bowel irritability.

▶ Avoid abrupt withdrawal because of significant discontinuation syndrome.

▶ Avoid prescribing to people who are at high risk for suicide; lethal dose is 1,000 mg or more (a week's supply of an average dose). *Combination of TCAs with MAOIs can cause lethal serotonin syndrome, hypertensive crisis, or both; adhere to 2-week washout period (5 weeks for fluoxetine) before switching between the two classes of medications.*

▶ Use caution if the person is taking both a TCA and an SSRI, because the SSRI can elevate TCA concentrations because of pharmacodynamic or pharmacokinetic interactions. Monitor TCA levels.

MAOIs

▶ Not first or second-line agents for MDD because of dangerous food and drug interactions (see Tables 9–5 and 9–6).

▷ *Hypertensive crisis* occurs when MAOIs are taken in conjunction with foods containing *tyramine*, a dietary precursor to norepinephrine.

▷ When MAO is inhibited, tyramine exerts a strong vasopressor effect, stimulating the release of catecholamines, epinephrine, and norepinephrine, which can increase blood pressure and heart rate.

▷ Hypertensive crisis is life-threatening and cannot be reversed unless more MAO is produced by the body.

> ▶ *Hypertensive crisis* and death also can occur when MAOIs are taken in conjunction with certain medications:
>> ▷ Meperidine
>> ▷ Decongestants
>> ▷ TCAs
>> ▷ Atypical antipsychotics
>> ▷ St. John's wort
>> ▷ L-tryptophan
>> ▷ Stimulants and other sympathomimetics
>> ▷ Asthma medications
>
> ▶ Symptoms of hypertensive crisis:
>> ▷ Sudden, explosive-like headache, usually in occipital region
>> ▷ Elevated blood pressure
>> ▷ Facial flushing
>> ▷ Palpitations
>> ▷ Pupillary dilation
>> ▷ Diaphoresis
>> ▷ Fever
>
> ▶ Treatment of hypertensive crisis:
>> ▷ Discontinue the MAOI.
>> ▷ Give phentolamine (binds with norepinephrine receptor sites, blocks norepinephrine).
>> ▷ Stabilize fever.
>> ▷ Reevaluate the person's diet and adherence, and reiterate medication guidelines as necessary.

▷ People on MAOIs must follow a tyramine-free diet and must avoid many medications, including most over-the-counter cold and allergy preparations.

▷ *Combining an MAOI with a serotonergic agent is contraindicated, because this may cause serotonin syndrome.*

> ▶ Symptoms of serotonin syndrome
>> ▷ Agitation, restlessness
>> ▷ Rapid heart rate and elevation in blood pressure

▷ Headache

▷ Sweating, shivering, and goose bumps

▷ Myoclonic jerking and loss of coordination

▷ Confusion, fever, seizures, unconsciousness

▶ Treatment of serotonin syndrome includes discontinuing the offending agents and supportive treatment of symptoms. Mild symptoms such as restlessness may respond to removal of the offending agent, close monitoring, and judicious use of a benzodiazepine. More severe symptoms constitute a medical emergency necessitating hospitalization and treatment such as cyproheptadine, anticonvulsants, and autonomic support.

▶ Can be fatal in overdose.

▶ Side-effect profile and stringent dietary restrictions often lead to poor client adherence.

▶ Clients who are on MAOIs must be taught to recognized the signs and symptoms of hypertensive crisis and serotonin syndrome and understand that they must seek immediate medical attention should they suspect either one of occurring.

▶ *Clinically significant side effects of MAOIs include*

▷ Insomnia

▷ Hypertensive crisis

▷ Weight gain

▷ Anticholinergic side effects

▷ Lightheadedness and dizziness

▷ Sexual dysfunction

▶ MAOIs are unsafe in many co-occurring disorders.

Other Antidepressants

▶ Other antidepressants used in the treatment of MDD may be classified as SNRIs, NDRIs, and SARIs. See Table 9–7 and Table 9–8.

▶ Psychotic features can be present with MDD and Bipolar I Disorder.

▷ Routinely assess for the presence of psychotic symptoms during periods of symptom exacerbation

▷ Features are usually mood-congruent.

▷ Can be managed with short-term use of antipsychotic medications (see Chapter 11)

▶ Comorbidities are common and include various medical conditions (as noted earlier in the chapter) as well as psychiatric comorbidities such as panic disorder, obsessive–compulsive disorder, and substance abuse or dependence.

▶ Altered appetite and sleep–rest patterns predispose clients with MDD to decreased overall health status.

▶ Increased mortality exists in people with MDD.

TABLE 9–7.
SNRIS

DRUG (CLASS)	BRAND NAME	DOSAGE FORMS DAILY DOSAGE	SIDE EFFECTS	COMMENTS
Venlafaxine (SNRI)	Effexor, Effexor XR	Capsule (XR), or tablet 75–375 mg/day XR 75–225 mg/d	Diaphoresis Headache Dizziness GI disturbances	Can raise BP QD for XR capsules b.i.d.–t.i.d. dosing for tablets Full SNRI effect at doses at or above 150 mg Safer in overdose than TCAs Has *significant* discontinuation syndrome if stopped abruptly Pregnancy Category C Lactation Category L3
Duloxetine (SNRI)	Cymbalta	Capsule 30–120 mg	Dizziness Headache GI disturbances	Once-daily dosing Can elevate BP Can elevate liver function tests Has *significant* discontinuation syndrome if stopped abruptly Pregnancy Category C Lactation Category L3
Vortioxetine (5HT-3 and 5HT7 antagonist, 5HT 1A agonist)	Brintellix	Tablet (5, 10, 20mg) 20 mg q.d.	Nausea Diarrhea Dizziness	Pregnancy Category C Lactation Category: Inadequate Information
Levomilnacipran (SNRI)	Fetzima	Tablet (20,40,80,120mg) 40-120 mg q.d.	Nausea and vomiting Constipation Sweating Palpitations Urinary hesitancy Hypertension Hypotension Decreased appetite	Pregnancy Category C Lactation Category: Inadequate Information

Nonpharmacological Management

▶ Electroconvulsive therapy (ECT)

▷ Grand mal seizure induced in anesthetized person

▷ Usual course is 6 to 12 treatments

▷ Mechanism of action:

▶ Neurotransmitter theory: Increases dopamine, serotonin, and norepinephrine

TABLE 9–8.
OTHER ANTIDEPRESSANT AGENTS

DRUG (CLASS)	BRAND NAME	DOSAGE FORMS DAILY DOSAGE	SIDE EFFECTS	COMMENTS
Bupropion (NDRI)	Wellbutrin	Tablet 150–450 mg/day	Headache Nervousness Tremors Tachycardia Insomnia Decreased appetite	Contraindicated if client has seizures, eating disorder SR offers b.i.d. dosing; XL offers once-daily dosing Can increase energy level Also used for attention-deficit hyperactivity disorder and smoking cessation Pregnancy Category C Lactation Category L3
Bupropion SR/XL	Wellbutrin SR	Sustained release 150–400 mg/day Extended release 150–450 mg/day		Caution with caffeine and in people with panic disorder
Mirtazapine (alpha2/5HT2 antagonist)	Remeron	Tablet 15–45 mg/day	Sedation Weight gain Increased cholesterol	Inverse relationship between dosage and sedation Pregnancy Category C Lactation Category L3
Nefazodone (SARI)	Serzone	Tablet 300–600 mg/day	Headache Drowsiness GI disturbances	*Must* monitor LFTs Can cause liver failure Safer in overdose than TCAs q.h.s. or b.i.d. dosing Potent P450 3A4 inhibitor Pregnancy Cateogory C Lactation Category L4 Avoid
Trazodone (SARI)	Desyrel	Tablet 200–600 mg/day	Sedation Nausea Headache Hypotension	Safer in overdose than TCAs Priapism possible Not well tolerated at antidepressant dosage because of sedation Most commonly used as hypnotic at 50–200 mg/h.s. May prolong QTc interval Pregnancy Category B Lactation Category L2

- ▶ Neuroendocrine theory: Releases hormones such as prolactin, thyroid-stimulating hormone, pituitary hormones, endorphins, and adrenocorticotropic hormone

- ▶ Anticonvulsant theory: Exerts an anticonvulsant effect, which then produces an antidepressant effect

▷ Situations in which ECT is used:

- ▶ Client preference

- ▶ Need for rapid response because of severity of illness

- ▶ MDD with psychotic features

- ▶ Risk of other treatment outweighs risk of ECT

- ▶ Treatment resistance

▷ Possible contraindications:

- ▶ Cardiac disease

- ▶ Compromised pulmonary status

- ▶ History of brain injury or brain tumor

- ▶ Anesthesia medical complications

▷ Adverse effects:

- ▶ Possible cardiovascular effects

- ▶ Systemic effects (e.g., headaches, muscle aches, drowsiness)

- ▶ Cognitive effects (e.g., memory disturbance and confusion)

▶ Transcranial magnetic stimulation (TMS)

▷ Option for clients who have not had adequate response to medications and psychotherapy (treatment-resistant depression)

▷ Involves placement of small wire coil on scalp to conduct electrical current, creating a magnetic field through the tissues of the head

▷ Performed in office setting, without anesthesia

▷ Sessions typically last 40 minutes and typical course is 5 sessions per week for 6 weeks.

▷ Side effects are minimal but may include headache, scalp discomfort, tingling or twitches to facial muscles, lightheadedness, and hearing discomfort from procedure noise.

▷ Seizures, although rare, have been reported.

▶ Vagal nerve stimulation (VNS)

▷ Option for clients who have not had adequate response to medications and psychotherapy (treatment-resistant depression)

▷ Pacemaker-like device implanted in left side of chest to stimulate left branch of nerve; transcutaneous devices being tested

▷ Generally done as outpatient procedure, but anesthesia is required

> ▷ Side effects generally occur as the pulse generator stimulates the vagal nerve and include voice changes, hoarseness, cough, throat or neck pain, chest spasms, dyspnea on exertion, tingling of skin, dysphagia

> ▷ Intended for use along with traditional treatments

▶ Phototherapy

> ▷ 2,500 to 10,000 lux light for 30 minutes up to 2 hours, 1 to 2 times daily (Sadock, Sadock, & Ruiz, 2015)

▶ Individual therapy (See Chapter 8. Nonpharmacological Treatment)

> ▷ Psychodynamic psychotherapy

> ▷ Cognitive behavioral therapy (CBT)

>> ▶ Modify perceptions

>> ▶ Decrease negativity

>> ▶ Increase sense of internal control

>> ▶ Enhance coping skills

>> ▶ Modify environmental factors contributing to illness

> ▷ Brief therapy (solution-focused therapy)

>> ▶ Focus on precipitant stressor

>> ▶ Cope with immediate impact of MDD on personal life

>> ▶ Modify contributory environmental factors

> ▷ Group therapy

>> ▶ Improve decision-making

>> ▶ Improve socialization skills

>> ▶ Improve assessment of individual strengths

>> ▶ Gain new coping skills

> ▷ Family therapy

>> ▶ Enhance family coping

>> ▶ Improve knowledge base

>> ▶ Plan for relapse

>> ▶ Gain insight into effects of MDD on family unit

>> ▶ Undertake psychoeducation for family members about the illness state of MDD

Clinical Management of Suicidality

▶ Pay significant attention to positive assessments for suicidality.

▶ Always assume client is serious when he or she vocalizes suicidal thoughts.

▶ Identify current stressors that may be contributing to crisis.

▶ Generally do not manage in community setting during acute suicidal ideation periods unless client is able to make "no harm" agreement.

▶ Consider hospitalization.

▶ Consider mobilizing available social resources.

   ▷ Risk factors for suicide:

      ▶ Ages 45 or older if male

      ▶ Ages 55 or older if female

      ▶ Divorced, single, or separated

      ▶ White

      ▶ Living alone

      ▶ Psychiatric disorder

      ▶ Physical illness

      ▶ Substance abuse

      ▶ Previous suicide attempt

      ▶ Family history of suicide

      ▶ Recent loss

      ▶ Male gender

Life Span Considerations: Children

▶ Core symptoms of MDD are the same for children. However, some symptoms are more pronounced in children.

   ▷ Irritability

   ▷ Somatic complaints

   ▷ Social withdrawal

▶ Some core symptoms are *less common* in children before onset of puberty:

   ▷ Psychosis

   ▷ Motor retardation

   ▷ Hypersomnia

   ▷ Increased appetite

▶ MDD often has a strong separation anxiety component in children.

▶ Children usually do not respond well to tricyclics; however, they do respond well to SSRIs.

▶ All antidepressants indicated for children, adolescents, and young adults carry a black box warning about an increase in suicidal thoughts; monitor closely for suicidal thoughts, behavior, agitation, and aggression in children taking antidepressants.

Life Span Considerations: Older Adults

▶ Persons with MDD admitted to a long-term-care facility have significantly shorter life spans than control population.

- ▶ 65% are more likely to die within the first year in a long-term-care facility.
- ▶ Cognition and memory symptoms of MDD in the older adult population often are confused with dementia-related symptoms (pseudodementia).
  - ▷ Clients with dementia usually have a premorbid history of slowly declining cognition.
  - ▷ In MDD, cognitive changes have a relatively acute onset and are significant when compared to premorbid functioning.
- ▶ It is important to complete a *functional assessment* for older adults.
  - ▷ Determines the degree to which the person's abilities and performance match the demands of his or her life
  - ▷ Determines the impact of illness on overall functioning
  - ▷ *Skill deficit*: Inability to perform a functional skill despite the physical ability, as in dementia
  - ▷ *Performance deficit*: Ability to perform a functional skill but lacks the motivation to do so, as in depression
- ▶ Reasons for performing functional assessment:
  - ▷ To correctly diagnose (for example, to differentiate depression from dementia)
  - ▷ To track client improvement or decompensation
  - ▷ To help families set realistic expectations
- ▶ Components of functional assessment:
  - ▷ Activities of daily living (ADLs): Basic self-care skills, such as bathing, dressing, eating, and toileting
  - ▷ Instrumental activities of daily living (IADLs): Complex activities needed for independent functioning, such as shopping, cooking, driving, and housekeeping
  - ▷ Executive functioning: Judgment and planning; ability to maintain calendar, manage money and appointments, and prioritize activities
- ▶ The degree of change over time and the speed of change are better observed with objective recording and when the assessment is measured at intervals such as every 6 months.

Follow-up

- ▶ Follow-up care practices for the PMHNP to consider
  - ▷ Include teaching client the goals, risks, benefits, and potential side effects of medication treatment
  - ▷ Continuously monitor client's response to medication; the treatment goal is complete remission of symptoms.
  - ▷ Utilize screening tool such as PHQ-9 in follow-up appointments.
  - ▷ Teach clients the symptoms of depression and that it is a chronic illness; establish a relapse plan for all clients.
  - ▷ Assess for suicidality during every client contact.

▷ Assess for the presence of psychotic symptoms during every client contact.

▷ Assess and manage client for side effects of treatment, including sexual side effects, in an attempt to increase medication compliance.

▷ Observe all clients treated with antidepressants for development of *serotonin syndrome* (overstimulation of serotonin receptors usually caused by drug–drug interactions).

▶ Drug combinations that can cause serotonin syndrome:

  ▷ SSRIs and MAOIs

  ▷ Drug and herbal interactions

  ▷ SSRIs and St. John's wort

▶ Symptoms of serotonin syndrome:

  ▷ Autonomic instability

  ▷ Altered sensorium

  ▷ Restlessness

  ▷ Agitation

  ▷ Myoclonus

  ▷ Hyperreflexia

  ▷ Hyperthermia

  ▷ Diaphoresis

  ▷ Tremor

  ▷ Chills

  ▷ Diarrhea and cramps

  ▷ Ataxia

  ▷ Headache

  ▷ Insomnia

▷ Monitor for adverse effects over time.

▷ Some SSRIs are known to increase blood glucose and contribute to hyperlipidemia, and others may elevate liver function tests.

▷ Discontinue SSRIs slowly to prevent *discontinuation syndrome*.

▶ Symptoms of discontinuation syndrome:

  ▷ Flu-like symptoms (due to cholinergic rebound; particularly problematic with TCAs)

  ▷ Fatigue and lethargy

  ▷ Myalgia

  ▷ Decreased concentration

  ▷ Nausea and vomiting

  ▷ Impaired memory

▷ Paresthesias, including "shock-like" sensations

▷ Irritability

▷ Anxiety

▷ Insomnia

▷ Crying without provocation

▷ Dizziness and vertigo

► Risk factors for discontinuation syndrome:

▷ Medications with short half-life

▷ Abrupt discontinuation

▷ Noncompliant, irregular use pattern

▷ High dose range

▷ Long-term treatment

▷ Prior history of discontinuation syndrome

► Expected course of MDD

▷ Evidence indicates the best treatment outcomes if medications are used in conjunction with appropriate therapy.

▷ Evidence indicates that clients should take an antidepressant agent for at least 12 months after remission of symptoms.

▷ Clients who have had 3 or more episodes of MDD usually require lifelong medication.

PERSISTENT DEPRESSIVE DISORDER (DYSTHYMIA)

Description

► A disorder similar to MDD but with less acute symptoms; with a more protracted, chronic disease course; and without any manifestations of psychotic symptoms

► Less discrete episodes of illness than MDD

► Symptoms often go undetected and therefore untreated for years

► Vegetative symptoms (e.g., sleep, appetite, weight changes) much less common in dysthymic disorder than in MDD

Etiology

► Similar to MDD

Incidence and Demographics

► Affects 5.4% of the U.S. population ages 18 or older, or 10.9 million Americans.

► People with dysthymia have an increased risk for developing MDD; 15% to 25% of people diagnosed with dysthymic disorder will have a lifetime episode of MDD.

▶ People with onset of symptoms before age 21 have a 75% likelihood of a lifetime episode of MDD.

▶ Women are 2 to 3 times more likely to develop dysthymic disorder than men.

Risk Factors

▶ Genetic predisposition

▶ A first-degree relative with MDD

▶ A first-degree relative with dysthymic disorder

▶ Female gender

Prevention and Screening

▶ At-risk family education

▶ Community education

▶ Stigma reduction

▶ Signs and symptoms of illness

▶ Treatment potential for control of symptoms

▶ Early recognition, intervention, and initiation of treatment

▶ Because of chronic nature of disorder, symptoms become a part of clients' day-to-day existence and often go unreported unless solicited by direct questioning

▶ Aggressive screening procedure required

Assessment

History

▶ Assess for the following:

  ▷ Chronically depressed mood that occurs for most of the day, more days than not, for at least 2 years

  ▷ Prominent presence of low self-esteem, self-criticism, and a perception of general incompetence compared to others

  ▷ Other common symptoms:

    ▶ Low energy and fatigue

    ▶ Poor concentration

    ▶ Difficulty with decision-making

    ▶ Feelings of hopelessness

    ▶ Feelings of inadequacy

    ▶ Mild anhedonia

    ▶ Social withdrawal

▶ Brooding about past issues

▶ Subjective irritability or anger

▶ Decreased productivity and activity

▷ Less common symptoms:

▶ Alteration in appetite

▶ Alteration in sleep–rest patterns

Physical Exam Findings

▶ Similar to MDD

Mental Status Exam Findings

▶ Similar to MDD

▶ Usually no vegetative findings

▶ Mood described as *sad, "down for all of my life"*

Diagnostic and Laboratory Findings

▶ Nonspecific

Polysomnographic Findings

▶ Similar to those found in MDD

Differential Diagnosis

▶ Similar to MDD

Clinical Management

Pharmacological Management

▶ Because of increased risk for development of MDD, dysthymia is often treated with antidepressant medications in a manner similar to MDD.

Nonpharmacological Management

▶ Similar to MDD

▶ Often good clinical outcomes with nonpharmacological management if client is willing

Common comorbidities

▶ MDD is often superimposed on dysthymia ("double depression")

▶ The subjective worsening of symptoms or onset of new symptoms such as vegetative ones often brings the person into treatment.

▶ When dysthymia precedes MDD, clinical management is more complex and outcomes can be less positive.

▶ Dysthymic disorder is associated with personality disorders.

   ▷ Borderline

   ▷ Histrionic

   ▷ Narcissistic

   ▷ Avoidant

   ▷ Dependent

Life Span Considerations

▶ Similar to MDD

▶ In children, prevalence rates of dysthymia are equal for boys and girls.

▶ Associated with several childhood disorders:

   ▷ Attention-deficit hyperactivity disorder

   ▷ Conduct disorder

   ▷ Anxiety disorders

   ▷ Learning disorders

▶ Period of symptoms required for diagnosis is only 1 year, compared with 2 years for adults.

▶ In children, the mood usually described as *irritable* rather than *sad* but may report both irritability and sadness

▶ Low self-esteem, poor social skills, and pessimism

Follow-up

▶ Similar to MDD

GRIEF AND BEREAVEMENT

Description

▶ Involve a wide range of normal responses that can become abnormal and excessive

▶ Involve normative emotional, cognitive, and behavioral reactions to death or loss of a significant person or object

▶ Unlike in major depression, self-esteem is usually preserved in the grieving person

▶ Involve nonnormative psychological responses to an identifiable stressor that can result in the development of clinically significant emotional or behavioral symptoms

   ▷ Stressor encompassing elements of perceived loss

   ▷ Develops *within 3 months* of stressor

      ▶ Single event

         ▷ End of relationship

         ▷ Death of relative or partner

▶ Recurring event

▷ Living with person with terminal illness

▶ Developmental event

▷ Leaving home to go away to school

▷ Getting married

▷ Becoming a parent

▷ Retiring from work

▶ PMHNP assessment is needed to separate normal, healthy grieving from pathological grieving, which may represent an adjustment disorder or major depression. The PMHNP must consider:

▷ Severity of response

▷ Duration of response

▷ Effects of response on normal daily functioning

▷ Person's perception of impact of stressor

▶ When severity or duration is excessive, the grieving may be abnormal.

▶ In the absence of other significant clinical symptoms, grief usually is classified as adjustment disorder:

▷ Adjustment disorder with depressed mood

▷ Adjustment disorder with anxiety

▷ Adjustment disorder with mixed anxiety and depression

▷ Adjustment disorder with disturbed conduct

Etiology

▶ Significant loss

▶ Limited coping skills

▶ Limited social supports

Incidence and Demographics

▶ Normal grief is universally experienced.

▶ Grief is common in older adults as their social sphere begins to decrease.

▶ 20% of older adults who lose a spouse experience depression within the first year of that loss.

▶ Lifetime prevalence for adjustment disorder is 2% to 8% in the U.S. population.

▶ Grief occurs in 12% of general hospital clients.

▶ Grief occurs in 50% of clients after cardiac surgery.

Risk Factors

▶ Limited social network

▶ Poor physical health

▶ Limited coping skills

Prevention and Screening

▶ Ask about losses.

▶ Identify at-risk persons.

▶ Do preventative counseling.

▶ Begin early recognition, intervention, and initiation of treatment.

    ▷ Routine screening at all healthcare settings.

Assessment

▶ Often clients will not disclose grieving or bereavement issues unless directly asked.

History

▶ Assess for the following:

    ▷ Recent losses

    ▷ Anniversary dates of past losses

    ▷ Reaction to loss

    ▷ Functional impairment

    ▷ Social and family support systems

    ▷ Insomnia

    ▷ Anorexia

    ▷ Presence of dysfunctional coping

        ▶ Suicidal thoughts

        ▶ Substance abuse

        ▶ Denial

Physical Exam Findings

▶ Nonspecific

Mental Status Exam Findings

▶ Depressed mood

▶ Anxious affect

▶ Crying uncontrollably

Diagnostic and Laboratory Findings

▶ CBC, chemistry profile, thyroid function tests, and B_{12} level to rule out metabolic causes or unidentified conditions

▶ Drug toxicity screening, if indicated by history

Differential Diagnosis

▶ Normal grieving

▶ Major depressive disorder (MDD)

▶ Anxiety disorders (see Chapter 10)

▶ Substance-related disorders (see Chapter 13)

Clinical Management

Pharmacological Management

▶ If needed

  ▷ Short-term use of anti-anxiety agents

    ▶ BNZs

  ▷ Short-term use of sleep-induction agents

    ▶ BNZs

    ▶ Nonbenzodiazepine hypnotic such as zolpidem

    ▶ Tricyclic or other sedating antidepressants

    ▶ Antihistamines

Nonpharmacological Management

▶ Encourage expression of grief and loss.

▶ Use support groups.

▶ Offer community resources.

▶ Offer psychoeducation on grief reactions and responses.

▶ With significant functional impairment, consider psychotherapy (e.g., crisis therapy, brief solution-focused therapy, CBT).

Life Span Considerations

▶ Can occur at any age

▶ Older adults are at greater risk because of higher numbers of losses that may become cumulative in their impact.

Follow-up

- ▶ Follow up weekly during acute period.
- ▶ Monitor for development of MDD.
- ▶ Monitor for impact on general health state.
- ▶ Maintain supportive follow-up over time.
- ▶ Be sensitive to nontraditional losses that may be significant to the person:
  - ▷ Loss of a pet
  - ▷ Loss of status in work or school setting

PREMENSTRUAL DYSPHORIC DISORDER

Description

- ▶ Dysphoric symptoms that occur in response to changing sex steroid hormones which occur during the ovulatory menstrual cycle.
- ▶ Symptoms generally begin during the luteal phase, approximately 1 week before onset of menses, and generally lift within a day or two after menses has begun.
- ▶ Common symptoms include:
  - ▷ Marked lability
  - ▷ Irritability
  - ▷ Depressed mood
  - ▷ Anxiety
  - ▷ Low energy
  - ▷ Sleep disturbances
- ▶ Symptoms occur repeatedly during each menstrual cycle and there must be a symptom-free period in the follicular phase, after menses has occurred.
- ▶ Symptoms may worsen as the woman becomes perimenopausal.
- ▶ Symptoms cause marked impairment in functioning and sense of well-being.
- ▶ A careful evaluation must be completed to rule out other mood disorder.
- ▶ Treatment may consist of hormonal contraceptives, SSRI antidepressants, or both.

BIPOLAR (BP) DISORDER

Description

- ▶ Complex brain-based illness with a primary characteristic of disturbance in mood
- ▶ Mood disturbance often of both polarities:
  - ▷ Depressive
  - ▷ Expansive or manic

▶ Several patterns:

  ▷ Single-polarity symptoms only (mania)

  ▷ Distinct symptom patterns of alternating polarity—manic symptoms alternating with depressive symptoms

  ▷ Mixed, co-occurring symptoms

▶ Presents with excessive or distorted degree of sadness or elation, or both

▶ Manifests with behavioral, affective, cognitive, and somatic symptoms

▶ May have precipitating event, situation, or concern but often occurs without any precipitating stressor identified

▶ Has complex genetic, biochemical, and environmental etiological factors

Etiology

▶ Multiple theories ranging from psychological to neurobiological

▶ Probable multifactorial etiological profile

  ▷ Biological theories

    ▶ GABA deregulation

    ▶ Increased noradrenergic activity

    ▶ Voltage-gated ion channel abnormalities

    ▶ Abnormalities lead to abnormal balances of intracellular and extracellular levels of neurotransmitters, which then cause subsequent disruption of electric signal transmission in brain regions.

    ▶ Kindling: Process of neuronal membrane threshold sensitivity dysfunction

      ▷ Long-lasting, epileptogenic changes induced by daily subthreshold brain stimulation

      ▷ Brain becomes overly sensitive to electrical stimuli

      ▷ Neuronal misfiring occurs

      ▷ Process becomes automatic; neuronal firing occurs even without stimuli.

Incidence and Demographics

▶ Less common than MDD

▶ 0.7% of general population at risk

▶ Affects 2.3 million American adults; 1.2% of the U.S. adult population older than age 18

▶ Mean age of onset is early 20s

▶ May present in childhood (rare) or adolescent years

▶ Prevalence for males and females is the same.

Risk Factors

▶ Genetic loading

▶ Family history of first-order relative having MDD or BP disorder

▶ 24% increased risk if relative has BP disorder Type I (see below)

▶ 5% increased risk if relative has BP disorder Type II (see below)

▶ 25% increased risk if relative has MDD

▶ For BP disorder Type II, similar to MDD

Prevention and Screening

▶ At-risk family education

▶ Community education

   ▷ Stigma reduction

   ▷ Signs and symptoms of illness

   ▷ Treatment potential for control of symptoms

▶ Early recognition, intervention, and initiation of treatment

   ▷ Significant and protracted prodromal symptom period usually noted before full onset of illness

   ▷ Usually mild manifestations of criteria symptoms before full clinical syndrome is apparent

   ▷ The longer time between onset of symptoms and diagnosis, the more difficult to interrupt cyclicity of illness.

   ▷ Depressive episodes predominate, making misdiagnosis common.

Assessment

History

▶ Assess for the following:

   ▷ Detailed history of present illness, including time frame, progression, and any associated symptoms

   ▷ Social history, including present living situation; marital status; occupation; education; and alcohol, tobacco, and illicit drug use

   ▷ Medication use, including prescription, over-the-counter, alternative, supplements, and home remedies

   ▷ Initial and periodic functional history and assessment

   ▷ Corroborative information from family member when possible

▶ Diagnostic criteria

   ▷ Period of abnormally or persistently elevated, expansive, or irritable mood, lasting for at least 1 week

▷ Mood episode has rapid development and escalation of symptoms over a few days

▷ Often precipitated by significant environmental stressor

▷ Mood disturbance may result in brief psychotic symptoms

▷ Manic episodes last days to several months

▷ Briefer duration and ending more abruptly than major depressive episodes

▷ In 60% of people, a major depressive episode immediately precedes or follows the manic episode

▷ Persistence of other suggestive symptoms:

  ▶ Decreased need for sleep

  ▶ Feels rested after 3 hours sleep on average

  ▶ Usually a marked difference from normal baseline sleep pattern

  ▶ Inflated self-esteem

  ▶ Grandiosity

  ▶ Increased goal-directed activities

  ▶ Excessive involvement in pleasurable activities with a high potential for painful consequences

  ▶ Unrestrained buying sprees

  ▶ Sexual indiscretions

  ▶ Unsound business ventures

  ▶ Excessive substance use or abuse

  ▶ Highly recurrent depressive episodes

▷ Recurrent shifts in polarity

  ▶ Major depressive episode shifting to a manic episode

  ▶ Manic episode shifting to a major depressive episode

  ▶ Major depressive episode shifting to a mixed episode.

▷ Expansive or elated mood symptoms

  ▶ Manic

    ▷ Symptoms as described above

  ▶ Hypomanic

    ▷ Similar to mania

    ▷ More brief in duration

    ▷ Episode not as severe as mania

    ▷ Does not require hospitalization

    ▷ Does not cause significant functional impairment

- ▶ Two common types
  - ▷ Type I
    - ▶ Clinical history characterized by occurrence of one or more manic or mixed episodes
  - ▷ Type II
    - ▶ Clinical history characterized by occurrence of one or more major depressive episodes accompanied by at least one manic or hypomanic episode
    - ▶ In a small subset of people with BP disorder, the recurrent shifts in polarity can occur more frequently—*rapid cycling.*
      - ▷ Occurrence of 4 or more mood episodes during the previous 12 months
      - ▷ Mood episodes are either major depressive or manic
      - ▷ Other than occurring more frequently, mood episodes are same as nonrapid-cycling episodes
      - ▷ 20% of people with BP disorder have rapid cycling
      - ▷ Most rapid cyclers are women (90%).
    - ▶ Identifying rapid cycling is important.
    - ▶ Antidepressants may accelerate the cycling.
    - ▶ Persons with rapid cycling have a poorer prognosis.

Physical Exam Findings

- ▶ Nonspecific
- ▶ Clinical findings consistent with thyroid dysfunction

Mental Status Exam Findings in Mania or Hypomania

- ▶ Appearance
  - ▷ Psychomotor restlessness or agitation
  - ▷ Frequent change of dress
  - ▷ Prone to bright-colored, often sexualized dress
  - ▷ Dramatic or flamboyant dress usually out of character for person when compared to nonsymptomatic periods
- ▶ Speech
  - ▷ Rapid
  - ▷ Loud
  - ▷ Pressured
  - ▷ Difficult to interrupt
  - ▷ Joking, irrelevant, amusing
  - ▷ Word clanging in severely ill clients

▶ Affect
  ▷ Labile
  ▷ Irritable
  ▷ Overly theatrical and dramatic

▶ Mood
  ▷ Euphoric
  ▷ Cheerful
  ▷ High
  ▷ Expansive
  ▷ Irritable

▶ Thought process
  ▷ Thoughts racing
  ▷ Flight of ideas
  ▷ Thoughts disorganized and incoherent in severely ill clients

▶ Thought content
  ▷ Inflated self-esteem
  ▷ Indiscriminate enthusiasm
  ▷ Inflated sense of abilities bordering on delusional
  ▷ Increased sexual content

▶ Orientation
  ▷ Fully oriented

▶ Memory
  ▷ Impaired short-term
  ▷ Impaired recall

▶ Concentration
  ▷ Highly distractible

▶ Abstraction
  ▷ Generally abstractive
  ▷ Can be concrete on proverb testing during psychotic episodes

▶ Judgment
  ▷ Poor
  ▷ Prone to imprudent behavioral choices with potential for negative consequences

▶ Insight
  ▷ The person usually does not recognize that he or she is ill
  ▷ Resists treatment options

Diagnostic and Laboratory Findings

▶ CBC, chemistry profile, thyroid function tests, and B_{12} level to rule out metabolic causes or unidentified conditions

▶ Drug toxicity screening if indicated by history

Differential Diagnosis

▶ If first onset of manic symptoms occurs after age 40, most likely symptoms are caused by another medical condition.

▶ Many medical conditions mimic manic symptoms:

  ▷ Endocrine disorders

  ▷ Hyperthyroidism

  ▷ Intoxication or withdrawal from illicit drug use:

    ▶ Amphetamines

    ▶ Cocaine

    ▶ Hallucinogens

    ▶ Opiates

▶ Medications:

  ▷ Captopril

  ▷ Cimetidine

  ▷ Corticosteroids

  ▷ Cyclosporine

  ▷ Disulfiram

  ▷ Hydralazine

  ▷ Isoniazid

▶ Mania can be precipitated by treatment of MDD or other unipolar mood disorders in susceptible persons.

  ▷ Antidepressants

  ▷ ECT

  ▷ Light therapy

Clinical Management

▶ Rule out or treat any conditions that may contribute to current symptom manifestation.

▶ Assess and identify client's level of acuity.

▶ Determine severity of illness.

▶ Determine duration of illness.

▶ Ascertain history of response to treatment.

▶ During acute manic episodes or significant depressive episodes, client may require brief hospitalization

  ▷ To ensure client safety,

  ▷ To ensure client adherence with treatment to reach stabilization, or

  ▷ To rapidly stabilize on medication.

▶ Clinical management during nonacute episodes occurs most often in community settings.

Pharmacological Treatment

▶ Pharmacological management should generally not entail the use of an antidepressant agent if a mood-stabilizing agent is not in place.

  ▷ Especially important in clients who are rapid-cycling

  ▷ May precipitate shift from depression to hypomania, mania, or dysphoric hypomania (mixed state)

▶ Mood-stabilizing agents

  ▷ Commonly used pharmacological agents

    ▶ Lithium

      ▷ Gold standard for treating manic episodes

      ▷ Evidence of antisuicidal effects

      ▷ Action largely unknown

      ▷ Long history of use; drug profile well established

      ▷ Evidence exists showing some effectiveness on depressive symptoms as well as on manic symptoms

      ▷ Has many clinically significant side effects; clients on this drug require careful monitoring (see Table 9–10)

      ▷ Narrow therapeutic window

      ▷ Therapeutic effect and potential for adverse side effects monitored by use of serum lithium level

        ▶ Drawn at trough level

        ▶ 12 hours post-dose

        ▶ Therapeutic serum range 0.5 to 1.2 mEq/l

        ▶ Level greater than 1.2 mEq/l increases risk for toxic side effects.

      ▷ Baseline labs before initiation of lithium to ensure safety and efficacy:

        ▶ Thyroid panel

        ▶ Serum creatinine

        ▶ Blood urea nitrogen (BUN)

        ▶ Pregnancy test

        ▶ ECG for clients older than age 50

TABLE 9–9.
CLINICALLY SIGNIFICANT SIDE EFFECTS OF LITHIUM

ORGAN SYSTEM AFFECTED	CLINICAL FINDING
Endocrine	Weight gain
	Impaired thyroid functioning
Central nervous system	Fine hand tremors
	Fatigue
	Mental cloudiness
	Headaches
	Coarse hand tremors with toxicity
	Nystagmus
Dermatological	Maculopapular rash
	Pruritus
	Acne
Gastrointestinal	GI upset
	Diarrhea
	Vomiting
	Cramps
	Anorexia
Renal	Polyuria with related polydipsia
	Diabetes insipidus
	Edema
	Microscopic tubular changes
Cardiac	T-wave inversions
	Dysrhythmias
Hematological	Leukocytosis

    ▷ Rapid-cycling clients seldom respond to lithium monotherapy

    ▷ Must educate client (and significant others) about side effects and signs and symptoms of lithium toxicity

  ▶ Anticonvulsant medication

    ▷ Carbamazepine

      ▶ Black box warning for carbamazepine: agranulocytosis and aplastic anemia

      ▶ Valproic acid/divalproex sodium

      ▶ Black box warning for valproic acid/divalproex sodium: hepatotoxicity and pancreatitis

    ▷ Lamotrigine

      ▶ Black box warning for lamotrigine: serious rash

    ▷ Baseline labs before carbamazepine or valproic acid/divalproex sodium

      ▶ CBC

      ▶ Liver function tests (LFTs)

TABLE 9–10.
DRUGS FOR MOOD DISORDERS: ANTICONVULSANTS

AGENT	BRAND NAME	DAILY DOSSAGE	THERAPEUTIC PLASMA LEVEL	SIDE EFFECTS	COMMENTS
Lithium carbonate	Eskalith Lithobid	1,200–2,400 mg/day (acute) 900–1,200 mg/day (maintenance)	0.8–1.2 mEq/l 0.6–1.2 mEq/l	*Common:* Nausea, fine-hand tremors, increased urination and thirst *Toxicity:* Slurred speech, confusion, severe GI effect	Established standard treatment for bipolar disorder Pregnancy Category D Lactation Category L3 Risk of hypothyroidism Avoid in pregnancy, especially 1st trimester Monitoring kidney functioning is essential Concurrent use of NSAIDs and angiotensin-converting enzyme inhibitors (ACEIs) may double lithium level
Carbamazepine	Tegretol	10–20 mg/kg/day	6–12 mcg/ml	*Common:* Nausea, dizziness, sedation, headache, dry mouth, constipation, skin rash *Rare:* Agranulocytos/aplastic anemia, Stevens-Johnson syndrome, particularly in Asians (screen for HLA-B 1502 allele before initiating)	Hepatic enzyme inducer Monitor LFTs Alternative to lithium or valproic acid Pregnancy Category D Lactation Category L2
Valproic acid, divalproex sodium	Depakene, Depakote	15–40 mg/kg/day	50–125 mcg/ml	*Common:* Nausea, diarrhea, abdominal cramps, sedation, tremor *Rare:* Increased liver enzymes, Stevens-Johnson syndrome (unlike carbamazepinedivalproex does not carry screening directive for HLA-B 1502 antigen at this time)	Depakote minimizes GI effects More effective than lithium for rapid cycling and mixed bipolar Loading dose: 20 mg/kg Pregnancy Category D Lactation Category L2

| Lamotrigine | Lamictal | 25–600 mg/day | Blood monitoring not necessary | *Common:* Dizziness, ataxia, somnolence, diplopia, nausea, headache, hepatotoxicity

Rare: Life-threatening rashes, including Stevens-Johnson syndrome (unlike carbamazepine, lamotrigine does not carry directive to screen for HLA-B 1502 antigen at this time), leukopenia | Indication for maintenance only

Helps in depressive phase of bipolar affective disorder

Titrate slowly: 25 mg p.o. q.d.x 2 weeks, then 50 mg p.o. q.d. x 2 weeks, etc. Concomitant use with divalproex may double lamotrigine level and should be factored into dosing

Concomitant use with carbamazepine may increase metabolism and should be factored into dosing

Often used in combination with lithium, second-generation antipsychotics, and antidepressants |

▷ Labs drawn 1 week after start of carbamazepine, valproic acid/divalproex sodium

  ► 12-hour trough serum drug level

  ► CBC

  ► LFTs

▷ Response to treatment with lithium or anticonvulsant medications is 1 to 2 weeks.

STEVENS JOHNSON SYNDROME (SJS)

SJS is a rare, potentially life-threatening immune reaction to a foreign antigen that can occur with exposure to any anticonvulsant drug. Treatment includes stopping the offending agent with supportive measures, often in a hospital burn unit. Signs and symptoms of SJS include:

► facial swelling

► tongue swelling

► macules, papules, and "burning," confluent erythematic rash

► skin sloughing

► prodromal headache, malaise, arthralgia, and painful mucous membranes may occur before rash occurs

Clinical Managment

Nonpharmacological Management

► Somatic treatments

  ▷ Treatment as previously discussed for MDD episodes

► Therapies

  ▷ Treatment as previously discussed for MDD episodes

► During acute phase of manic episode:

  ▷ Monitor and help client meet nutritional needs.

  ▷ Help client meet sleep–rest needs.

  ▷ Monitor for safety.

► During less acute periods:

  ▷ CBT

  ▷ Behavioral therapies

  ▷ Interpersonal therapies

  ▷ Supportive groups

  ▷ Milieu therapy

    ► Provides for structure and safety needs

    ► Provides socialization and interpersonal support

    ► Encourages independence

- ▶ Client and family education
  - ▷ Explain underlying pathology of illness.
  - ▷ Discuss signs and symptoms.
  - ▷ Help identify strategies for living with illness.
- ▶ Help understand and make decisions regarding care options
- ▶ Relapse prevention plan
- ▶ Overall health promotion

Common Comorbidities

- ▶ Hypothyroidism
- ▶ Substance abuse

General Health Considerations

- ▶ High-risk activities from manic behavior
  - ▷ Sexual
    - ▶ Client education for sexually transmitted infections (STIs)
    - ▶ Assessment and monitoring for STIs
  - ▷ Financial and legal
    - ▶ Client access to community resources
- ▶ Nutritional counseling
- ▶ Client health education

Life Span Considerations

- ▶ Adolescent manic episodes present differently from adult episodes.
  - ▷ More psychotic features
  - ▷ Often associated with antisocial behavior
  - ▷ Often associated with substance abuse
  - ▷ Prodromal period of significant behavioral problems
    - ▶ School truancy
    - ▶ Failing grades

Follow-up

- ▶ Clients initially should be seen weekly to titrate medications and monitor serum blood levels of pharmacological agents.
- ▶ Treatment duration and success rates vary with individual characteristics and motivation.

▶ Clients and significant others should be taught symptoms of mania and depression and that the disorders are chronic illnesses.

▶ Relapse is common and occurs frequently.

▶ Relapse plans need to be developed.

▶ Client teaching should include risks, benefits, potential side effects, and signs and symptoms of medication toxicity.

▶ Educate about potential dietary and fluid intake effects on lithium level

▶ Lithium and divalproex sodium are teratogenic.

▷ Women of child-bearing years need effective contraceptive care while on BP disorder treatment medication.

▶ Routine use of lab tests to monitor for therapeutic serum levels of anticonvulsants and lithium is needed.

▷ Routine evaluation of CBC, renal function, and thyroid and parathyroid function (thyroid-stimulating hormone and calcium levels) is needed for clients taking lithium long-term.

▶ Assessment for suicidality should occur during every client contact.

▶ All clients should be observed for development of adverse effects of pharmacological management.

▶ Standardized rating scales help to monitor clinical status, establish baseline functioning, and monitor disorder course over time:

▷ Young Mania Rating Scale (YMRS; Young, Biggs, Ziegler, & Meyer, 1978)

▷ A daily mood chart that tracks mood, energy, and specific information about sleep is helpful in informing both diagnosis and treatment

CYCLOTHYMIC DISORDER

Description

▶ Chronic, fluctuating mood disorder with symptoms similar to but less severe than BP disorder

▶ Numerous periods of hypomanic and dysthymic symptoms.

Etiology

▶ Similar to BP disorder

Incidence and Demographics

▶ Lifetime prevalence 0.4% to 1%

▶ Insidious onset

▶ Chronic course

▶ Begins early in life

▶ 15% to 50% of persons with cyclothymic disorder subsequently develop BP disorder.

Risk Factors

▶ Genetic loading

▶ Family history

▶ BP disorder Type I

▶ Substance abuse

Prevention and Screening

▶ At-risk family education

▶ Community education

▷ Stigma reduction

▷ Signs and symptoms of illness

▷ Treatment potential for control of symptoms

▶ Early recognition, intervention, and initiation of treatment

▷ Significant and protracted prodromal symptom period usually noted before full onset of illness

▷ The longer the time period between onset of symptoms and diagnosis, the more difficult to interrupt cyclicity of illness.

Assessment

History

▶ Assess for the following:

▷ Fluctuating mood episodes

▷ Affected people can function well during hypomanic episodes

▷ May experience clinically significant distress or impaired function related to cyclicity

▷ Unpredictable mood changes

▷ Often regarded by others as *temperamental, moody, unpredictable, inconsistent,* and *unreliable*

▷ No psychotic episodes

Physical Exam Findings

▶ Similar to MDD and BP disorder

Mental Status Exam Findings

▶ Similar to MDD and BP disorder but with less severity of symptoms

Diagnostic and Laboratory Findings

▶ Similar to MDD and BP disorder

Differential Diagnosis

▶ Nonpsychiatric

  ▷ Similar to MDD and BP disorder

▶ Psychiatric

  ▷ BP disorder

  ▷ Dysthymia

  ▷ Substance abuse

Clinical Management

Pharmacological Management

▶ Similar to MDD and BP disorder

▶ Because of increased risk for development of BP disorder, commonly treated with medication

Nonpharmacological Management

▶ Similar to MDD and BP disorder

Life Span Considerations

▶ Usually begins in adolescence

▶ Onset in later life usually suggests general medical condition such as multiple sclerosis.

Follow-up

▶ Similar to MDD and BP disorder

CASE STUDY

Ms. M., a 35-year-old homemaker and mother of two children, presents to the PMHNP on refer-ral from her primary care provider. Accompanied by her husband, Mary describes worsening insomnia and poor energy. The symptoms are affecting her ability to take care of her children and the household. Husband reports that Ms. M. often has crying spells, is not eating, and cannot seem to concentrate. When questioned further, husband reports that Ms. M. has mentioned not wanting to live, but he thought that she was just having a bad day.

Past Psychiatric History

▶ Reports depression off and on since late adolescence

▶ No history of treatment

▶ Husband adds that Ms. M. had "the baby blues" for several months after the births of both of their children

Past Medical History

▶ Seasonal allergies and stress-induced asthma

▶ No significant surgical history, except for a tonsillectomy when she was a child

▶ Normal pregnancies and deliveries

▶ No chronic health problems identified

Family History

▶ Significant for grandmother and father, who had "breakdowns."

▶ Father had alcoholism.

Social History

Ms. M. is a homemaker and has two children, ages 8 and 10. She and her husband moved to the area 6 months ago. She does not smoke or use drugs but drinks socially. She has an MA degree in English and had planned to go back to school to get her teaching certificate when her children began high school.

Mental Status Exam

Client appears disheveled. Hair is not combed. She appears very tired. She avoids eye contact, talks very softly, and is slow to respond to questions. She hardly moves during the interview. Affect is constricted and sad. She says she has no energy, and her mood is "very sad." She does not hear voices or have hallucinations. Her thoughts are appropriate and organized. She does admit to having episodic thoughts of suicide and has a vague plan to ingest an overdose of aspi-rin, acetaminophen, and alcohol when the children are with their father but has no clear timeline or planned intent. She is unable to do serial number testing and shows impaired short-term memory. She exhibits a few problems with immediate recall. She has difficulty concentrating but no difficulty with abstractions. She is oriented times 3, and shows good judgment and insight. She has above-average intelligence.

Current Medications

Ms. M. takes cetirizine for allergies and is now on ethinyl estradiol/norgestimate contraceptive pills.

Labs

- ▶ Platelets 230/mm^3
- ▶ WBC 6,000/mm^3
- ▶ Hematocrit 40%, hemoglobin 13.0
- ▶ NA 140, K 4.0, Cl 101, CO_2 26, BUN 15, creatinine 0.9, glucose 102
- ▶ TSH 1.1, T3 179, T4 1.3

There are several issues to consider in planning care for Ms. M.

1. What is the most probable diagnosis?

2. What further assessment is needed?

3. What target symptoms does the client display that are consistent with the probable diagnosis?

4. What medications would be considered?

5. If client had psychotic features with her depression, how would this change the treatment plan?

6. What nonmedication treatment would be indicated for a client with MDD with psychotic features?

7. How would the plan differ if client had a heart condition and was taking no other medications?

8. Assume Ms. M. has started an antidepressant and returns after 2 weeks on the medication. Her speech has normalized and is now more spontaneous. If Ms. M now tells you that she feels "better" and that her energy and motivation have improved, but that she is still having difficulty falling and staying asleep, would your diagnosis change?

9. What further assessment should be done?

10. How would you change the treatment plan?

11. If Ms. M. returns for her follow-up appointment reporting irritable mood, racing thoughts, rapid speech and inability to sleep, should your diagnosis and treatment plan change?

ANSWERS TO CASE STUDY DISCUSSION QUESTIONS

1. The client's most probable diagnosis is consistent with major depressive disorder.

2. Further assessment needed is to ensure that the client meets the DSM-5 criteria for major depression. Complete physical assessment and use common symptom rating scale such as Beck's Depression Inventory or PHQ-9. Complete assessment for any other physical health states. The PMHNP should explore what "inability to sleep" means in specific detail.

3. The target symptoms for this client include: depressed mood most of the day nearly every day, lack of energy, suicidal ideation, MSE findings consistent with MDD.

4. The medications to be considered for this client are SSRIs as this class of antidepressant medication is often considered the first-line agent for treatment of MDD.

5. If the client had psychotic symptoms, clinical management would include the short-term use of an antipsychotic agent to control psychotic symptoms. If used, an atypical antipsychotic is usually best tolerated.

6. For clients with severe MDD, with psychosis ECT might be considered.

7. If the client had cardiovascular disease, the PMHNP must look at compatibility issues to ensure that the medication choice for treatment of MDD does not have significant risk for adverse cardiac side effects. TCAs are contraindicated.

8. If the client presented for a follow-up appointment stating that she is feeling better, but still has residual symptoms of sleep problems your diagnosis would not change because the symptoms Ms. M. reports are consistent with a depressive episode that is beginning to resolve.

9. Further assessment of this client should include an assessment for mood, anhedonia, suicidal ideation, and activities over the past 2 weeks and for any indication that the antidepressant may be fueling a switch from depression to hypomania or mixed state.

10. In this client, if the treatment plan changes, monitor for further improvements. Teach Ms. M about sleep hygiene measures. Discuss expected outcomes and the importance of monitoring for any significant increase in goal-directed activities, decreased need for sleep, racing thoughts, and shift in mood to euphoria or irritability. Begin psychotherapy.

11. If Ms. M. returns for a follow-up appointment reporting irritable mood, racing thoughts, rapid speech and inability to sleep, yes, your treatment plan should change. Rule out unspecified bipolar disorder, bipolar II disorder, and bipolar I disorder. The antidepressant dose should be lowered and a medication with mood stabilizing properties should be added. The client should be monitored closely and reevaluated within several days.

REFERENCES AND RESOURCES

American Psychiatric Association. (1998). *Practice parameters for the assessment and treatment of children and adolescents with bipolar disorder.* Washington, DC: Author.

American Psychiatric Association. (2007). *Practice parameter for the assessment and treatment of children and adolescents with depressive disorders.* Washington, DC: Author.

American Psychiatric Association. (2013). *Diagnostic and statistical manual of mental disorders* (5th ed., text rev.). Washington, DC: Author.

American Psychiatric Association. (2000). *Practice guidelines for the treatment of patients with major depressive disorder.* Washington, DC: Author.

Beck, A. T. (1979). *Cognitive therapy of depression.* New York, NY: Guilford Press.

Beck, A. T., Ward, C. H., Mendelson, M., Mock, J., & Erbaugh, J. (1961). An inventory for measuring depression. *Archives of General Psychiatry, 4,* 561–571.

Beydoun, A. (2001). Innovative treatment strategies with anticonvulsants: A focus on bipolar disorder. *Primary Psychiatry, 8*(6), 49–52.

Clewell, T. (2004). Mourning beyond melancholia: Freud's psychoanalysis of loss. *Journal of the American Psychoanalytic Association,* 52(1), 43–67.

Freidrich, M. (1999). Lithium: Proving its mettle for 50 years. *JAMA: Journal of the American Medical Association, 281,* 2271–2275.

Gilbert, P. (2006). Evolution and depression: Issues and implications [Abstract]. *Psychological Medicine,* March(3), 287–297. doi:10.1017/S0033291705006112.

Giles, D. E., Kupfer, D. J., Rush, A. J., & Roffwarg, H. P. (1998). Controlled comparison of electrophysiological sleep in families of probands with unipolar depression. *American Journal of Psychiatry, 155,* 192–196.

Gloaguen, V., Cottraux, J., Cucherat, M., & Blackburn, I. M. (1998). A meta-analysis of the effects of cognitive therapy in depressed patients. *Journal of Affective Disorders, 49*(1), 59–62.

Green, J. (2001). Helping patients understand depression and its treatment. *Primary Psychiatry, 8*(11), 49–53.

Hirschfeld, R., Holzer, C., Calabrese, J., Weissman, M., Reed, M., Davies, M., ... Hazard, E. (2003). Validity of the mood disorder questionnaire: A general population study. *American Journal of Psychiatry, 160,* 178–180.

Hoyert, D. L., Kochanek, K. D., & Murphy, S. L. (1998). *Deaths: Final data for 1997* (National Vital Statistics Report, DHHS Publication No. PHS-99-1120). Hyattsville, MD: National Center for Health Statistics.

Judd, L., Paulus, M., Schettler, P., Akiskal, H., Endicott, J., Leon, A.,... Keller, M. (2000). Does incomplete recovery from first lifetime major depressive episode herald a chronic course of illness? *American Journal of Psychiatry, 157*(9), 1501–1504.

Kedzior, K. K. & Reitz, S. K. (2014). Short-term efficacy of repetitive transcranial magnetic stimulation (rTMS) in depression—Reanalysis of data from meta-analyses up to 2010. *BioMedCentral Psychology, 2(1):39.*

Ketter, T. A., Miller, S., Dell'Osso, B., Calabrese, J. R., Frye, M. A., & Citrome, L. (2014). Balancing benefits and harms of treatments for acute bipolar depression. *Journal of Affective Disorders,* 169 S1, 24-33.

Kleimann, A., Schrader, V., Stubner, S., Greil, W., Kahl, K.G., Bleich, S.,... S. (2015). Psychopharmacological treatment of 1650 in-patients with acute mania-data from the AMSP study. *Journal of Affective Disorders, 191,* 164-171.

Klein, D. N., Schwartz, J. E., & Rose S. (2000). Five-year course and outcome of dysthymic disorder: A prospective, naturalistic follow-up study. *American Journal of Psychiatry, 157,* 931–939.

Kimrell, T., Little, R., & Dunn, T. (1999). Frequency dependence of antidepressant response to left prefrontal repetitive transcranial magnetic stimulation (rTMS) as a function of baseline cerebral glucose metabolism. *Biological Psychiatry, 46,* 1603–1613.

Lowe-Ponsford, F. L., & Nutt, D. J. (2001). Pathophysiology of depression. *Primary Psychiatry, 8*(11), 43–48.

McBride, A., & Austin, J. (1996). *Psychiatric–mental health nursing: Integrating the behavioral and biological sciences.* Philadelphia, PA: W. B. Saunders.

Monroe, S. M., Rohde, P., & Seeley, J. R. (1999). Life events and depression in adolescence: Relationship loss as a prospective risk factor for first onset of major depressive disorder. *Journal of Abnormal Psychology, 108,* 606–614.

McQuade, R., & Young, A. (2000). Future therapeutic targets in mood disorders: The glucocorticoid receptor. *British Journal of Psychiatry, 177,* 390–395.

Ornstein, S., Stuart, G., & Jenkins, R. (2000). Depression diagnosis and antidepressant use in primary care practices. *Journal of Family Practice, 49*(1), 68–71.

Sadock, B. J., Sadock, V. A., & Ruiz, P. (2015). *Kaplan and Sadock's synopsis of psychiatry: Behavioral sciences/clinical psychiatry* (11th ed.). Philadelphia, PA: Wolters Kluwer.

Saeed, M. (2001). Assessment and management of the suicidal patient in the managed care era. *Primary Psychiatry, 8*(6), 38–45.

Seligman, M. (1972). Learned helplessness. *Annual Review of Medicine, 23,* 407–412.

Siu, A., & U.S. Preventative Services Task Force. (2016). Screening for depression in adults US Preventative Services Task Force recommendation statement. *JAMA, 315*(4), 380–387.

Shaffer, D., & Craft, L. (1999). Methods of adolescent suicide prevention. *Journal of Clinical Psychiatry, 60*(Suppl. 2), 70–74.

Stuart, G. W., & Laraia, M. (2004). *Principles and practice of psychiatric nursing* (8th ed.). St. Louis, MO: Mosby.

Young, J. W., & Dulcis, D. (2015). Investigating the mechanism(s) underlying switching between states in bipolar disorder. *European Journal of Pharmacology, 759,* 151–162.

Young, R. C., Biggs, J. T., Ziegler, V. E., & Meyer, D. A. (1978). A rating scale for mania: Reliability, validity, and sensitivity. *British Journal of Psychiatry, 133,* 429–435.

CHAPTER 10

ANXIETY DISORDERS, OBSESSIVE–COMPULSIVE DISORDER, AND TRAUMA- AND STRESSOR-RELATED DISORDERS

This chapter reviews the psychiatric–mental health nurse practitioner's (PMHNP's) evaluation of and treatment of people who have anxiety-related disorders. Anxiety disorders are among the most common of all psychiatric illnesses, and can initially manifest as a number of physical illness states. Often only after extensive, unnecessary assessment and diagnostic evaluation is a client's problem correctly identified as an anxiety disorder. Because of the high degree of somatic symptomatology, it is common for clients to present to a primary care setting and thus receive initial care from a primary care provider.

Anxiety is a very common and normal human emotion. PMHNPs caring for clients who present for evaluation of anxiety must be able to distinguish between normal levels of anxiety and pathological levels that are symptomatic of an underlying brain-based illness. Pathological levels of anxiety require treatment and generally will not fully abate without therapeutic intervention. Untreated high levels of anxiety predispose people to other serious health problems; therefore, pathological levels of anxiety should not go untreated (Narrow, Rae, & Regier, 1998).

▶ Normal emotion of anxiety

  ▷ Anxiety is one of the most common human emotions.

  ▷ Anxiety exists on a continuum ranging from the absence of anxiety at one end to pathological levels that produce significant symptoms of psychiatric disorder at the other (see Table 10–1).

  ▷ Anxiety can be a normal, healthy reaction to life stressors that motivates a person to deal with events and emotions.

  ▷ Anxiety can be pathological if it is disproportionate to events, if it is sustained over a significant time frame, if it significantly impairs functioning, or if it is apparently unrelated to any identifiable event or situation in a person's life.

  ▷ High pathological levels of anxiety interfere with perceptions, memory, judgment, and motor responses.

TABLE 10–1.
ASSESSING LEVELS OF ANXIETY

LEVEL OF ANXIETY	DEFINITION	PHYSIOLOGICAL SIGNS AND SYMPTOMS	PSYCHOLOGICAL SIGNS AND SYMPTOMS
Level I: Mild	Normative level experienced by all, which functions to motivate	Vital signs normal, pupils constricted, minimal increase in muscle tone	Perceptual field broadened, heightened awareness of environment
Level II: Moderate	Normative level experienced by most in response to significant stressors	Vital signs normal, mild increased heart rate, moderate increase in muscle tone	Subjective feeling of tension or worry, narrowed perceptions
Level III: Severe	Pathological level	Autonomic nervous system triggered, fight-or-flight response, pupils dilated, vital signs increased, diaphoresis, muscles rigid, hearing decreased, pain threshold increased, urinary frequency, diarrhea	Perceptual field greatly narrowed, difficulty with problem-solving, distorted perception of time, selective inattention, dissociative sensations, automatic behavior
Level IV: Panic	Pathological level	Severe symptoms markedly increased: client is pale, hypotensive, has poor eye–hand coordination, muscle pains, marked decrease in hearing, dizziness, shortness of breath	Scattered perceptions, unable to attend to environmental stimuli, illogical thinking, may exhibit hallucinations or delusions

▷ Cultural differences can affect behavioral manifestations of anxiety.

   ▶ "Ataques de nervios" is a Latino cultural syndrome usually provoked by disruptions in family bonds and may be manifested by trembling, crying, and screaming. The attacks are usually experienced in the presence of others and the person often feels relief afterward.

   ▶ "Khyal" (wind) attacks are a common manifestation among Cambodian and other Asian cultures, and commonly manifest in neck soreness and tinnitus.

▷ Older adults often express anxiety as somatic concerns and anxiety disorders may overlap with medical conditions.

▷ Psychotherapy is the first-line treatment for children and adolescents who are diagnosed with an anxiety disorder.

▷ The role of the PMHNP in assessing anxiety is to separate normal versus pathological levels of anxiety, to intervene to lower the level of anxiety, and to improve overall functioning.

ANXIETY DISORDERS

Description

▶ Anxiety disorders are the most common group of psychiatric disorders and are characterized by the degree of anxiety experienced by the client, by the duration

TABLE 10–2.
DSM-5 ANXIETY, OBSESSIVE–COMPULSIVE DISORDER (OCD), AND TRAUMA- AND STRESSOR-RELATED DISORDERS

ANXIETY DISORDERS	OBSESSIVE–COMPULSIVE AND RELATED DISORDERS	TRAUMA AND STRESSOR-RELATED DISORDERS
• Panic Disorder • Agoraphobia • Specific Phobia • Social Anxiety (Social Phobia) • Selective Mutism • Generalized Anxiety Disorder	• Obsessive–Compulsive Disorder • Body Dysmorphic Disorder • Hoarding Disorder • Trichotillomania (Hair-Pulling Disorder) • Excoriation (Skin-Picking Disorder) • Substance- or Medication-Induced Obsessive–Compulsive and Related Disorder	• Reactive Attachment Disorder • Disinhibited Social Engagement Disorder • Posttraumatic Stress Disorder • Acute Stress Disorder • Dissociative Identity Disorder • Dissociative Amnesia • Depersonalization or Derealization Disorder

and severity of the anxiety, and by the typical behavioral manifestation of anxiety observed in the client. Anxiety ranges from acute states to chronic disorders and is accompanied by multiple somatic symptoms.

▶ People most often present first in primary care settings with nonspecific physical concerns.

▷ Panic attacks are often confused with cardiac and respiratory disorders, so careful differential diagnostic assessment is essential.

▶ Frequent comorbidity exists with substance abuse, depression, and eating disorders.

▶ Symptoms significantly impair functioning and occur more days than not for a period of at least 6 months, with the person reporting little or no volitional control over the symptoms.

▶ Nine specific anxiety disorders are identified in the *Diagnostic and Statistical Manual of Mental Disorders* (DSM-5; American Psychiatric Association, 2015) and are described in more detail in this chapter.

Etiology

▶ Multiple theories range from psychological to neurobiological; however, most likely there is a multifactorial etiological profile.

▷ *Psychodynamic Theory*

▶ This theory is based on work of Sigmund Freud (1856–1939), who believed that anxiety initially occurs in response to the stimulation of birth and need of the infant to adapt to the changed environment.

▶ Subsequent anxiety results from intrapsychic conflict.

▶ The process of unconscious repression of sexual drive is at the core of much of the conflict.

▶ Conflict exists between instinctual needs of the *id* and the *superego* (conscience); anxiety signals the person of the need to deal with the id–superego conflict.

▶ Conflict is unconscious, but anxiety is consciously perceived.

▶ Conflict entails fear of punishment and of doing wrong.

▶ Defense mechanisms are unconsciously used by the person to deal with the conflict.

▶ The behavioral manifestations of anxiety disorders stem from the pathological overuse of defense mechanisms.

▷ *Interpersonal Theory*

▶ This theory is based on work of Harry Stack Sullivan (1892–1949), who believed that humans are goal-directed toward attainment of satisfaction and security needs.

▶ Satisfaction and security needs are normally met in interpersonal interactions.

▶ Anxiety arises when a person's needs are unmet.

▶ Anxiety is first experienced in an infant's interactions with his or her mother.

▶ Subsequent anxiety arises because of interpersonal conflict.

▶ Conflict occurs when a person perceives his or her needs will not be met because of rejection, feelings of inferiority, or inability to engage with significant others.

▶ Sense of self becomes based on the person's perception of how others view him or her.

▷ *Neurobiological Theory*

▶ Pathological levels of anxiety result from neurobiological deficits in normal brain functioning.

▶ Deficits are genetically mediated by and involve predominantly the limbic system, midline brainstem area, and sections of the cortex.

▶ Deficits predispose the person to abnormal stress responses, with hyperactivity of autonomic nervous system causing symptoms such as increased heart rate and blood pressure, diaphoresis, papillary dilation, tremors, and increased respiratory rate.

▶ Problems with the hypothalamic pituitary adrenal (HPA) axis:

▷ Threat is perceived, and amygdala signals the hypothalamus to secrete corticotrophin-releasing hormone (CRH).

▷ The amygdala also activates the sympathetic nervous system to start the fight-or-flight response.

▷ The pituitary is stimulated to release adrenocorticotropic hormone (ACTH).

> ▷ The adrenal glands are then stimulated to release cortisol, which shuts off the alarm system and restores the body to homeostasis.

▶ In anxiety disorders, the amygdala may not be able to shut off the response (overactive amygdala), or there may not be enough cortisol to stop the fight-or-flight response.

▶ Neurobiological deficits result in low levels of the neurotransmitter gamma-aminobutyric acid (GABA), the chemical responsible for inhibitory responses of neurons, and in high levels of norepinephrine, the chemical associated with the fight-or-flight response

▶ Neurotransmitters involved in suppressing the HPA axis are serotonin and GABA.

Incidence and Demographics

▶ Anxiety disorders are common, with a lifetime prevalence of 28.8% among the general U.S. population.

▶ Except for obsessive–compulsive disorder (OCD) and social phobia, anxiety disorders are more common in girls and women than in boys and men.

▶ Most anxiety disorders manifest in adolescence and early adulthood (Narrow, Rae, & Regier, 1998).

▶ Median age at onset is 11 years of age.

Risk Factors

▶ Genetic loading (National Institute of Mental Health, Genetics Workgroup, 1998)

> ▷ A first-degree relative of a person with panic disorder is up to 8 times more likely than general population to develop panic disorder.

> ▷ If a first-degree relative of a person developed panic disorder before age 20, that person is up to 20 times more likely than general population to develop panic disorder.

▶ Limited range of coping skills.

▶ History of trauma

▶ High levels of parental distress affect a child's ability to cope with traumatic events

Prevention and Screening

▶ At-risk family education

▶ Community education

> ▷ Stigma reduction

> ▷ Signs and symptoms of illness

> ▷ Treatment potential for control of symptoms

▶ Early recognition, intervention, and initiation of treatment

  ▷ Teach at-risk persons to recognize and manage anxiety levels.

  ▷ Help at-risk persons reduce anxiety through improved coping activities.

Assessment

History

▶ Assess for the following:

  ▷ Detailed history of present illness, including time frame and progression, any associated symptoms

  ▷ Social history, including present living situation; marital status; occupation; education level

  ▷ Medication use, including prescription, over-the-counter, alternative, supplements, and home remedies

  ▷ Clients initially may be more troubled by, and complain more often of, physical symptoms and may not identify anxiety as a concern.

  ▷ Explore the client's subjective sensations of being nervous, tense, worried, anxious, or stressed out.

  ▷ Identify current environmental stressors as experienced by the client.

  ▷ Determine if anxiety is normative or pathological.

  ▷ *Pathological* levels of anxiety indicative of underlying anxiety disorder:

    ▶ Anxiety is perceived of as distressing and out of the control of the person..

    ▶ Anxiety is unlinked and not seen as caused by life events.

    ▶ Anxiety is accompanied by somatic complaints, which is more uncommon in normal anxiety levels.

    ▶ Anxiety interferes with social, occupational, and recreation activities and with activities of daily living.

  ▷ Determine the level of the client's anxiety using the 4-point scale of mild to panic levels (1 = mild to 4 = panic; see Table 9–1).

  ▷ Use standardized rating scales such as the Hamilton Rating Scale for Anxiety (HAM-A; Hamilton, 1959) for establishing and monitoring the client's anxiety level over time.

  ▷ Assess general level of health and presence of concomitant illnesses.

  ▷ Assess for *dysfunctional coping:*

    ▶ Alcohol use or abuse

    ▶ Illicit substance use or abuse

    ▶ Caffeine use

    ▶ Increased nicotine use

    ▶ Misuse of anti-anxiety medications

▷ Assess for specific psychological symptoms of anxiety:

▶ Fear of dying, losing one's mind, or a sense of unreality

▶ Belief that he or she is very ill, with no findings to support this belief

▶ Narrowed perceptions

▶ Limited eye contact

Physical Exam Findings

▶ Possible physical manifestations:

▷ Diaphoresis

▷ Headaches

▷ Dizziness and lightheadedness

▷ Missing hair on scalp, eyebrows, or eye lashes (for trichotillomania or excoriation disorders)

▷ Pupillary dilation

▷ Increased muscle tone

▷ Palpitations, often with tightness in chest

▷ Tachycardia

▷ Hypertension

▷ GI problems such as nausea, diarrhea, or abdominal discomfort

Mental Status Exam Findings

▶ Appearance

▷ Psychomotor restlessness

▷ Tremors

▷ Hand wringing

▶ Speech

▷ Overproductive

▷ Rapid

▷ Distractible speech patterns

▷ Thought blocking

▶ Mood

▷ Nervous

▷ Worried

▶ Affect

▷ Anxious

▷ Worried

▷ Tearful

▶ Thought process

▷ Overall organized

▷ Goal-directed

▷ Redirectable

▶ Thought content

▷ Thematic for worry

▷ Mild perseveration on topics of concern

▶ Orientation

▷ Usually fully oriented

▶ Memory

▷ Impaired short-term and immediate memory

▷ Forgetful

▶ Concentration

▷ Inattentive

▷ Decreased concentration

▶ Abstraction

▷ Abstract on proverbs and similarities

▶ Judgment

▷ Intact

▶ Insight

▷ Intact or limited insight

Diagnostic and Laboratory Findings

▶ Obtain baseline labs such as complete blood count (CBC), chemistry profile, thyroid function tests, and B_{12} level to rule out metabolic causes or unidentified conditions.

▶ Obtain drug toxicity screening if indicated by history.

▶ In some cases, clients may have labs reflecting compensated respiratory alkalosis:

▷ Decreased carbon dioxide levels

▷ Decreased bicarbonate levels

▷ Normal pH

Differential Diagnosis

▶ Many medical conditions can cause worry, fear, and normal levels of anxiety (see Table 10–3).

▶ Ensure that client symptoms meet criteria for anxiety disorders.

General Clinical Management

▶ Rule out or treat any conditions that may contribute to pathological levels of anxiety.

TABLE 10–3.
MEDICAL CONDITIONS THAT MAY MIMIC ANXIETY DISORDERS

GENERAL CATEGORY OF DISORDER	SPECIFIC ILLNESS
Cardiovascular	Congestive heart failure
	Mitral valve prolapse
	Myocardial infarct
	Arrhythmias, especially tachycardic arrhythmias
	Pulmonary embolism
	Coronary artery disease
Respiratory	Asthma
	Chronic obstructive pulmonary disorder
	Pneumonia
Endocrine	Hyperthyroidism
	Hyperparathyroidism
	Cushing's disease
Neurological	Seizure disorders
	Transient ischemic attacks
	Cerebral vascular accident
	Encephalitis
	Central nervous system (CNS) neoplasms
Metabolic	Hypoglycemia
	Vitamin B deficiency
	Porphyria
Substance abuse or dependency	Intoxication with CNS stimulants (e.g., cocaine, amphetamines, caffeine)
	Withdrawal from CNS depressants (e.g., alcohol, marijuana)

Pharmacological Management

▶ Most of the medications known to improve symptoms of anxiety act directly or indirectly on the GABA system.

   ▷ Selective serotonin reuptake inhibitors (SSRIs)

      ▶ Considered *first-line agents* for chronic anxiety disorders

      ▶ Action on serotonin system and indirectly on GABA system

      ▶ Carry no risk of dependency

      ▶ Cannot be used p.r.n.

      ▶ Generally well tolerated

      ▶ Takes time to reach symptom control (usually 3–4 weeks)

      ▶ Best when combined with psychotherapy

      ▶ Black box warning for increased suicidality in children, adolescents, and young adults

▷ Benzodiazepines (BNZs)

  ▶ Potentiate the effect of GABA

  ▶ Rapid onset of action

  ▶ Can be used p.r.n.

  ▶ Limit to lowest possible dose and short-term use if possible, because long-term use may lead to tolerance, dependence, memory impairment, and depression.

  ▶ Use should be limited to period of excessive symptoms, period of high stress, or in unremitting symptoms.

  ▶ Use with extreme caution in clients with history of substance dependence.

    ▷ Effective but carry risk for addiction, especially in persons who have a history of substance abuse.

  ▶ The use of benzodiazepines has been associated with Alzheimer's disease.

  ▶ BNZs with *longer half-lives* require less frequent dosing, have less severe withdrawal, and have less rebound anxiety.

  ▶ BNZs with longer half-lives are more useful for continuous, moderate to severe anxiety or as bridge medications while waiting for efficacy of SSRI:

    ▷ Clonazepam (Klonopin)

    ▷ Diazepam (Valium)

  ▶ BNZs with *shorter half-lives* require more frequent dosing, have more severe withdrawal, and have more rebound anxiety:

    ▷ Alprazolam (Xanax)

    ▷ Lorazepam (Ativan)

  ▶ Advantages of BNZs with short half-lives

    ▷ BNZs with short half-lives are often useful for intermittent or infrequent moderate to severe anxiety

      ▶ Less daytime sedation

      ▶ Less drug accumulation

      ▶ Quick onset of action

      ▶ Useful for treatment of insomnia

  ▶ Disadvantages of BNZs with short half-lives:

    ▷ Increased risk of addiction

▷ Tricyclics (TCAs)

  ▶ Effective but affect multiple receptors and have problematic side-effect profiles

  ▶ Side effects often affect compliance

TABLE 10–4.
NON-BENZODIAZEPINE ANXIOLYTICS FOR ADULTS

GENERIC	BRAND	DOSAGE RANGE	SIDE EFFECTS	COMMENTS
Buspirone	Buspar	20–60 mg daily	Dizziness, insomnia, tremors, akathisia, stomach upset, dry mouth	Helpful adjunct for anxiety
Tiagabine	Gabitril	4–56 mg daily	Dizziness, somnolence, stomach upset, tremors, dry mouth	Helpful adjunct for anxiety Off-label use
Gabapentin	Neurontin	300–3,600 mg daily	Ataxia, decreased coordination, sedation, disequilibrium	Used for anxiety, neuropathic pain, fibromyalgia, and as an anti-craving medication Off-label use
Propranolol	Inderal	10–20 mg daily p.r.n.	Bradycardia, hypotension	Performance anxiety Off-label use

▷ Non-BNZ anxiolytics (see Table 10–4)

  ▶ Buspirone (BuSpar)

    ▷ Must be taken regularly, not as p.r.n.

  ▶ Tiagabine (Gabitril)—off-label use

  ▶ Gabapentin (Neurontin)—off-label use

  ▶ Beta blockers (propranolol, atenolol)—off-label use

    ▷ Usually adjunctive use with other pharmacological agent

Life Span Considerations

▶ In children, alpha-agonists are often used for anxiety.

  ▷ Clonidine (Catapres), .003–.01 mg/kg/d, off-label use

  ▷ Guanfacine (Tenex), .015–.05 mg/kg/d), off-label use

Nonpharmacological Management

▶ Behavioral therapy

  ▷ Systematic desensitization

  ▷ Exposure therapy

  ▷ Relaxation therapies

  ▷ Biofeedback

▶ Cognitive behavioral therapy (CBT)

▶ Interpersonal therapies

▶ Community self-help groups

▶ Alternative therapies as adjunctive treatments

Comorbidities

▶ Anemia

▶ Cardiac disorders, especially in clients with dysrhythmias

▶ Endocrine disorders

 ▷ Cushing's disease

 ▷ Hyperthyroidism

 ▷ Hypoglycemia

▶ Pulmonary conditions

 ▷ Chronic obstructive pulmonary disorder

 ▷ Asthma

 ▷ Pulmonary embolism

 ▷ Pneumothorax

▶ Adverse medication reactions

 ▷ Caffeine

 ▷ Nicotine

 ▷ Anticholinergics

 ▷ Antihistamines

 ▷ Antipsychotics

 ▷ Steroids

 ▷ Bronchodilators

 ▷ Anesthetics

▶ Mood disorders

▶ Substance abuse–related disorders

General Health Considerations

▶ Chronic anxiety is wearing on the body; therefore, assess for effects on the cardio-vascular system.

▶ Perform a general assessment for a healthy lifestyle.

Follow-up

▶ General considerations

 ▷ Clients should initially be seen weekly or biweekly to titrate medications.

 ▷ Client teaching should include risks, benefits, and potential side effects of medication treatment.

 ▶ If the client is taking BNZs, monitor for appropriate use and potential dependence.

 ▶ If the client is taking SSRIs, monitor for common side effects and adverse effects.

> ▷ Clients should be taught symptoms of anxiety and the fact that disorders are chronic illnesses; a relapse plan should be established for all clients.

> ▷ Assessment for suicidality should occur during symptom exacerbation periods.

> ▷ Because of frequent comorbidity with major depressive disorder, assess frequently for depression levels using standardized rating scales (see below).

> ▷ Medication should be combined with therapy to reach maximum control of symptoms.

> ▷ Clients may need encouragement to continue treatment, especially after initial symptom relief occurs.

▶ Standardized rating scales for anxiety disorders

> ▷ Zung's Self-Rating Anxiety Scale (Zung, 1971)

> ▷ Hamilton Rating Scale for Anxiety (HAM–A; Hamilton, 1959)

> ▷ Yale-Brown Obsessive Compulsive Scale (Y-BOCS; Goodman et al., 1989).

PANIC DISORDER

Description

▶ Panic disorder is experienced as discrete episodes or attacks with sudden onset of intense apprehension, fearfulness, or terror, often associated with sense of impending doom.

▶ Attacks occur without warning and in the absence of any real danger.

▶ Attacks build to a peak of intensity within a short, self-limiting time, usually within 10 minutes of onset.

▶ Panic disorder is more common in women than in men.

Assessment

History

▶ Assess for the following:

> ▷ *Diagnostic criteria* of panic disorder:

> > ▶ Discrete episode in which client experiences 4 or more of the following symptoms having a sudden onset and peaking within 10 minute of onset:

> > > ▷ Paresthesias

> > > ▷ Chills or hot flushing

> > > ▷ Fear of losing control or of going crazy

> > > ▷ Fear of dying

> > > ▷ Shortness of breath or smothering sensation

> > > ▷ Palpitations, pounding, or accelerated heart rate

> > > ▷ Chest pain, tightness, or discomfort

> ▷ Sweating

> ▷ Trembling or shaking

> ▷ Nausea or abdominal distress

- ▶ After first attack, persistent concern over having another attack, worry over the consequences of initial attack, or a significant behavioral change related to attack

- ▶ With high somatic sensations, clients are often sensitive to new somatic experiences or perceptions.

- ▶ Often intolerant of or concerned with common side effects of medication treatments

▷ Discouraged or ashamed about "failure" to control emotions and over concern about dying when no other pathology identified

- ▶ In two-thirds of cases, major depression occurs first, followed by panic disorder symptoms.

- ▶ In one-third of cases, panic disorder symptoms precede major depression symptoms.

Physical Exam Findings

- ▶ Nonspecific, especially when client not experiencing panic attack
- ▶ Nonspecific cardiac-related complaints during panic episodes often bring client into treatment:
  - ▷ Chest pain
  - ▷ Numbness and paresthesia
  - ▷ Shortness of breath

Mental Status Exam Findings

- ▶ General findings of anxiety as described earlier
- ▶ Findings very pronounced during panic episodes and less pronounced during non-panic periods
- ▶ High level of anticipatory anxiety between panic episodes

Diagnostic and Laboratory Findings

- ▶ None specific

Differential Diagnosis

- ▶ Rule out general medical conditions known to produce similar symptoms, including
  - ▷ Hyperthyroidism
  - ▷ Hyperparathyroidism
  - ▷ Pheochromocytosis
  - ▷ Vestibular dysfunction

    ▷ Seizure disorders

    ▷ Cardiac arrhythmias such as supraventricular tachycardia (SVT)

    ▷ Use of CNS stimulants, including

        ▶ Cocaine

        ▶ Amphetamines

        ▶ Caffeine

    ▷ Another anxiety disorder such as posttraumatic stress disorder (PTSD) or phobias

    ▷ Separation anxiety disorder

    ▷ Consider general medical disorder if

        ▶ First episode of panic attack symptoms occurs after age 45

        ▶ Panic symptoms are atypical, such as

            ▷ Vertigo

            ▷ Loss of consciousness

            ▷ Incontinence

            ▷ Headache

            ▷ Slurred speech

            ▷ Amnesic pattern after attacks

▶ Differentiated from other anxiety conditions by

    ▷ Sudden onset of attack

    ▷ Discrete, self-limiting nature of symptoms

    ▷ Paroxysmal symptom profile

    ▷ Level 3–4 anxiety symptoms with somatic symptoms that are experienced as distressing and severe by the client

Clinical Management

▶ Follow guidelines of general clinical management of anxiety disorders.

Pharmacological Management

▶ SSRIs

▶ BNZs, usually used for short-term symptom control or "bridge" medication when starting an SSRI or other antidepressant

    ▷ Buspar effective as an adjunct to an antidepressant

    ▷ Other non-benzodiazepine anxiolytic meds used as adjuncts

Nonpharmacological Management

▶ CBT

▶ Individual or group therapy

▶ Exposure therapy

▶ Relaxation therapies

Common Comorbidities

▶ Frequent with major depressive disorder

▶ Estimated between 10% and 65%, depending on source:

▷ Social phobia

▷ OCD

▷ Substance abuse

AGORAPHOBIA

Description

▶ Agoraphobia is characterized by avoidance of places or situations from which escape may be difficult or embarrassing or in which help may not be available in the event of perceived need, such as a panic attack. Up to 50% of people meeting criteria for agoraphobia report panic attacks or panic disorder preceded onset of agoraphobia.

▶ The anxiety usually leads to avoidant behavior that impairs a person's ability to travel, to work, or to carry out responsibilities of daily living.

▶ Differential diagnosis is assisted by the awareness that people with agoraphobia feel better and report less significant concerns with anxiety when accompanied by a trusted companion.

▶ When people meet criteria for agoraphobia and panic or other anxiety disorder, both diagnoses should be assigned.

Assessment

History

▶ Assess for the following:

▷ Clinical presentation meets *diagnostic criteria* for agoraphobia:

▶ Presence of agoraphobic anxiety related to fear of developing panic-like symptoms

▶ Never met criteria for panic disorder

▶ Avoidant behavior as a result of the agoraphobic anxiety

Physical Exam Findings

▶ Nonspecific for agoraphobia

Mental Status Exam Findings

▶ Consistent with finding for anxiety

▶ Thought content consistent with criteria for agoraphobia

Diagnostic and Laboratory Findings

▶ Nonspecific for agoraphobia

Clinical Management

▶ Follow guidelines of general clinical management of anxiety disorders

Pharmacological Management

▶ SSRIs

▶ BNZs for short-term use

▶ Beta blockers (off-label use) used for discrete episodes of social anxiety

Nonpharmacological Management

▶ CBT

▶ Supportive group therapy

▶ Desensitization therapy

Common Comorbidities

▶ Panic disorder

SPECIFIC PHOBIAS (SIMPLE PHOBIAS)

Description

▶ In specific phobias is a clinically significant level of marked and persistent fear that is clearly observable and is, by client perception, clearly related to specific objects or situations.

▶ In adults, but not in children, exists the conscious recognition that the fear is excessive or unreasonable.

▶ In children, the degree of insight to the unreasonable nature of the fear increases as age increases.

Risk Factors

▶ Traumatic past exposure

▷ Having been bitten by dog, having choked on food, and so forth.

▶ Observation of another's trauma

▷ Seeing others be bitten by dog, seeing others choking on food, and so forth.

▶ Excessive informational transmission

▷ Repeated graphic parental warnings of dangers of certain events or situations.

▶ Genetic loading

▷ Having family member with specific phobia

▷ Blood-injection-injury type is most familial

▷ Subtype aggregation patterns noted within families; for example, if a person's first-degree relative has animal subtype, the risk is highest for him or her to develop animal subtype

Assessment

History

▶ Assess for the following:

 ▷ The content of phobias, which can vary with culture, ethnicity, and age

 ▷ Phobic diagnosis should occur only when accompanied by significant functional impairment, such as full avoidance of school related to fear of encountering a spider.

 ▷ Exposure to the specific feared object or situation immediately provokes the onset of clinically significant levels of anxiety

  ▶ This anxiety may fit the criteria for cued panic attack.

  ▶ The level of anxiety is directly related to how physically close the object or situation is to the person and the degree to which escape from the object or situation is possible.

  ▶ Children manifest fear and anxiety as crying, freezing, tantrums, or excessive clinging behavior.

  ▶ Children normatively express a transient fear of animals and other natural objects.

 ▷ Person engages in avoidant behavior to prevent reaction to object or situation or endures object or situation with dread.

  ▶ Avoidant behavior is distressful and has implications for social, recreational, and occupational or school functioning.

▶ Assess for subtypes:

 ▷ There are five common subtypes: situational, natural environment, blood injection injury, animal, and other.

  ▶ A person can experience more than one subtype at a time.

  ▶ A phobia to one object or situation in a subclass predisposes a person to another phobia within the same subclass (e.g., fear of rats increases the risk for fear of spiders).

  1. *Situational Type:* Cued by specific situations; examples include driving, enclosed spaces, tunnels or bridges, or flying

   ▷ Most common adult form

   ▷ In older adults, fear of closed-in situations most common

   ▷ Bimodal peak of onset

    ▶ First peak, childhood

    ▶ Second peak, mid-20s

2. *Natural Environment Type:* Fear cued by objects in the natural environment; examples include storms, lightning, water, or heights

   ▷ Second most common adult form

   ▷ Onset usually during childhood

3. *Blood-Injection-Injury Type:* Cued by seeing blood or an injury or by receiving an injection or other invasive medical procedure

   ▷ Third most common adult form

   ▷ Strong vasovagal component that can produce other somatic sensations

      ▶ May exacerbate underlying cardiac or respiratory disorders

      ▶ Person often presents with fainting as chief complaint

      ▶ Experiences paroxysmal tachycardia and hypertension followed by deceleration of heart rate and drop in blood pressure

      ▶ Clinical presentation and disease natural history similar to panic disorder with agoraphobia

4. *Animal Type:* Fear cued by animals or insects; examples include rats, snakes, or spiders

   ▷ Fourth most common adult form

   ▷ Onset usually during childhood

5. *Other Type:* Fear cued by range of other stimuli; examples include fear of choking, vomiting, or fear of a specific illness

   ▷ In children, often manifests as fear of loud sounds or costumed characters

Physical Exam Findings

▶ Nonspecific

Mental Status Exam Findings

▶ Consistent with finding for anxiety

▶ Thought content consistent with criteria for phobia

Diagnostic and Laboratory Findings

▶ Nonspecific

Differential Diagnosis

▶ Avoidance behavior in PTSD, OCD, separation anxiety disorder, or psychotic disorders

Clinical Management

▶ Follow guidelines of general clinical management of anxiety disorders

Pharmacological Management

▶ SSRIs

▶ TCAs

▶ Short term use of BNZs

Nonpharmacological Management

▶ CBT

▶ Biofeedback

▶ Desensitization therapy

SOCIAL ANXIETY (PHOBIA) DISORDER

Description

▶ Social anxiety disorder is a marked and persistent fear of social or performance situations in which embarrassment may occur.

▶ Anxiety levels often are sufficient to fit criteria for a situationally bound panic attack.

▶ The disorder has an estimated 3% to 13% prevalence rate among the U.S. population.

▶ Rates are equal for the genders.

Assessment

History

▶ Assess for the following:

▷ Some degree of social anxiety is common and normative in adolescence.

▷ Social phobia should be diagnosed only if symptoms persist for longer than 6 months.

▷ Onset is in the mid-teens, often following stressful or humiliating experience, and tends to remit with age.

▶ Differential diagnosis is assisted by awareness that people with social phobia do *not* feel better or experience decreased anxiety when accompanied by a trusted companion.

▷ Common descriptive features:

▶ Hypersensitivity to criticism

▶ Negative self-evaluations

▶ Sensitivity to rejection

▶ Low self-esteem

▶ Inferiority feelings

▶ Lack of assertiveness

▷ Protracted anticipatory anxiety may occur days or weeks before the feared social situation.

▷ Levels of subjective distress and impaired functioning can be significant and have been associated with suicidal ideation.

Physical Exam Findings for a Person Who Is Acutely Anxious

▶ Sweating

▶ Tremors

▶ Palpitations

▶ Muscle tension

▶ Diarrhea

▶ Blushing

Mental Status Exam Findings

▶ Consistent for anxiety

▶ Thought content consistent with criteria for social anxiety

Diagnostic and laboratory findings

▶ Nonspecific

Clinical Management

▶ Follow guidelines of general clinical management of anxiety disorders.

Pharmacological Management

▶ SSRIs

▶ BNZs, for short-term use

▶ Beta blockers

▷ Used for discrete episode relief

▷ For example, before having to attend a scheduled social function

Nonpharmacological Management

▶ CBT

▶ Exposure therapy

▶ Relaxation therapy

GENERALIZED ANXIETY DISORDER (GAD)

Description

▶ In GAD, excessive worry, apprehension, or anxiety about events or activities occurs more days than not for a period of at least 6 months.

▷ The person finds it hard to control the anxiety.

     ▷ No clear link exists to life events or stressors.

     ▷ Worry and anxiety interfere with activities of daily living.

     ▷ The nature and focus of worry shift frequently.

     ▷ A pattern of waxing and waning of symptoms exists.

▶ Symptoms worsen as life events stress the person.

Assessment

History

▶ Assess for the following:

     ▷ In GAD, anxiety and worry are out of proportion to the actual likelihood or effect of the feared event.

     ▷ People report subjective distress caused by the constant worry but do not always describe the worry as excessive.

     ▷ Excessive anxiety and worry last for more days than not for at least 6 months.

     ▷ The person finds it difficult to control anxiety.

▶ Differential diagnosis

     ▷ PTSD

     ▷ Adjustment disorder with anxiety

     ▷ Obsessions in OCD

     ▷ Anxiety associated with another disorder such as hypochondriasis or social phobia

Physical Exam Findings

▶ Nonspecific

▶ Associated with other health states

     ▷ Irritable bowel syndrome

     ▷ Migraine and other headache disorders

▶ Physical signs of anxiety

     ▷ Muscle tension

     ▷ Generalized muscle ache and soreness

     ▷ Tremors

     ▷ Twitching

     ▷ Subjective complaints of shakiness

     ▷ Shortness of breath

     ▷ Autonomic hyperarousal signs

     ▷ Tachycardia

    ▷ Increased respiratory rates

    ▷ Dizziness

    ▷ Numbness

    ▷ Easily fatigued, often experienced as activity intolerance

    ▷ Muscle tension and increased tone

    ▷ Sleep disturbance

Mental Status Exam Findings

▶ Appearance

    ▷ Psychomotor restlessness

▶ Mood

    ▷ Anxious

    ▷ Feeling keyed up or on edge

    ▷ Irritability

▶ Concentration

    ▷ Difficulty concentrating

▶ Thought content

    ▷ Thematic for the anxiety and worry

    ▷ Descriptive of the significant distress and impairment in daily functioning caused by GAD

Diagnostic and Laboratory Findings

▶ Nonspecific

Clinical Management

Pharmacological Management

▶ SSRIs

▶ Buspar

▶ BNZs as p.r.n. agents

Nonpharmacological Management

▶ Good candidates for therapy as single treatment modality

▶ CBT

▶ Relaxation therapies

▶ Stress management

▶ Supportive counseling

Common Comorbidities

▶ Mood disorders

▶ Other anxiety disorders

▶ Substance-related disorders

Life Span Considerations

▶ Children

▷ Anxiety is common in children, but it is important to assess normal versus pathological levels.

▷ Anxiety is manifested in excessive worry over competence or quality of performance in school, work, sports, or other activities.

▷ Common worry often manifests as anxiety over punctuality or catastrophes such as earthquakes or war.

▷ Often accompanied by

▶ Overly conforming behavior

▶ Perfectionist self-expectations

▶ Excessive seeking of approval of others

▶ Need for frequent reassurance about performance

SEPARATION ANXIETY DISORDER

▶ Developmentally inappropriate and excessive distress occurring after the age of 4 when faced with separation from a major attachment figure.

▶ Refer to Chapter 15: Disorders of Childhood and Adolescence

▶ May persist into adulthood and in the DSM-5 it can be diagnosed in adulthood

OBSESSIVE–COMPULSIVE DISORDER (OCD)

Description

▶ OCD is the presence of anxiety-provoking obsessions or compulsions that function to reduce the person's subjective anxiety level.

▷ Obsession

▶ Defined as recurrent and persistent thoughts, impulses, or images that are experienced and cause anxiety and distress

▶ Experienced as intrusive and inappropriate

▶ Ego-dystonic experience in which a person feels the content of obsession is alien to his or her belief structure and not the kind of common thought, impulse, or image he or she usually experiences

▷ Compulsion

▶ Defined as repetitive behaviors or mental actions that a person feels driven to perform in response to an obsession.

Risk Factors

▶ Genetic predisposition

  ▷ Familial transmission pattern

   ▶ Disease rates higher in people with a first-degree relative who has OCD than in the general population.

   ▶ Rates are also higher in people with a first-degree relative who has Tourette's syndrome than in the general population.

   ▶ PANDAS (pediatric autoimmune neuropsychiatric disorders associated with streptococcal infections) should be considered in all children with sudden-onset OCD symptoms

Assessment

History

▶ Assess for the following:

  ▷ Diagnostic criteria:

   ▶ Presence of *either* obsessions *or* compulsions

   ▶ The person recognizing that the obsession or compulsion is excessive or unreasonable

   ▶ The obsession or compulsion is causing marked distress, is time-consuming, or interferes with normal daily activity.

  ▷ Common obsessions include:

   ▶ Repeated thoughts about contamination, dirt, or germs

   ▶ Repeated doubts, such as having hit someone with a car or having left an oven on, without evidence

   ▶ Need to have things in a specific order, with marked distress when that order is disturbed

   ▶ Aggressive or horrific thoughts

   ▶ May occur in pregnancy and postpartum periods and manifest as intrusive thoughts about something happening to their baby or doing something to their baby; the thoughts are highly ego-dystonic

   ▶ Sexual imagery

  ▷ Obsessions usually do not involve real-world worries such as concern over finances.

  ▷ The person recognizes that the thoughts, impulses, or images are a product of his or her own mind.

  ▷ The person attempts to ignore or suppress thoughts, impulses, or images or to override them with other thoughts or actions.

  ▷ People often avoid situations in which the content of obsession may be encountered (e.g., avoiding public restrooms to avoid contamination)

▷ Common compulsions include

- ▶ Repetitive actions, usually behavioral, and often called *rituals*
    - ▷ Handwashing
    - ▷ Excessive cleaning
    - ▷ Checking to see, for example, if the lights are turned off, the stove is turned off, or the doors are locked
    - ▷ Needing to place objects in certain order
- ▶ Common mental actions include
    - ▷ Counting
    - ▷ Silently repeating words
    - ▷ Praying
- ▶ Behaviors or mental acts are not experienced as pleasurable and are intended to prevent or reduce distress and subjective anxiety.
    - ▷ If the person resists the compulsion, anxiety and subjective tension usually increase.
    - ▷ Some people believe the compulsion can prevent some dreaded event or situation that is experienced as an obsession, such as sexual or horrific images.

Physical Exam Findings

- ▶ Nonspecific
- ▶ Dermatitis may be present related to excessive handwashing or overuse of caustic cleaning agents.
- ▶ Hypochondriasis and somatic fixation common

Mental Status Exam Findings

- ▶ Consistent with finding for anxiety
- ▶ Thought content dominated by obsessions
- ▶ Behavioral manifestations of rituals may be noted

Diagnostic and Laboratory Findings

- ▶ Nonspecific

Differential Diagnosis

- ▶ Body dysmorphic disorder
- ▶ Eating disorders
- ▶ Trichotillomania
- ▶ Hypochondriasis

▶ Obsessive–compulsive personality disorder

▶ Tic or stereotypic movement disorder

Clinical Management

▶ Follow guidelines of general clinical management of anxiety disorders.

Pharmacological Management

▶ SSRIs (clients often need higher dosing range for adequate symptom control)

▶ TCAs (clomipramine)

▶ Second-generation antipsychotics such as risperidone are off-label but have data supporting their adjunctive use with SSRI medication

Nonpharmacological Management

▶ CBT

▶ Exposure therapy

Common Comorbidities

▶ Major depression

▶ Eating disorders

▶ Other anxiety disorders

Life Span Considerations

▶ Children

  ▷ Common in childhood, usually with prepubertal onset

  ▷ More common in boys than in girls

  ▷ Washing, checking, and ordering are the most common behavioral manifestations.

  ▷ Common comorbidities in children:

    ▶ Learning disorders

    ▶ Disruptive behavioral disorders

    ▶ Tourette's syndrome

  ▷ Associated in children with Group A beta-hemolytic streptococcal infections (e.g., scarlet fever, strep throat)

▶ Older adults

  ▷ More obsessions than compulsions usually present

  ▷ Obsessive content characteristically about dying

  ▷ Compulsions characteristically about washing and cleaning

POSTTRAUMATIC STRESS DISORDER (PTSD)

Description

▶ PTSD is the reexperiencing of an extremely traumatic event accompanied by symptoms of increased arousal and avoidance of stimuli associated with the trauma.

▶ The traumatic event can be experienced directly or witnessed.

   ▷ Common *experienced* trauma includes

      ▶ Military combat

      ▶ Violent personal assault such as robbery or rape

      ▶ Kidnapping or hostage situation

      ▶ Terrorist attack

      ▶ Torture

      ▶ Prolonged sexual abuse

      ▶ Natural or human-made disasters

   ▷ Common *witnessed* trauma includes

      ▶ Observing the death of or significant injury to another

      ▶ Unexpectedly witnessing of any of the above traumas

      ▶ Learning of the sudden or unexpected death of or significant injury to family member or close friend

▶ A relationship exists between the person's physical proximity to the traumatic event and the likelihood of symptom onset.

Risk Factors

▶ Experienced or witnessed trauma

▶ Genetic predisposition

   ▷ Assumed to have strong genetic etiological component and tends to run in families

   ▷ History of major depression in first-degree relative related to increased risk of developing PTSD

Assessment

History

▶ Assess for the following:

   ▷ Symptoms cannot predate exposure to trauma.

   ▷ Presenting symptoms and history can be delineated as one of *three subtypes:*

      ▶ *Acute*: Duration of symptoms less than 3 months

      ▶ *Chronic:* Symptoms lasting 3 months or longer

      ▶ *Delayed onset:* At least 6 months between traumatic event and the onset of symptoms

Physical Exam Findings

- ▶ Nonspecific
- ▶ Increased rates of somatic complaints
- ▶ Insomnia frequently chief complaint on presentation for evaluation
- ▶ Distractibility in motor tasks
- ▶ Measurable increased autonomic symptoms
    - ▷ Tachycardia
    - ▷ Diaphoresis
    - ▷ Increased respiratory rates
    - ▷ Pupillary dilation
    - ▷ Increased startle response

Mental Status Exam Findings

- ▶ Consistent with finding for anxiety
- ▶ Thought content consistent with criteria for PTSD and often dominated by traumatic experience
- ▶ May demonstrate some psychotic findings during flashback episodes.

Diagnostic and Laboratory Findings

- ▶ Diagnostic criteria (symptoms for 1 month or longer):
    - ▷ Exposure to a traumatic event
        - ▶ The person experienced, witnessed, or was confronted with an event involving the actual or threatened death or serious injury, **and** the person's response involved intense fear, helplessness, or horror.
    - ▷ The traumatic event is persistently reexperienced in one or more of the following ways:
        - ▶ Recurrent and intrusive, distressing recollection of the event, including images, thoughts, and perceptions
        - ▶ May be experienced as flashbacks
        - ▶ Rare cases involve dissociative states lasting hours to days
        - ▶ Recurrent distressing dreams about the event
        - ▶ Acting or feeling as if the traumatic event were reoccurring
        - ▶ Intense psychological distress at exposure to cues that symbolize or resemble aspects of the traumatic event
        - ▶ Physiological reactivity on exposure to cues that symbolize or resemble aspects of the traumatic event
    - ▷ Three or more avoidance symptoms
        - ▶ Persistent avoidance of stimuli associated with the traumatic event and numbing of responsiveness
        - ▶ Efforts to avoid talking about or thinking about traumatic event

▶ Avoidance of activities, places, or people that arouse recollections of traumatic event

▶ Inability to recall important aspects of event

▶ Marked decreased interest or participation in activities

▶ Feelings of detachment or estrangement from others

▶ Restricted range of affect

▶ Sense of foreboding and of shortened future, premature death, or no expectation for success or happiness

▷ Two or more increased arousal symptoms

   ▶ Persistent symptoms of increased arousal

      ▷ Difficulty falling asleep

      ▷ Irritability or outburst of anger

      ▷ Difficulty concentrating

      ▷ Hypervigilance

      ▷ Exaggerated startle response

▷ Symptoms causing significant distress or impairment in activities of daily functioning

▷ Symptoms usually occur within 3 months of trauma

▷ Duration of symptoms highly variable

   ▶ Symptoms remit within 3 months in one-half of cases

   ▶ Common waxing and waning of symptoms related to internal and external cues that resemble the trauma

Diagnostic and Laboratory Findings

▶ Nonspecific

Differential Diagnosis

▶ Adjustment disorder

▶ Brief psychotic disorder

▶ Acute stress disorder

▶ Intrusive thoughts in OCD

Clinical Management

▶ Follow guidelines of general clinical management of anxiety disorders.

Pharmacological Management

▶ SSRIs

▶ TCAs

- ▶ BNZs are not recommended in the treatment of PTSD
- ▶ Antipsychotics may be useful during episodes of flashbacks.
- ▶ Alpha antagonists (e.g., Prazosin) may be used for treating nightmares (off-label use).

Nonpharmacological Management

- ▶ CBT
- ▶ Exposure Therapy with Response Prevention (ERP)
- ▶ Supportive group therapy
- ▶ Relaxation therapies
- ▶ Eye movement desensitization and reprocessing

Common Comorbidities

- ▶ Major depression
- ▶ Dysthymia
- ▶ Substance abuse or dependence

Life Span Considerations

- ▶ Can occur at any age, including childhood
  - ▷ Children
    - ▶ Expression of fear and horror occurs in disorganized or agitated behavior.
    - ▶ Repetitive play behaviors show themes or aspects of trauma.
    - ▶ Frightening dreams, but without recognized content, are common.
    - ▶ In young children, learning that a traumatic event occurred to a parent or a caregiver may be the precipitating factor.

DISSOCIATIVE DISORDERS

- ▶ Dissociative amnesia, depersonalization or derealization, and dissociative identity disorder (DID)
- ▶ *Dissociation* is a defense mechanism that protects a person from overwhelming anxiety by emotionally separating.
  - ▷ Dissociation causes gaps or interruption in the person's memory
- ▶ *Depersonalization or derealization:* A persistent feeling of oneself not being real, or the environment not being real; reality testing remains intact
  - ▷ Depersonalization and derealization are generally perceived as uncomfortable.
  - ▷ Etiology of depersonalization and derealization can be physical or psychological.
  - ▷ Physical causes are seizures, migraine headaches, psychedelic drugs, and alcohol.
  - ▷ Psychological causes are severe anxiety and traumatic stress.

- ▶ *DID* is characterized by two or more distinct personality states ("alters").
    - ▷ Personality states are generally split off from one another, leading to gaps in recall of everyday events.
    - ▷ Symptoms cause significant distress and impaired functioning.
    - ▷ Comorbid with PTSD.
    - ▷ Etiology is a history of severe physical or sexual trauma, or both, in childhood.

BODY DYSMORPHIC DISORDER

- ▶ Preoccupation with one or more perceived defects or flaws in physical appearance
- ▶ Engages in repetitive behaviors (checking mirror, reassurance-seeking, etc.) in response to appearance concerns
- ▶ Preoccupation causes considerable distress
- ▶ Insight ranges from good to poor to absent (fixed delusion)

HOARDING DISORDER

- ▶ Persistent difficulty discarding possessions, regardless of actual value
- ▶ Experiences marked distress in response to pressure to discard
- ▶ Results in accumulation of possessions that compromise living space or ability to function, including maintaining a safe environment for self or others
- ▶ Insight ranges from good to poor to absent (fixed delusion)

TRICHOTILLOMANIA

- ▶ Recurrent pulling out of one's hair despite repeated attempts to stop
- ▶ Causes significant distress or impairment in functioning
- ▶ Hair-pulling is not an attempt to improve a perceived defect or flaw

EXCORIATION DISORDER

- ▶ Recurrent skin picking that results in lesions despite attempts to stop
- ▶ Results in significant distress or impairment
- ▶ Behavior not better explained by physiologic response to substance (e.g., methamphetamine use) or intentional attempt at self-harm

CASE STUDY

Mr. J. is a 47-year-old school custodian with a long history of GAD. He reports he had been doing well until about 4 weeks ago, when he was traveling overseas with his church group for a caring mission in South America. Mr. J. noted that he began feeling "depressed by seeing all the poverty and despair in those places." He began to have difficulty falling and staying asleep. He experienced disturbing dreams about what he was seeing during the day. The sleep disturbances persisted upon his return home, and he started feeling anxious and could not concentrate during his work day.

One week ago, Mr. J. began to feel overwhelmed by anxiety. He was unable to go to work. He experienced discreet "attacks" of rapid heart rate, sweating, and difficulty breathing. He went to a local emergency department several times, was evaluated, and each time was given "a shot" and sent home. The emergency department doctor also suggested he contact a therapist. He was not convinced that his distress was due to anxiety. On the third visit to the emergency department, the doctor gave Mr. J. a prescription for alprazolam 0.5 mg #30 with the directions "take as needed for anxiety" and referred him back to his primary care provider. Although Mr. J. initially felt the medication was helping, he has continued to have difficulty falling and staying asleep and has continued to have "bad dreams." He needed 4 tablets of alprazolam yesterday before finally falling asleep until this morning. He now believes "the medicine isn't working. There is something really wrong with me and nobody believes me. My wife and the people at the hospital think it's all in my head. I know I'm anxious, but what if there's also something wrong with my heart? Doctors miss things all the time…." Mr. J. now presents to the PMHNP at the hospital-based outpatient psychiatry department.

Mental Status Exam

- ▶ Appearance: Well-nourished, well-dressed
- ▶ Motor: Some motor restlessness
- ▶ Speech: Some pressure
- ▶ Affect: Anxious
- ▶ Mood: Depressed
- ▶ Thought process and content: Thematic for fear of serious cardiac etiology not being adequately assessed or treated. There is no evidence of an overt delusional process.
- ▶ Abstractive on proverbs
- ▶ Memory: Impaired
- ▶ Concentration: Impaired

Social History

- ▶ Married and has 3 children
- ▶ Works as high school custodian
- ▶ Overweight at 280 lbs., with sedentary lifestyle
- ▶ Smokes 2 packs a day
- ▶ Does not drink alcohol for religious reasons
- ▶ Wife very concerned and supportive

Past Psychiatric History

▶ Hospitalized in 1998 for "nerves"

▶ At that time started on paroxetine (Paxil) 20 mg/d

▶ After 3 months, dose was raised to 40 mg q.d. and he remained on that dose for the next 18 months, when he tapered off the drug under his primary care provider's supervision.

▶ Has had no significant exacerbation of symptoms since initial treatment

Past Medical History

▶ History of seizure disorder since childhood; well-controlled with levetiracetam (Keppra)

Current Medications

▶ Alprazolam 0.5 mg p.o. p.r.n. q 4 hrs.

Labs

▶ Electrocardiogram (EKG), CBC, thyroid function tests, and chemistry panel done in emergency department and all within normal limits

Screening Tools

▶ Current level of anxiety: moderate–severe

In planning care for this client, the PMHNP has many issues to consider:

1. What is the most likely diagnosis?

2. How will the PMHNP separate comorbidity from complications of current diagnosis?

3. What medication adjustments would the PMHNP make?

4. How will the PMHNP address the family issues?

5. How often will the PMHNP plan to see the client?

Given the level of Mr. J.'s initial distress, you decide to restart paroxetine and continue using alprazolam as a bridge medication while waiting for a therapeutic response to the antidepressant.

6. What considerations should be given to using a benzodiazepine in a client with panic disorder?

Mr. J. has now been taking paroxetine 20 mg for the past 2 weeks. He has not had a panic attack since beginning treatment with the scheduled dose of benzodiazepine that was started when he started the paroxetine. He no longer worries that he has a heart condition. He falls asleep quickly, but continues to have some mild middle-phase insomnia that lasts up to one hour. He eventually falls back to sleep, but wakes up feeling anxious. He is tearful at times during the day, and worries that the panic attacks will recur if he stops taking the benzodiazepine.

7. How should the PMHNP adjust the treatment plan?

8. Mr. J. has been taking paroxetine 40 mg q.d. for the past month. He is now taking clonazepam 0.5 mg q.a.m. and q.h.s. for the past 2 weeks after he experienced sedation while taking 0.5 mg q.a.m. and 1.0 mg q.h.s. He continues to experience mild–moderate anxiety periodically most days. How should the PMHNP alter the treatment plan?

9. At what point should the PMHNP begin to taper the client off the clonazepam?

ANSWERS TO CASE STUDY DISCUSSION QUESTIONS

1. Mr. J meets criteria for panic disorder. It is not unusual for people who have panic attacks to misinterpret the symptoms as cardiac or other etiology. The PMHNP must also assess for a mood disorder as symptoms anxiety and mood symptoms often overlap.

2. The PMHNP should perform a complete assessment which includes a physical examination, mental status examination, and lab studies. The client's current medications should be evaluated and the chronology of symptoms should be compared to any changes in his health status.

3. After assessing the efficacy of Mr. J's treatment history, the PMHNP should consider restarting paroxetine.

4. Several approaches might be appropriate, including using psychoeducation for the family, providing supportive counseling, or involving the family in family therapy.

5. Mr. J. should be seen frequently until symptoms are stable. Weekly appointments during the initial phase of treatment would be ideal.

6. Before starting a benzodiazepine, the PMHNP should assess the client's history of recent and remote substance use or abuse. Potential risks versus benefits of short-term use must also be discussed along with the expectation that the medication will be tapered once the antidepressant is therapeutic. The PMHNP should discuss the expected therapeutic outcome of using an SSRI or other antidepressant. When using a benzodiazepine, consider using scheduled dosing to prevent onset of panic symptoms. Clients who have severe anxiety often underdose or overdose medications to address their symptoms. Discuss expectations that the client will not adjust his dose of medication without direction. Short-acting benzodiazepines require dosing more frequently than long-acting benzodiazepines and may contribute to the client connecting the feeling of being anxious with taking a pill.

7. The PMHNP should consider switching to a long-acting benzodiazepine that may be scheduled in the a.m. and h.s. to provide better nighttime and early morning coverage. The NP should discuss the expected outcome of each medication with the client. The PMHNP should increase the paroxetine dose in increments back to the dose that was previously therapeutic (40 mg).

8. As long as he is not having considerable side effects, increase the paroxetine to 50 mg q.d. Continue weekly psychotherapy. Continue clonazepam.

9. Although benzodiazepines should be used for as brief a period as possible, discontinuing the medication too quickly may result in relapse. Unless otherwise indicated by side effects, benzodiazepine taper should begin after the client is at an adequate dose of antidepressant and he is no longer having significant anxiety symptoms

REFERENCES AND RESOURCES

American Nurses Association, American Psychiatric Nurses Association, & International Society of Psychiatric-Mental Health Nurses. (2014). *Psychiatric–mental health nursing: Scope and standards of practice* (2nd ed.). Silver Spring, MD: Nursesbooks.org

American Psychiatric Association. (2015). *Diagnostic and statistical manual of mental disorders* (5th ed.). Washington, DC: Author.

Davidson, J. R. (2000). Trauma: The impact of post-traumatic stress disorder. *Journal of Psychopharmacology, 14*(Suppl. 1), 5–12.

Fernandez-Lewis, R., Hinton, D., Laria A., Patterson, E., Hofmann, S., Craske, M. G., … Liao, B. (2010) Culture and the anxiety disorders: Recommendations for DSM-V. *Depression and Anxiety, 27,* 212–229.

Goodman, W. K., Price, L. H., Rasmussen, S. A., Mazure, C., Fleischmann, R. L., Hill, C. L., … Charney, D. S.. (1989). The Yale-Brown obsessive–compulsive scale I: Development, use, and reliability. *Archives of General Psychiatry, 46,* 1006–1011.

Grant, J. E., Fineberg, N., Van Ameringen, M., Cath, D., Visser, H., Carmi, L., … (2015) New treatment models for compulsive disorders. *European Neuropsychopharmacology,* doi:10.1016/j.euroneuro.2015.11.008.

Guess, K. (2006). Posttraumatic stress disorder: Early detection is key. *The Nurse Practitioner, 31*(3), 1–8.

Hamilton, M. (1959). The assessment of anxiety states by rating. *British Journal of Medical Psychology, 32*(1), 50–55.

Hembree, E. (2002). Psychosocial treatment of post-traumatic stress disorder. *Primary Psychiatry, 9*(2), 49–52.

Hoskins, M. (2015). Pharmacotherapy for post-traumatic stress disorder: systematic review and meta-analysis. *British J of Psychiatry,* (2), 93-100.

Kessler, R. C., Chin, W. T., Merikangas, K. R., Demler, O. M., & Walters, E. E. (2005). Prevalence, severity and comorbidity of 12-month DSM-IV disorders in the National Comorbidity Survey Replication. *Archives of General Psychiatry, 62,* 617–627.

Lopez, I., Rivera, F., Ramirez, R., Guarnaccia, P., Canino, G., & Bird, H. (2009). Ataques de Nervios and their psychiatric correlates in Puerto Rican children from two different contexts. *Journal of Nervous and Mental Disease, 197*(12), 923–929.

Margolin, G., & Gordis, E. B. (2000). The effects of family and community violence on children. *Annual Review of Psychology, 51,* 445–479.

Meredith, P. V., & Horan, N. M. (2000). *Adult primary care.* Philadelphia, PA: W. B. Saunders.

Narrow, W. E., Rae, D. S., & Regier, D. A. (1998). *NIMH epidemiology note: Prevalence of anxiety disorders. One-year prevalence best estimates calculated from ECA and NCS data.* Washington, DC: National Institute of Mental Health.

National Institute of Mental Health, Genetics Workgroup. (1998). *Genetics and mental disorders* (NIH Publication No. 98-4268). Rockville, MD: Author.

Raines, A. M., Allan, N. P., Oglesby, M. E. & Short, N. A. (2015). Specific and general facets of hoarding: a bifactor model. *Journal of Anxiety Disorders,* (34), 100–106.

Regier, D. A., Rae, D. S., & Narrow, W. E. (1998). Prevalence of anxiety disorders and their comorbidity with mood and addictive disorders. *British Journal of Psychiatry* (Suppl. 34), 24–28.

Stark, E. A., Parsons, E. E., Van Hartevelt, T. J., Charquero-Ballester, M., McManners, H., Ehlers, A., … Kriingelbach, M. L. (2015). Post-traumatic stress influences the brain even in the absence of symptoms: A systematic, quantitative meta-analysis of neuroimaging studies. *Neuroscience and Biobehaviora Reviews, 56,* 207–221.

Yehuda, R. (1999). Biological factors associated with susceptibility to posttraumatic stress disorder. *Canadian Journal of Psychiatry, 44*(1), 34–39.

Yehuda, R. (2000). Biology of posttraumatic stress disorder. *Journal of Clinical Psychiatry,* *61*(Suppl. 7), 14–21.

Zung, W. W. K. (1971). A rating instrument for anxiety disorders. *Psychometrics, 12,* 371–379.

CHAPTER 11

SCHIZOPHRENIA SPECTRUM AND OTHER PSYCHOTIC DISORDERS

This chapter describes a category of severe mental illnesses that have a researched biological basis to the disorders. Schizophrenia, the prototypic disorder of this category of illnesses, is multifaceted and affects a person's ability to function in many spheres of daily life. Of the psychotic disorders, schizophrenia is the illness that has been heavily researched and the one we know the most about.

The other disorders that compose this category of illnesses will be presented after the in-depth discussion of schizophrenia. Almost all of the information provided for schizophrenia and for the clinical management of this disorder will pertain to the other psychotic disorders presented in this chapter.

GENERAL DESCRIPTION OF PSYCHOTIC DISORDERS

▶ These brain-based psychiatric disorders are grouped together because of similarity in frequent psychotic symptoms. Each disorder has a different etiology.

▶ Psychotic disorders are some of the most debilitating classes of psychiatric disorders, as determined by the degree of functional impairment and financial burden of severe mental illness.

▶ *Psychotic* implies inability to test reality.

   ▷ Manifests in symptoms (see Table 11–1) such as

      ▶ Hallucinations

      ▶ Delusions

      ▶ Disorganized thinking and speech

      ▶ Referential thinking

      ▶ Abnormal motor behavior

      ▶ Negative symptoms

▶ Psychotic disorders are generally known to have a strong genetic component.

TABLE 11–1.
SYMPTOMS OF PSYCHOSIS

CLINICAL MANIFESTATION	DEFINITION	TYPE
Hallucinations	False sensory experience without stimuli being present	(Arranged in order of commonality) Auditory Visual Tactile Olfactory Gustatory Note: Hypnogogic* and hypnopompic* experiences are considered normative and do not fall under the true definition of hallucinations.
Delusions	A false belief firmly maintained despite evidence to the contrary	Persecutory Religious Grandiose Somatic Jealous Erotomanic
Disorganized thinking (often referred to as *formal thought disturbance* or *disorder*)	Problems with information organization and interpretation that is best assessed in the speech patterns of clients	Loose association Derailment Speaks tangentially Word salad
Disorganized behavior	Unusual behavior ranging from childlike silliness to anger	Silliness Unpredictable anger Difficulties with activities of daily living Disheveled Odd or unusual dress Inappropriate sexual activity Stereotypic motor activities
Referential thinking and delusions of control	Belief that events, actions, or situations in the environment hold special significance or meaning	Thought insertion Thought withdrawal Thought control Thought broadcasting
Illusional	Misperception of actual environmental stimuli	Auditory Visual Tactile Olfactory Gustatory

Hypnopompic hallucination = a false perception that occurs when one is waking up; *hypnogogic hallucination* = a false perception that occurs when one is falling asleep; both are not considered pathological hallucinations.

SCHIZOPHRENIA

Description

▶ Schizophrenia causes significant disturbance in many areas of functioning:

▷ Cognition

▷ Perception

▷ Emotion

▷ Behavior

▷ Eye movement

▷ Socialization

Etiology

▶ Multiple theories exist, ranging from psychological to neurobiological.

▶ The etiological profile is probably multifactorial.

▶ *Neurobiological theory*

▷ Implicates three areas of neurobiological functioning: genetics, neurodevelopment, and neurobiological defects

▶ Genetics

▷ Studies of twins have identified schizophrenia as having a strong genetic component.

▷ Incidence increases from 1% risk of illness in general population to 50% risk in monozygotic twin of a person with schizophrenia.

▷ 15% risk in dizygotic twin of a person with schizophrenia.

▷ 40% risk in children if both parents have schizophrenia.

▷ No one specific gene has yet been identified.

▷ A polygenic SNIP defect is believed to exist.

▷ Chromosomes 6p24–22 have been implicated (Sadock, Sadock, & Ruiz, 2015).

▶ Neurodevelopment

▷ Genetic defects are believed to cause abnormal neuronal cell development, connection, organization, and migration.

▶ These include inadequate synapse formation, excessive pruning of synapses, and excitotoxic death of neurons.

▷ Intrauterine insults may contribute to etiological picture:

▶ Prenatal exposure to toxins, including viral agents

▶ Oxygen deprivation

▶ Maternal malnutrition, substance use, or other illness

▶ Neurobiological defect

▷ Several abnormal brain structures have been identified in people with schizophrenia:

▶ Enlarged ventricles

▶ Smaller frontal and temporal lobes

▷ Reduced symmetry in temporal, frontal and occipital lobes

▶ Cortical atrophy

▶ Decreased cerebral blood flow

▶ Hippocampal and amygdala reduction (Sadock, Sadock, & Ruiz, 2015).

▷ Abnormalities lead to suspected impaired neuronal communication:

▶ Suspected alterations in chemical neuronal signal transmission

▷ Excess dopamine in mesolimbic pathway

▷ Decreased dopamine in the mesocortical pathway

▷ Excess glutamate

▷ Decreased gamma-aminobutyric acid (GABA)

▷ Decreased serotonin

Incidence and Demographics

▶ Geographic and historical variations in incidence give insight into etiological factors; higher rates seen in:

▷ Urban-born

▷ First-born

▷ Lower socioeconomic status

▷ Born in winter and early spring

▶ Schizophrenia tends to occur less often in women than in men.

▷ *Men*: Onset ages 18–25 years

▶ Tend to have more negative symptoms than women

▶ Tend to have poorer prognosis, more hospitalizations, and less responsiveness to medications than women

▷ *Women:* Onset ages 25–35 years

▶ Usually have less premorbid dysfunction than men

▶ Usually experience more dysphoria than men

▶ Tend to have paranoid delusions and more hallucinations than men

▶ Age of onset has pathophysiological and prognostic significance.

▷ *Earlier age of onset*

▶ Tend to be men

▶ Have poorer premorbid functioning

▶ Have more evidence of structural brain abnormalities

▶ Have more prominent negative symptoms

▶ Have more cognitive impairment

▶ Have poorer prognosis

▷ *Later age of onset*

▶ Tend to be women

▶ Have less evidence of structural abnormalities

▶ Have less cognitive impairment

▶ Have better prognosis

Possible Risk Factors

▶ Genetic loading

▷ First-order relative with schizophrenia

▶ Prenatal exposure to flu or virus

▶ Prenatal malnutrition

▶ Obstetrical complications

▶ Central nervous system (CNS) infection in early childhood

Prevention and Screening

▶ At-risk family education

▶ Community education

▷ Stigma reduction

▷ Signs and symptoms of illness

▷ Treatment potential for control of symptoms

▶ Early recognition, intervention, and initiation of treatment

▷ Significant and protracted prodromal symptom period usually noted before full onset of illness

▷ Usually mild manifestations of criteria symptoms:

▶ Odd or unusual beliefs but not to delusional proportion

▶ Feel unliked or picked on but not to delusional proportion

▶ Odd speech patterns but not illogical

▷ Digressions

▷ Tangentiality

▶ Overly concrete or abstractive

- ▶ Odd behavior but not disorganized
    - ▷ Collects odd or worthless items
    - ▷ Mumbles to self
    - ▷ Isolates self and avoids interaction with others

Assessment

History

- ▶ Assess for the following:
    - ▷ There exists no single pathognomonic symptom of schizophrenia, but rather a constellation of symptoms.
    - ▷ Schizophrenia is a disease of information processing.
    - ▷ The symptoms are behavioral and cognitive.
    - ▷ The illness is associated with marked social or occupational functioning.
    - ▷ Prominent dysfunctions exist in many spheres of daily living.
        - ▶ Interpersonal relationships
            - ▷ 60% to 70% of clients do not marry
        - ▶ Social or occupational functioning
            - ▷ "Downdrift" functionality is noted over time.
                - ▶ Lower academic achievement compared to unaffected siblings
                - ▶ Difficulty holding a job
                - ▶ Underemployed relative to intellectual capacity
        - ▶ Self-care deficits
            - ▷ Poor hygiene
            - ▷ Difficulty with financial management
            - ▷ Limited independent living skills
    - ▷ Characteristic symptom clusters for the illness (see Table 11–2) include
        - ▶ Positive symptom cluster
        - ▶ Negative symptom cluster
        - ▶ Associated symptoms
- ▶ DSM-5 (American Psychiatric Association, 2013) diagnostic criteria for schizophrenia:
    - ▷ Two or more of the following frequently are present during a 1-month period and at least one must be delusions, hallucinations, or disorganized speech:
        - ▶ *Delusions:* Bizarre and unorganized type; examples include delusions that manifest as loss of control over mind or body:
            - ▷ Thought withdrawal
            - ▷ Thought insertion

TABLE 11–2.
POSITIVE AND NEGATIVE SYMPTOM CLUSTERS OF SCHIZOPHRENIA

SYMPTOM CLUSTER	EXPLANATION	CLINICAL MANIFESTATIONS
Positive symptoms	Symptoms that respond positively to and that can be controlled by antipsychotic medications Reflect excesses or distortions of normal brain functioning Caused by increased dopamine in the mesolimbic pathway	Hallucinations Delusions Referential thinking Disorganized behavior Hostility Grandiosity Mania Suspiciousness
Negative symptoms	Symptoms less responsive to antipsychotic medications but respond better to atypical antipsychotic medications Represent a decrease or loss of normal functioning Caused by decreased dopamine in the mesocortical pathway	Affective flattening Alogia or poverty of speech Avolition Apathy Abstract-thinking problems Anhedonia Attention deficits
Associated symptoms	Symptoms not required to be present to diagnose the disorder but often are present and a focus of treatment	Inappropriate affect Dysphoric mood Depersonalization Derealization High anxiety

▶ *Hallucinations:* Bizarre and unorganized type; examples include hallucinations that are improbable or readily apparent as not likely to have occurred

▶ *Disorganized speech*

▶ Grossly disorganized behavior

▶ Negative symptoms

▶ Significant impairment usually is evident by social or occupational dysfunction.

▶ Duration of symptoms lasts for at least 6 months.

▷ The course of illness is variable.

    ▶ Many clients have a fairly stable illness course.

    ▶ Some clients have clear episodic remissions and exacerbation periods.

    ▶ Negative symptoms tend to appear first as the illness develops.

    ▶ Positive symptoms appear to decrease over time, but negative symptoms persist.

    ▶ Negative symptoms are more debilitating.

▶ Factors predictive of good prognosis:

▷ High level of premorbid functioning

▷ Acute onset

▷ Later age of onset

▷ Clear precipitating event

▷ Married or partnered

▷ Good support system

▷ Positive symptoms

▷ Short interval between treatment and onset of first symptoms

▶ The sooner the client is treated, the better the prognosis.

▶ Longer untreated premorbid period is associated with a poorer prognosis.

▷ Absence of structural brain abnormalities

▷ Family history of mood disorders

▷ No family history of schizophrenia

▶ Subtype identification is of limited clinical value, because illness course, response to treatment, and prognosis appear unrelated to subtype (see Table 11–3).

Physical Exam Findings

▶ Abnormal smooth pursuit eye movements

▶ Abnormal saccadic eye movement

▶ Poor eye–hand coordination

▷ Client identified as "clumsy" or "awkward"

TABLE 11–3.
SUBTYPES OF SCHIZOPHRENIA*

SUBTYPE	CHARACTERISTIC
Paranoid	Prominent delusions or auditory hallucinations Lack of prominence of disorganized speech or behavior
Disorganized	Prominence of disorganized speech, behavior, and flat or inappropriate affect
Catatonic	Prominence of motor symptoms, including immobility as evidenced by catalepsy or stupor, excessive motor movement that is purposeless and not influenced by environmental stimuli, extreme negativity, mutism, oddities of posturing, echolalia,* and echopraxia*
Undifferentiated	Presence of symptoms consistent with schizophrenia but not a prominence of symptoms consistent with any of the other subtypes
Residual	Absence of prominent delusions, hallucinations, disorganized speech, and disorganized or catatonic behavior, and the continued presence of disturbance as indicated by presence of negative symptoms

*Subtypes are no longer diagnosed in the DSM-5. *Echolalia* = repetition of the last-heard words of other people; e*chopraxia* = imitation of observed behavior or movements.

- ▶ Presence of neurological nonlocalizing "soft signs":
  - ▷ *Astereognosis*: Loss of ability to judge the form of an object by touch
  - ▷ Twitches, tics, or rapid eye blinking
  - ▷ *Dysdiadochokinesia*: Impairment of the ability to perform rapidly alternating movements
  - ▷ Impaired fine-motor movement
  - ▷ Left–right confusion
  - ▷ Mirroring
- ▶ Presence of neurological localizing "hard signs":
  - ▷ Weakness
  - ▷ Decreased reflexes
- ▶ Other abnormalities that may be noted:
  - ▷ Highly arched palate
  - ▷ Narrow or wide-set eyes
  - ▷ Subtle malformations of the ears

Mental Status Exam Findings

- ▶ Appearance
  - ▷ Odd
  - ▷ Unusual
  - ▷ Peculiar
- ▶ Speech
  - ▷ Bizarre content
  - ▷ Disorganized
  - ▷ Tangential
  - ▷ Loose association
- ▶ Affect
  - ▷ Blunted
  - ▷ Flat
  - ▷ Inappropriate
- ▶ Mood
  - ▷ Blandness
  - ▷ Impoverished
- ▶ Thought process
  - ▷ Psychotic
    - ▶ Hallucination
    - ▶ Delusion

► Referential

► Thought control, insertion, or withdrawal

► Thought content

► Thematically matched to psychotic content

► May be impoverished

► Cognition

▷ Illogical

▷ Disorganized

► Orientation

▷ Usually intact

► Memory

▷ May have impaired short-term

► Concentration

▷ Impaired during acute episodes

► Abstraction

▷ Concrete on formal testing

► Judgment

▷ Impaired for self-welfare

Diagnostic and Laboratory Findings

► No specific diagnostic lab findings exist.

► Abnormalities noted in structural studies

▷ Enlargement of lateral ventricles

▷ Widened cortical sulci

▷ Diffuse decrease in volume of white and gray matter

▷ Decreased volume of temporal lobe

▷ Decreased volume in hippocampus, amygdala, and thalamus (Sadock, Sadock, & Ruiz, 2015)

► Abnormalities noted in functional studies

▷ Hypofrontality

▷ Decreased cerebral blood flow and metabolism

▷ Diffuse hypometabolic action in cortical–subcortical circuitry

Differential Diagnosis

► Nonpsychiatric disorders

▷ Epilepsy

▷ CNS neoplasm

▷ AIDS

▷ Acute intermittent porphyria

▷ B_{12} deficiency

▷ Heavy-metal poisoning

▷ Huntington's disease

▷ Neurosyphilis

▷ Systemic lupus erythematosus

▷ Wernicke-Korsakoff syndrome

▷ Wilson's disease

▶ Psychiatric disorders

▷ Bipolar affective disorder

▷ Substance-induced psychotic disorder

▶ Amphetamines

▶ Hallucinogens

▶ Alcoholic hallucinosis

▶ Barbiturate withdrawal

▶ Cocaine

▶ PCP (phencyclidine or angel dust)

▷ Mood disorders with psychotic features (see Chapter 9)

▷ Schizoaffective disorder (see below)

▷ Schizophreniform disorder (see below)

▷ Brief psychotic disorder (see below)

▷ Delusional disorder (see below)

▷ Schizotypal personality disorder (see Chapter 14)

▷ Schizoid personality disorder (see Chapter 14)

▷ Paranoid personality disorder (see Chapter 14)

Clinical Management

▶ Assess for acuity level

▷ During acute psychotic episodes, client may require brief hospitalization to

▶ Ensure client safety,

▶ Rapidly stabilize client's symptom level in a controlled environment, and/or

▶ Monitor treatment adherence with the goal of stabilization and recovery.

▶ Clinical management during nonacute episodes occurs most often in community settings.

TABLE 11–4.
ATYPICAL ANTIPSYCHOTICS

AGENT	BRAND NAME	DOSAGE FORMS; DAILY DOSAGE	SIDE EFFECTS	COMMENTS
Clozapine	Clozaril	Tablet or oral disintegrated tablet; 25–900 mg/d	*Common:* Tachycardia, drowsiness, dizziness, hypersalivation (sialorrhea), weight gain, hyperlipidemia *Rare:* Agranulocytosis, myocarditis, neuroleptic malignant syndrome	Only drug for treatment-resistant schizophrenia Must be enrolled in a clozapine risk evaluation and management strategy program (clozapine REMS program) Risk for neutropenia is monitored by the absolute neutrophil count (ANC) only, not in conjunction with the white blood cell count During first 6 months: weekly; during second 6 months: every 2 weeks; then monthly if ANC normal ANC levels less than 500/µl suspend drug Clients can be rechallenged if the prescriber determines benefits outweigh the risks Monitor for myocarditis Dose-related seizure risk Significant weight gain and risk of diabetes Rare hyperprolactinemia Monitor weight, body mass index (BMI), waist circumference Monitor serum lipids and glucose Assess family and personal history of cardiovascular disease
Quetiapine	Seroquel and Seroquel XR	Tablet; 50–800 mg/d	*Common:* Sedation and hypotension (orthostatic hypotension), weight gain *Rare:* Cataract formation	Transient and asymptomatic elevated liver function tests (LFTs) Monitor for cataract development Divided doses: b.i.d. or t.i.d. No prolactin elevation Monitor weight, BMI, waist circumference Monitor serum lipids and glucose Assess family and personal history of cardiovascular disease

Drug	Brand names	Formulation/dosage	Side effects	Monitoring/considerations
Olanzapine	Zyprexa, Zyprexa Zydis, Zyprexa Relprevv	Tablet and intramuscular injection (acute); 5–20 mg/d. Injection; 150–405 mg every 2–4 weeks	Sedation, weight gain, hyperlipidemia, elevated glucose, elevated LFTs, mild prolactin elevation. Long-acting preparation (Zyprexa Relprevv) requires that clients be monitored for 3 hours postinjection due to risk of postinjection delirium sedation syndrome	Significant weight gain. Monitor weight, BMI, waist circumference. Monitor serum lipids and glucose. Assess family and personal history of cardiovascular disease
Risperidone	Risperdal, Risperdal Consta	Tablet, liquid, and orally disintegrated tablets; 2–8 mg. Injectable; 25–50 mg IM every 2 weeks	Hypotension, galactorrhea, nausea, insomnia	Doses >6 mg associated with a higher incidence of extrapyramidal symptoms. Less weight gain than with clozapine or olanzapine. Greatest prolactin elevation among atypical psychotics. Monitor weight, BMI, waist circumference. Monitor serum lipids and glucose. Assess family and personal history of cardiovascular disease
Ziprasidone	Geodon	Tablets; 40–200 mg/d. Injectable; 10–20 mg IM (acute treatment)	Hypotension, sedation, dizziness. *Rare:* Prolongation of QTc interval, skin reaction, drug reaction with eosinophilia and systemic symptoms (DRESS)	Requires QTc monitoring. Avoid coadministration with other drugs known to prolong QTc. Taking with food increases absorption twofold. Use caution when administering with clients at risk for hypokalemia, hypomagnesemia, after myocardial infarction, or with congestive heart failure. Monitor weight, BMI, waist circumference. Monitor serum lipids and glucose. Assess family and personal history of cardiovascular disease

CONTINUED

AGENT	BRAND NAME	DOSAGE FORMS; DAILY DOSAGE	SIDE EFFECTS	COMMENTS
Paliperidone	Invega, Invega Sustenna (monthly injection) Invega Trinza (3-month injection)	Tablets; 3–12 mg/d Injection; 39 mg–234 IM Injection every three months; 273 mg, 410 mg, 546 mg, or 819 mg IM	Orthostatic hypotension, hyperprolactinemia, GI upset, dizziness, headache	Extended-release risperidone
Aripiprizole	Abilify	Tablets; 5–30 mg/d Injection (acute agitation); 5.25–15 mg IM, (long-acting) or 200–400 mg IM monthly	Headache, agitation, anxiety, insomnia, somnolence, akathisia, gastrointestinal (GI) problems	Is a partial agonist of D2 receptors Monitor weight, BMI, waist circumference Monitor serum lipids and glucose Assess family and personal history of cardiovascular disease
Iloperidone	Fanapt	12–24 mg/day in divided doses	Orthostatic hypotension, sedation, dizziness	Titrate slowly due to the alpha 1 antagonist properties Might be helpful for posttraumatic stress disorder hyperarousal symptoms due to alpha 1 blocking Monitor weight, BMI, waist circumference Monitor serum lipids and glucose Assess family and personal history of cardiovascular disease

Asenapine	Saphris	5–10 mg p.o. b.i.d. sublingual	Akathisia, somnolence	Monitor weight, BMI, waist circumference Monitor serum lipids and glucose Assess family and personal history of cardiovascular disease
Lurasidone	Latuda	40–160 mg daily	Akathisia, sedation, and nausea	Should be taken with food to increase absorption Use with caution at lower doses in clients with renal and hepatic impairment Monitor weight, BMI, waist circumference Monitor serum lipids and glucose Assess family and personal history of cardiovascular disease
Brexpiprazole	Rexulti	2–4 mg p.o. once daily	Akathisia, weight gain	Monitor serum lipids and glucose Assess family and personal history of cardiovascular disease (July 2015 approval)
Cariprazine	Vraylar	1.5–6 mg p.o. daily	EPSE, akathesia, gl upset, restlessness, somnolence	Monitor serum lipids and glucose Assess family and personal history of cardiovascular disease (September 2015 approval)
Aripiprazole lauroxil	Aristada	Once a month IM injection; 441 mg, 662 mg, or 882 mg	Akathisia	Monitor serum lipids and glucose Assess family and personal history of cardiovascular disease (October 2015 approval)

Note. All atypical antipsychotic medications have a warning: increase in mortality in older adults with dementia-related psychosis

Pharmacological Management

▶ Pharmacological therapy is the primary treatment modality, augmented by nonpharmacological treatments.

▶ Most clients will require lifelong medication.

▶ Client and family education is important for treatment adherence.

▶ Adjunctive medications may be used to achieve full symptom control:

▷ Antidepressants

▷ Anxiolytics

▷ Anticonvulsants

▶ *Atypical antipsychotics* (see Table 11–4)

▷ Primary first-line treatment agents

▷ First introduced in the 1990s

▷ Have fewer significant neurological side effects compared to typical antipsychotic medication

▷ Effectively treat positive *and* negative symptoms

▷ Function as serotonin-dopamine antagonists (SDAs)

▶ D_2 and 5HT2a blockade

▷ Expensive (some generics now available)

▷ Fewer clinically significant side effects related to EPS and TD compared to typical antipsychotics

▶ Can cause extrapyramidal side effects (EPSE; see five common types in Table 11–5) but with lower risk compared to typical antipsychotics

▶ Lower incidence of tardive dyskinesia (TD; see below).

▷ Improved compliance

▷ Mode of action:

▶ In addition to the dopaminergic blockade found in first-generation antipsychotics, second-generation drugs capitalize on the interplay between dopamine and serotonin. Serotonin binds to 5HT2a heteroreceptors on dopamine (DA) neurons, thus further shutting off release of DA. By antagonizing (blocking) the 5HT2a heteroreceptors on DA neurons, DA release in the nigrostriatal, tuberoinfundibular, and mesocortical pathways is enhanced.

▶ *Dopamine pathways:* These explain both the therapeutic effects *and* the side effects of the atypical antipsychotics.

▷ *Mesolimbic pathway:* SDAs block dopamine in this pathway, causing decreased positive symptoms.

▷ *Mesocortical pathway:* SDAs increase dopamine in this pathway, causing decreased negative symptoms.

TABLE 11–5.
EXTRAPYRAMIDAL SIDE EFFECTS (EPSE)

SIDE EFFECT	DEFINITION
Akathisia	Motor restlessness; inability to remain still; rocking, pacing, or constant motion of unilateral limb; also can manifest as a subjective sense of restlessness without objective finding *Note:* Often mistaken for increasing anxiety
Akinesia	Absence of movement, difficulty initiating motion, subjective feeling of lack of motivation to move *Note:* Often mistaken for laziness or lack of interest
Dystonia	Muscle spasm; spasticity of muscle group, especially back or neck muscles; subjectively painful *Note:* Often mistaken for agitation or unusual, stereotypic movements characteristic of schizophrenia
Pseudo-Parkinson's	Presence of symptoms of Parkinson's disease produced by D2 blockade; includes shuffling gait, motor slowing, mask-like facial expression, pill-rolling, tremors, and muscle rigidity *Note:* Mask-like facial expression often confused as affective blunting or flattening
Tardive dyskinesia	Involuntary abnormal muscle movement of the mouth, tongue, face, and jaw that may progress to limbs; can be irreversible; can occur as an acute process at initiation of medications or as a chronic condition at any point in treatment

▷ *Nigrostriatal pathway:* Dopamine has a reciprocal relationship with acetylcholine (ACh). When serotonin is blocked by the SDA, dopamine increases; therefore, ACh decreases, which causes decreased EPSE. (EPSE is caused by increased ACh.)

▷ *Tuberoinfundibular pathway:* Dopamine inhibits prolactin. The blockade of dopamine by SDAs cause prolactin to increase, causing galactorrhea and gynecomastia.

▶ Hyperprolactinemia associated with the antipsychotics may cause sexual problems, galactorrhea, amenorrhea, gynecomastia, and bone demineralization in postmenopausal women not on estrogen.

▶ *Typical antipsychotics* (first-generation; see Table 11–6)

▷ Cross-classified as neuroleptics because of significant side effects

▷ First introduced in the 1950s

▷ Useful for treating positive symptoms by blocking dopamine in the mesolimbic pathway

▷ Can make negative symptoms worse by blocking dopamine in the mesocortical pathway

▷ Therapeutic effect related primarily to D_2 receptor blockade

▷ Generic (inexpensive)

▷ Can be used as sustained-released injectable agents

▶ Decanoate long-acting injectable dose forms of typical antipsychotics:

▷ Prolixin-D (limited availability due to low production)

▷ Haldol-D

TABLE 11–6.
TYPICAL ANTIPSYCHOTICS

AGENT	BRAND NAME	DOSAGE FORMS; DAILY DOSAGE	SIDE EFFECTS	COMMENTS
Chlorpromazine	Thorazine	Tablet, SR, liquid; 50–2,000 mg/d	*High:* Sedation, hypotension *Moderate:* EPSE, anticholinergic	Allergic dermatitis Photosensitivity ECG changes—QTc monitoring
Mesoridazine	Serentil	Tablet, liquid, injection; 100–400 mg/d	*High:* Anticholinergic, sedation, hypotension *Low:* EPSE	ECG changes—QTc monitoring
Thioridazine	Mellaril	Tablet, liquid; 50–800 mg/d	*High:* Anticholinergic, sedation, hypotension, prolonged QT interval *Low:* EPS	ECG changes—QTc monitoring Irreversible retinal pigmentation at doses >800 mg/d Decreased libido Retrograde ejaculation
Fluphenazine	Permitil Prolixin	Tablet, liquid, injection; 2–40 mg/d, 12.5–75 mg/IM every 2 weeks (decanoate)	*Very high:* EPSE *Low:* Anticholinergic, sedation, hypotension	
Perphenazine	Trilafon	Tablet, liquid, injection; 8–64 mg/d	*High:* EPSE *Low:* Anticholinergic, sedation, hypotension	
Trifluoperazine	Stelazine	Tablet, injection; 5–80 mg/d	*High:* EPSE *Low:* Anticholinergic, sedation, hypotension	
Haloperidol	Haldol	Tablet, liquid, injection; 2–40 mg/d, 50–300 mg IM, every month (decanoate)	*Very high:* EPSE *High:* Anticholinergic, sedation *Low:* Hypotension	In older adults, monitor for oculogyric crisis and pneumonia
Loxapine	Loxitane	Capsule, liquid; 20–250/d	*High:* EPSE *Moderate:* Sedation, hypotension *Low:* Anticholinergic	
Molindone	Moban	Tablet, liquid; 50–225 mg/d	*High:* EPSE *Low:* Anticholinergic, hypotension *Very low:* sedation	Little or no weight gain
Thiothixene	Navane	Capsule, liquid, injection ; 5–60 mg/d	*High:* EPSE *Low:* Anticholinergic, sedation, hypotension	

▷ *High potency:* Have a greater risk of EPSE but less risk of sedation and anticholinergic symptoms

▷ *Low potency:* Have a greater risk of sedation and anticholinergic side effects but less risk of EPSE

▷ Caffeine and nicotine cause diminished antipsychotic effect; dose may need to be higher

TABLE 11–7.
MEDICATIONS USED TO TREAT EPSE

EFFECTIVE DRUG; CROSS-CLASSIFICATION	AKINESIA	AKATHISIA	DYSTONIA	PSEUDO-PARKINSON'S	TARDIVE DYSKINESIA
Cogentin (benztropine) 0.5 mg–2 mg p.o. t.i.d.; *Anticholinergic*	X	X	X	X	
Kemadrin (procyclidine) 2.5 mg–5 mg p.o. b.i.d.–q.i.d.; *Anticholinergic*	X	X	X	X	Best treatment strategy is prevention through careful monitoring.
Artane (trihexyphenidyl) 2–5 mg p.o. t.i.d.; *Anticholinergic*	X	X	X	X	
Benadryl (diphenhydramine) 25 mg p.o. q.i.d.; *Antihistamine*	X		X	X	
Symmetrel (amantadine) 100–200 mg p.o. b.i.d.; *Dopamine agonist*	X			X	
Inderal (propranolol) 20–40 mg p.o. t.i.d.; *Beta blocker*		X			If present, treat by reducing current dose, or change client to atypical agent.
Catapres (clonidine) 0.1 mg p.o. t.i.d.; *Alpha 2 agonist*		X			
Klonopin (clonazepam) 1 mg p.o. b.i.d.; *Benzodiazepine*		X	X		
Ativan (lorazepam) 1 mg p.o. t.i.d.; *Benzodiazepine*		X	X		

▷ Because of multiple clinically significant side effects, are not considered first-line treatment agents

▶ Side effects leading to poor adherence

▶ High client teaching needs

▶ EPSE most common side effect (see Table 11–6)

    ▷ Caused by D_2 receptor antagonism (when dopamine receptors are blocked, ACh increases, which causes EPSE; a reciprocal relationship exists between ACh and dopamine)

    ▷ Treated by use of anti-Parkinson drugs (cross-classified; see Table 11–7)

        ▶ Anticholinergics

        ▶ Antihistamines

        ▶ Dopamine agonists

        ▶ Benzodiazepines (BNZs)

    ▷ Tardive dyskinesia (TD)

        ▶ TD is a potentially irreversible movement disorder that may occur in people who are treated for more than 1 year with typical antipsychotics.

        ▶ Symptoms consist of abnormal, involuntary movements such as lip smacking, chewing, tongue protrusion, or twisting movements of the trunk or limbs.

        ▶ Perioral movements are most common.

        ▶ Treatment involves discontinuation of the offending agent and often starting an atypical antipsychotic.

▷ Clients on typical antipsychotics should have routine abnormal involuntary muscle movement screening (see below) every 6 months.

▶ Client and family education on the detection of early signs and symptoms of abnormal movements

▶ If abnormal movements are noted, consider reducing the dosage or switching to an atypical antipsychotic.

▶ Risk factors include

    ▷ Long-term treatment with neuroleptics

    ▷ Older age

    ▷ Female gender

    ▷ Presence of mood or cognitive disorder

▶ Assessment of abnormal movement rating scales

    ▷ Abnormal Involuntary Movement Scale (AIMS)

    ▷ Dyskinesia Identification System Condensed User Scale (DISCUS)

    ▷ Simpson-Angus Rating Scale (SAS)

- ▶ Neuroleptic malignant syndrome (NMS)
  - ▷ Rare but potentially life-threatening
  - ▷ Can occur at any point during treatment.
  - ▷ Most common with typical but has been reported with atypical antipsychotics
  - ▷ Risk factors include
    - ▶ Rapid dose escalation
    - ▶ Use of high-potency typical antipsychotic
    - ▶ Parenteral administration of antipsychotics
  - ▷ Assess for the following abnormal labs:
    - ▶ Elevated CPK (creatine phosphokinase)
    - ▶ Elevated WBCs (white blood cell count)
    - ▶ Elevated LFTs (liver function tests)
  - ▷ Assess for symptoms known to occur first:
    - ▶ Altered sensorium
    - ▶ Hyperthermia
    - ▶ Hyperreflexia
  - ▷ Assess for symptoms of autonomic instability:
    - ▶ Hypotension
    - ▶ Extreme muscular rigidity
    - ▶ Hyperthermia
    - ▶ Tachycardia
    - ▶ Diaphoresis
    - ▶ Tachypnea
    - ▶ Coma and potentially death
- ▶ Treatment
  - ▷ Seek immediate medical care for treatment
  - ▷ Discontinue antipsychotic medication(s)
  - ▷ Administration of Dantrium (dantrolene) or Parlodel (bromocriptine) for antipsychotic inducted dopamine receptor blockade
  - ▷ Antipyretic (Acetaminophen) and cooling blanket for hyperthermia
  - ▷ Intravenous hydration
  - ▷ Benzodiazepine for muscular rigidity (catatonic symptoms)
- ▷ Other common side effects related to effects on receptors other than dopamine:
  - ▶ Alpha adrenergic blockade
    - ▷ Cardiovascular side effects
    - ▷ Orthostatic hypotension

▶ Muscarinic cholinergic blockade

▷ Dry mouth

▷ Blurred vision

▷ Constipation

▷ Urinary retention

▶ Endocrine side effects

▷ Weight gain

▷ Increased prolactin levels

▶ Neurological side effects

▷ Lowering of seizure threshold

▶ Other side effects

▷ Photosensitivity

▷ Agranulocytosis

Nonpharmacological Management

▶ Individual therapy

▷ Usually supportive rather than insight-oriented

▶ Focuses on establishing reality testing

▶ Builds daily-life skills

▶ Assists client in establishing and meeting life goals

▷ Cognitive behavioral therapy (CBT) for management of hallucinations and delusions.

▶ Group therapy

▷ Focuses on problem-solving

▷ Focuses on education

▶ Medication groups

▶ Life skills groups

▶ Proactive crisis management planning to deal with potential relapse needs

▷ Identify symptom triggers.

▷ Identify symptoms that indicate relapse.

▷ Identify past pattern of relapse to help predict future relapses.

▷ Identify self-care interventions.

▷ Identify point at which professional intervention is required.

▷ Identify support network of family and friends.

▷ Identify other resources to be mobilized when symptom level increases.

▶ Assertive community treatment (ACT)

▷ Evidence-based case management program

▷ Multidisciplinary treatment team

- ▶ Illness management recovery (IMR)

  - ▷ Evidence-based recovery program

- ▶ Education modules

  - ▷ Recovery strategies, information on mental illness, building supports, using medication, drugs and alcohol, coping, reducing relapse, mental health system, advocacy, and stress-vulnerability model (Whitley, Gingerick, Lutz, & Mueser, 2009).

- ▶ Milieu therapy

  - ▷ Provides for structure and safety needs

  - ▷ Provides socialization and interpersonal support

  - ▷ Encourages independency

- ▶ Client and family education

  - ▷ Explain underlying pathology of illness.

  - ▷ Discuss signs and symptoms.

  - ▷ Assist in identifying strategies for living with illness.

  - ▷ Assist in understanding and making decisions about care options.

  - ▷ Develop relapse prevention plan.

  - ▷ Promote overall health.

Common Comorbidities

- ▶ Rates of substance abuse and dependency are high.

  - ▷ 20% to 40% comorbidity

- ▶ Nicotine dependence is especially high.

  - ▷ 80% to 90% comorbidity

  - ▷ Tend to use cigarettes with highest nicotine content

- ▶ Drug interaction with antipsychotic medications

  - ▷ May need to reduce doses when client quits or cuts back.

- ▶ Other common psychiatric comorbidities are anxiety disorders (see Chapter 10), especially panic disorder and obsessive–compulsive disorder.

General Health Considerations

- ▶ Schizophrenia is significantly associated with shorter-than-expected life span when compared to the general population.

- ▶ Persons with a severe mental illness (SMI) prematurely lose 10 to 25 years of life compared to the general population.

  - ▷ Reasons are unclear but may include overall general lack of routine health care and high levels of comorbidity (see below)

- ▶ Suicide

  - ▷ Suicide rates are high; assess for suicidal ideations at every visit.

  - ▷ 10% commit suicide.

▷ 20% to 40% attempt suicide.

▷ Known risk factors for suicide include

▶ Male gender

▶ Ages 45 or younger

▶ Presence of depressive symptoms

▶ Hopelessness

▶ Unemployed

▶ Noncompliance

▶ Recent hospitalization

▶ Postpsychotic period

▶ Comorbid substance abuse

▶ General medical illnesses

▷ Clients need access to ongoing primary care.

▷ High rates of cardiometabolic illnesses

▷ Monitor client for development of metabolic syndrome, diabetes, hypertension, hyperlipidemia, respiratory illnesses, and cardiac illnesses.

▶ Monitor weight gain, lipids, and blood glucose.

▶ Provide weight management and nutritional assistance.

▶ Use the body mass index (BMI) as the accepted standard for determining if a client's weight places him or her at risk of developing serious health problems.

▶ BMI categories

▷ *Underweight:* BMI 18.5 or less

▷ *Normal weight:* BMI 18.5–24.9

▷ *Overweight:* BMI 25.0–29.9

▷ *Obese:* BMI 30.0–39.9

▷ *Severely obese:* BMI 40 and higher.

▶ Risks related to BMI

▷ Clients who are overweight to obese as determined by BMI have

▶ 2.9 times increased risk for diabetes

▶ 2.9 times increased risk for hypertension

▶ 2.1 times increased risk of coronary artery disease

▶ 3.0 times increased risk for endometrial cancer

▶ 2.7 times increased risk for colon cancer

Life Span Considerations

▶ Children

▷ Hallucinatory and delusional content less rich, elaborate, and bizarre

▷ Visual hallucinations more common than auditory

▶ Older adults

▷ More women than men with rare late onset

▷ Although exhibiting prodromal social isolation, are more often married

▷ Prognosis usually better; more responsive to medications due to dominance of positive symptom cluster (see below)

▷ Black box warning on all atypical antipsychotic medications: increase in mortality in older adults with dementia-related psychosis

▷ Risk factors

▶ Postmenopausal states

▶ Presence of human leukocyte antigen

▶ Positive family history

▷ Symptoms

▶ Predominance of positive symptoms

▶ High levels of persecutory delusions and hallucinations

▶ Lower levels of disorganized behavior

▶ Preservation of social and occupational interest

▶ Fewer negative symptoms

Follow-up

▶ Chronic illness

▷ Usually requires lifelong treatment

▷ Case management necessary to coordinate aspects of care.

▶ Relapse periods

▷ Develop relapse plan with client and family.

▶ Multiple health needs

▷ Perform frequent assessment of general health status.

▷ Address comorbid nicotine addiction.

▶ Preventative care

▷ Monitor routine labs to screen for complications of treatment:

▶ Serum glucose and lipid panels

▶ Weight, BMI, and waist-to-hip ratio

▶ Liver and kidney function (based on medication)

▶ Complete blood count

▶ American Diabetes Association, American Psychiatric Association, American Association of Clinical Endocrinologists, & North American Association for the Study of Obesity ADA APA SGA Guidelines (2004)

▶ Perform annual eye exam if on typical antipsychotic agent or Seroquel (quetiapine)

    ▷ Clinical outcome measures

        ▶ Standardized rating scales include:

            ▷ Positive and Negative Syndrome Scale (PANNS)

            ▷ Brief Psychiatric Rating Scale (BPRS)

            ▷ Scale for Assessment of Positive Symptoms (SAPS)

            ▷ Scale for Assessment of Negative Symptoms (SANS)

SCHIZOPHRENIFORM DISORDER

Description

▶ Closely resembles schizophrenia

▶ Two differences from schizophrenia:

    ▷ Total duration of the illness is at least 1 month but less than 6 months, including prodrome, active illness period, and residual symptom phase

    ▷ Does not require impaired social or occupational functioning for diagnosis, although these may be present

Etiology

▶ Similar to schizophrenia

Demographics

▶ Little is known

▶ Fivefold increase in men than women

▶ Lifetime prevalence rate of 0.11 percent

Risk Factors

▶ Similar to schizophrenia

Prevention and Screening

▶ Identification of individuals at high risk and monitoring

▶ Relative with Schizophrenia and Bipolar Disorder

Assessment

History

▶ Assess for the following:

▷ Two or more of the following frequently present during a 1-month period

▶ Delusions

▶ Hallucinations

▶ Disorganized speech

▶ Grossly disorganized behavior

▶ Presence of negative symptoms

▷ Duration of symptoms for at least 1 month and for no longer than 6 months

▷ Almost all information provided for schizophrenia pertains to this disorder, except:

▶ Occurs much less often than schizophrenia; incidence is 0.03% of general U.S. population.

▶ Approximately one-third recover completely within 6 months.

▶ Remaining two-thirds develop schizophrenia or schizoaffective disorder (see below).

Physical Exam Findings

▶ Similar to schizophrenia

Mental Status Exam Findings

▶ Similar to schizophrenia

Diagnostic and Laboratory Findings

▷ Similar to schizophrenia

Clinical Management

▶ Similar to schizophrenia

▶ Assess for acuity level.

▶ During acute psychotic or affective episodes, client may require brief hospitalization to

▷ Ensure client safety.

▷ Rapidly stabilize client's symptom level in a controlled environment.

▷ Ensure client compliance with treatment to reach stabilization.

▶ Clinical management during nonacute episodes occurs most often in community settings.

Pharmacological Management

▶ Similar to schizophrenia

Nonpharmacological Management

▶ Similar to schizophrenia

Follow-up

▶ Similar to schizophrenia

SCHIZOAFFECTIVE DISORDER

Description

▶ An uninterrupted period of illness in which the person experiences psychotic symptoms similar to those seen in schizophrenia as well as mood symptoms similar to major depressive disorder (MDD) or bipolar (BP) disorder (see Chapter 9).

Etiology

▶ Cause is unknown

▶ The disorder may be a psychotic spectrum disorder, mood spectrum disorder, or both

Prevalence and Demographics

▶ Less than 1%.

▶ Equal number males and females.

▶ Depressed type of the disorder is more common in older persons.

▶ Men with the disorder tend to exhibit more antisocial behaviors.

Risk Factors

▶ Family history of schizophrenia or bipolar disorder

Prevention and Screening

▶ Screening persons with a positive family history

Assessment

History

▶ Assess for the following:

▶ Symptoms of schizophrenia—two or more of the following frequently present during a 1-month period:

▷ Delusions

▷ Hallucinations

▷ Disorganized speech

- ▷ Grossly disorganized behavior
- ▷ Presence of negative symptoms but usually less severe than those in schizophrenia
- ▶ Symptoms of one or more of mood disorders (see Chapter 9):
  - ▷ Major depressive episode
  - ▷ Manic episode
  - ▷ Mixed-mood episode
- ▶ Presence of delusions or hallucinations for at least 2 weeks in the absence of prominent mood symptoms
- ▶ Subtypes
  - ▷ Two subtypes differentiated by type of mood-related symptoms:
    - ▶ *Depressive*: When prominent mood symptoms are of the depressive type only
    - ▶ *Bipolar*: When predominant mood symptoms are manic or mixed type

Physical Exam Findings

- ▶ Similar to schizophrenia

Mental Status Exam Findings

- ▶ Similar to schizophrenia

Diagnostic and Laboratory Findings

- ▶ Similar to schizophrenia

Clinical Management

Pharmacological Management

- ▶ Similar to schizophrenia
- ▶ Similar to MDD or BP disorder (see Chapter 9)

Nonpharmacological Management

- ▶ Similar to schizophrenia
- ▶ Similar to MDD or BP disorder (see Chapter 9)

Follow-up

- ▶ Similar to schizophrenia
- ▶ Similar to MDD or BP disorder (see Chapter 9)

DELUSIONAL DISORDER

Description

▶ Presence of one or more nonbizarre delusions lasting for at least 1 month

▶ Psychosocial functioning and daily behavior not at all impaired except as they surround content of delusion

▶ Seldom any other symptoms; in rare cases may have hallucinations or mood disturbances

Etiology

▶ Cause is unknown

Prevalence and Demographics

▶ 0.2% to 0.3% of population in the United States

▶ Mean onset is about 40 years of age

▶ Men are more likely to have paranoid delusions

▶ Women are more likely to have delusions of erotomania

Risk Factors

▶ Person with disorders of the limbic system and basal ganglia

Prevention and Screening

▶ Unknown

Assessment

History

▶ Assess for the following:

▷ Presence of delusions

▶ Well-organized and potentially believable

▶ Any unusual behavior is explainable if content of delusion understood

▷ Subtypes (categorized by thematic content of delusion)

▶ Erotomanic

▷ Delusional content focused on false belief that another person is in love with the client

▷ Usually focused on idealized or spiritual love and only infrequently has strong sexual content

- ▷ Focus of love usually a famous or powerful person who does not usually know the client
  - ▶ In rare cases, person may know client
- ▷ Leads to obsessive behaviors such as surveillance or stalking
- ▶ Grandiose
  - ▷ Delusional content focuses on the client having some great talent, skill, or knowledge
  - ▷ May have strong religious component, such as prophecy or deity connections (special connection to God)
- ▶ Jealous
  - ▷ Delusional content focuses on false belief that client's spouse or partner is being unfaithful with someone else.
  - ▷ Belief has no connection with realistic evidence.
  - ▷ Usually seen in men.
  - ▷ Client may try to control behavior of spouse or partner in an attempt to prevent imagined infidelities.
- ▶ Persecutory
  - ▷ Delusional content focuses on clients' belief that others are out to harm them, spy on them, or otherwise do them harm
  - ▷ Often angry and hostile at perceived persecution
- ▶ Somatic
  - ▷ Delusional content focuses on bodily functions and sensations
  - ▷ Often belief that a body part is infected, absent, emits a strange odor, or is misshapen or malformed.
- ▶ Mixed
  - ▷ No clear predominant theme for the delusional content
- ▷ Related symptoms that can be present but are not required for diagnosis include
  - ▶ May become depressed over protracted problems with thematic content
  - ▶ May become involved in legal difficulties related to behaviors based on delusional content
  - ▶ May be subjected to or request unnecessary medical tests and procedures

Physical Exam Findings

- ▶ Nonspecific

Mental Status Exam Findings

- ▶ Normal except for delusions
  - ▷ Abstraction
    - ▶ May be concrete on proverbs during delusional episodes

▷ Thought process

► Presence of delusions

► Perseveration on topics related to delusion

▷ Thought content

► Thematic for type of delusion

Diagnostic and Laboratory Findings

► Nonspecific

Clinical Management

Pharmacological Management

► Similar to schizophrenia

Nonpharmacological Management

► Similar to schizophrenia

BRIEF PSYCHOTIC DISORDER

Description

► Disorder with sudden onset of psychotic symptoms lasting at least 1 day but less than a month

Etiology

► Unknown cause

Incidence and Demographics

► Unknown incidence

► Occurs more in younger clients (20 to 30 years of age)

Risk Factors

► Family history of psychotic disorder

Prevention and Screening

► Unknown

Assessment

History

- ▶ Assess for the following:
  - ▷ Age of onset in adolescence or early adulthood
  - ▷ Positive-type psychotic symptoms:
    - ▶ Delusions
    - ▶ Hallucinations
    - ▶ Grossly disorganized behavior
    - ▶ Disorganized speech
  - ▷ Can occur with or without identified stressor
  - ▷ Person always returns to premorbid level of functioning

Physical Exam Findings

- ▶ Nonspecific

Mental Status Exam Findings

- ▶ Similar to schizophrenia

Diagnostic and Laboratory Findings

- ▶ Nonspecific

Clinical Management

Pharmacological Management

- ▶ Similar to schizophrenia

Nonpharmacological Management

- ▶ Similar to schizophrenia
- ▶ Acute episode requires frequent monitoring for safety needs because of the following:
  - ▷ Confusion
  - ▷ Rapid shifting in emotions
  - ▷ Impaired judgment
  - ▷ Inability to meet nutritional and hygiene needs

SHARED PSYCHOTIC DISORDER (FOLIE Á DEUX)

Description

- ▶ Characterized by development of a delusion in a client who has a close relationship with another person who already has a psychotic disorder with a prominent delusion

Etiology

▶ Cause is unknown

Incidence and Demographics

▶ Unknown

Risk Factors

▶ Unknown

Prevention and Screening

▶ Unknown

Assessment

History

▶ Assess for the following:
  ▷ Client in close contact with a person who already has a delusion and
    ▶ That person usually has schizophrenia.
    ▶ That person usually is the dominant person in the relationship.
    ▶ That person gradually imposes his or her delusion on the client.
    ▶ Usually the relationship is long-term and very close.
  ▷ Aside from the delusional content, the client's behavior is otherwise normal.

Physical Exam Findings

▶ Nonspecific

Mental Status Exam Findings

▶ Similar to schizophrenia

Diagnostic and Laboratory Findings

▶ Nonspecific

Clinical Management

Pharmacological Management

▶ Similar to schizophrenia

Nonpharmacological Management

▶ Similar to schizophrenia

▶ Chronic disease course

▶ Poor prognosis if relationship continues, especially if person with delusion goes untreated

▶ Good prognosis if the client can be separated from person with the delusion

CASE STUDY

Casey is a 23-year-old client who has been recently diagnosed with schizophrenia. He experienced his first psychotic break at age 22 while serving in the military. Casey lives at home with his parents and is reluctant to accept his diagnosis, stating "I got bad weed" in the service and "will be fine once the weed leaves my body." He has been adherent with appointments but only intermittently takes his Risperdal (3 mg p.o.) twice a day. His parents are threatening to kick him out of the house if he does not start accepting treatment.

Casey has a history of juvenile-onset diabetes and has struggled to maintain a diabetic diet and to control his weight. When asked to identify his current goals, Casey wishes to find a good wife, have children, and settle down to a normal life. There are many issues to consider in planning care with this client.

1. What is the top priority for the psychiatric–mental health nurse practitioner (PMHNP)?

2. What medications changes would the PMHNP consider for Casey?

3. What is the relationship between his diabetes and schizophrenia?

4. How will his comorbid illness affect the PMHNP's care planning?

5. What routine ongoing monitoring will he require?

ANSWERS TO CASE STUDY DISCUSSION QUESTIONS

1. The top priority for the PMHNP is to build a therapeutic alliance with Casey

2. Medication changes appropriate for Casey include switching to an alternative atypical antipsychotic medication that has a lower risk for weight gain and elevated glucose levels

3. The relationship between diabetes and schizophrenia is that individuals with schizophrenia have a twofold increase of developing diabetes which is considered an independent risk factor.

4. Because clients with schizophrenia are at high risk for developing cardiometabolic illness as comorbidities, the care plan must address both his physical health, specifically his diabetes management, and his mental health.

5. The routine monitoring required for Casey includes ongoing monitoring for atypical antipsychotic medication should include serum glucose or A1c, lipid profile, and complete blood count, weight, height, body mass index.

REFERENCES AND RESOURCES

American Diabetes Association, American Psychiatric Association, American Association of Clinical Endocrinologists, & North American Association for the Study of Obesity. (2004). Consensus development conference on antipsychotic drugs and obesity and diabetes. *Diabetes Care, 27*(2), 596–601.

American Psychiatric Association. (2013). *Diagnostic and statistical manual of mental disorders* (5th ed.). Washington, DC: Author.

Rector, N. A., & Beck, A. (2002). A clinical review of cognitive therapy for schizophrenia. *Current Psychiatric Reports, 4,* 284–292.

Richardson, C., Faulkner, G., McDevitt, J., Skrinar, G., Hutchinson, D., & Piette, J. (2005). Integrating physical activity into mental health services for persons with serious mental illness. *Psychiatric Services, 56*(3), 324–331.

Sable, J. A. (2002). Antipsychotic treatment for late-life schizophrenia. *Current Psychiatric Reports, 4,* 299–306.

Sadock, B. J., Sadock, V. A., & Ruiz, P. (2015). *Kaplan & Sadock's synopsis of psychiatry: Behavioral sciences/clinical psychiatry* (11th ed.). New York, NY: Wolters Kluwer.

Staal, W. G., Hulshoff Pol, H., Schnack, G., van Haren, N. E., Seifert, N., & Kahn, R. (2001). Structural brain abnormalities in chronic schizophrenia at the extremes of the outcome spectrum. *American Journal of Psychiatry, 158,* 1140–1142.

Stahl, S. M. (2014). *The prescriber's guide Stahl's essential psychopharmacology* (5th ed.). New York, NY: Cambridge University Press.

Tamminga, C. (2001). Treating schizophrenia now and developing strategies for the next decade. *CNS Spectrums, 6,* 987–991.

Tandon, R., & Jibson, M. D. (2001). Pharmacologic treatment of schizophrenia: What the future holds. *CNS Spectrums, 6,* 980–986.

U.S. Food and Drug Administration/Protecting and Promoting Your Health. (2013). *FDA Drug Safety Communication: FDA is investigating two deaths following injection of long-acting antipsychotic Zyprexa Relprevv (olanzapine pamoate)*. Retrieved from www.fda.gov/Drugs/DrugSafety/ucm356971.htm

Whitley, R., Gingerich, S., Lutz, W., & Mueser, K. (2009). Implementing the illness management and recovery program in community mental health settings: Facilitators and barriers. *Psychiatric Services, 60*(2), 202–209.

CHAPTER 12

NEUROCOGNITIVE DISORDERS

Cognitive disorders often are thought of as disorders of older adults. Although most common in this population, cognitive disorders can occur at any age. Very young or very old people with cognitive disorders have multiple health needs. Older adult clients usually have more than one chronic illness, and psychiatric disorders can be accompanied by other comorbidities.

Psychiatric–mental health nurse practitioners (PMHNPs) must approach clients with cognitive disorders by conducting a multisystem assessment.

COGNITIVE DISORDERS

Description

▶ Cognitive disorders cause a clinically significant deficit in cognition that represents a major change from the person's previous baseline level of functioning.

▶ Two common disorders are

▷ Delirium

▷ Dementia

Etiology

▶ Cognitive disorders are a complex general medical condition resulting in changes in multiple domains including memory, interpersonal relationships, and behavior. Cognitive disorders can result from injury, medical condition, substance use or abuse, a reaction to medications or other ingested agents, or a combination of some or all of these factors.

DELIRIUM

Description

▶ Delirium is a syndrome and not a disease, with an acute onset that causes short-term changes in cognition.

► The hallmark symptom is a disturbance of consciousness accompanied by changes in cognition.

► Subtypes of delirium

▷ Hyperactive: Agitated, restless, hyperalert

▷ Hypoactive: Lethargic, slowed, apathetic

▷ Mixed: Cycles between hyperactive and hypoactive

Etiology

► Due to changes in one of the following:

▷ General medical condition

▷ Substance induced

▷ Multiple physical health problems

▷ Medication, sleep deprivation, or other causes

Incidence and Demographics

► Common, especially in older adults

► Often overlooked and mistaken for other medical conditions or dementia

► In persons with psychiatric disorders, often mistaken for worsening of psychotic symptoms instead of a distinct condition

► Prevalence varies based on age, client setting, and sample

▷ Highest in hospitalized older adults

▷ 0.4% in general U.S. population ages 18 years or older

▷ 1% to 2% in those ages 65 or older

▷ 6% to 56% of hospitalized clients

▷ 15% to 53% in postoperative older adults

▷ 70% to 87% of older adults in the intensive care unit

▷ 60% in nursing home patients

▷ 25% in clients with cancer

▷ 80% in terminal clients nearing death

► Poor prognosis

▷ 1 year mortality rate of clients with delirium is up to 40%

Risk Factors

► Advancing age

► Multisystem medical illness

▷ The more physically ill the client, the higher the risk.

▶ Substance abuse

▶ Visual or hearing impairment

▶ Past episode of delirium or preexisting brain disorder or cognitive impairment

Prevention and Screening

▶ At-risk family education

▶ Community education

   ▷ Stigma reduction

   ▷ Signs and symptoms of illness

   ▷ Treatment potential for control of symptoms

▶ Use of the Confusion Assessment Method (CAM) instrument

▶ Early recognition, intervention, and initiation of treatment

   ▷ Whenever a client's clinical presentation changes rapidly from baseline, consider delirium as one possible differential diagnosis.

Assessment

History

▶ Assess for the following:

   ▷ Key findings

      ▶ Disturbance of consciousness develops over a short time, usually hours to days.

      ▶ This disturbance tends to fluctuate during the day.

   ▷ Sleep–rest cycle disturbances

      ▶ Reversal of the sleep–wake cycle is common: clients are awake at night and sleep during the day.

   ▷ Impaired recent and intermediate memory

   ▷ Psychomotor agitation

      ▶ The client exhibits purposeless, random actions.

   ▷ Course of illness may resolve within hours to days

      ▶ The more quickly the underlying physiological disturbance is recognized and treated, the more rapidly the delirium will resolve.

      ▶ Symptoms, when unrecognized, may persist for months.

      ▶ Most symptoms resolve within 3 to 6 months.

Physical Exam Findings

▶ Evidence that significant clinical symptoms are a consequence of direct physiological processes, substance use or abuse, or general medical condition

▶ Usually nonspecific neurological abnormalities

▷ Tremors

▷ Incoordination

▷ Urinary incontinence

▷ Myoclonus

▷ Nystagmus

▷ Asterixis—a flapping motion of the wrists

▷ Increased muscle tone and reflex

Mental Status Exam Findings

▶ General appearance

▷ Unconcerned with appearance

▷ Disheveled

▷ Highly inattentive

▶ Speech

▷ Impaired

▷ Disorganized

▷ Rambling

▷ Incoherent

▷ Slurred

▶ Affect

▷ Rapid, unpredictable shifts in affective state without known precipitation

▶ Lethargic

▶ Agitated

▶ Mood

▷ Difficult to elicit from client

▶ Thought process

▷ Disorganized

▷ Distractible

▷ Perceptual disturbances

▶ Illusions most common

▶ Hallucinations are typically visual and accompanied by illusions

▶ Thought content

▷ Disorganized, distorted thought

▷ Delusions and hallucinations are common.

▶ Orientation

▷ Disorientation is usually the first symptom to appear

▷ Client usually disoriented to time and place

▶ Memory

▷ Impaired recent and immediate memory

▶ Concentration

▷ Grossly impaired

▶ Abstraction

▷ Grossly impaired

▶ Judgment

▷ Grossly impaired

Diagnostic and Laboratory Findings

▶ Findings consistent with underlying physiological etiology

▶ Workup includes standard tests

▷ Blood chemistry

▷ Complete blood count (CBC)

▷ Thyroid function tests

▷ Syphilis

▷ Human immunodeficiency virus (HIV) antibody test

▷ Urinalysis

▷ Chest radiograph

▷ Serum or urine drug screen

▶ Electroencephalogram (EEG) abnormalities

▷ Generalized slowing

▷ Generalized increased activity if delirium is related to alcohol withdrawal

Differential Diagnosis

▶ Dementia (see below)

▶ Substance intoxication or withdrawal (see Chapter 13)

▶ Schizophrenia (see Chapter 11)

▶ Schizophreniform disorder (see Chapter 11)

▶ Mood disorders with psychotic features (see Chapter 9)

Clinical Management

▶ Undertake treatment of underlying condition or disorder.

▶ Avoid the use of new medications whenever possible, because using them can cloud the diagnostic picture.

Pharmacological Management

- ▶ Symptomatic treatment
- ▶ Agitation and psychotic symptoms
  - ▷ Antipsychotic agents
    - ▶ Haloperidol (Haldol)
    - ▶ Atypical antipsychotic agents
    - ▶ Anxiolytic agents for insomnia

Nonpharmacological Management

- ▶ Monitor for safety needs.
- ▶ Determine reality orientation frequently.
- ▶ Pay attention to basic needs:
  - ▷ Hydration
  - ▷ Nutrition
- ▶ Client should be neither sensory-deprived nor overstimulated.
- ▶ It is helpful to have in the client's room familiar people; familiar pictures or decorations; a clock or calendar; and regular orientation to person, place, or time.

General Health Considerations

- ▶ Delirium is associated with high morbidity and mortality.
- ▶ High morbidity results from injury or its associated problems related to inactivity:
  - ▷ Pneumonia
  - ▷ Hydration and nutritional deficits
- ▶ Safety concerns exist.
- ▶ Mnemonic: DELIRIUM (Dick & Morency, 2011)
  - ▷ **D**rugs
  - ▷ **E**lectrolyte abnormality
  - ▷ **L**ow oxygen saturation
  - ▷ **I**nfection
  - ▷ **R**educed sensory input
  - ▷ **I**ntracranial
  - ▷ **U**rinary or renal retention
  - ▷ **M**yocardial

Life Span Considerations

- ▶ Children
  - ▷ Especially susceptible
  - ▷ Related to immature brain development

▷ Often mistaken for uncooperative behavior

 ▶ If a child is not soothed by common methods (e.g., parental presence), delirium is suspected.

  ▷ Most common in febrile states

  ▷ Medications known to affect cognition

   ▶ Especially common with anticholinergic medications

▶ Older adults

 ▷ Susceptibility related to physiological changes of aging

 ▷ Older men more prone than older women for unknown reasons

DEMENTIA

Description

▶ Dementia is a group of disorders characterized by gradual development of multiple cognitive deficits:

 ▷ Impaired executive functioning

 ▷ Impaired global intellect with preservation of level of consciousness

 ▷ Impaired problem-solving

 ▷ Impaired organizational skills

 ▷ Altered memory

▶ Various forms of dementia share common symptoms but have different underlying pathology.

 ▷ Dementia of Alzheimer's type (DAT)

  ▶ Most common type

  ▶ Gradual onset and progressive decline without focal neurological deficits

  ▶ Hallmark amyloid deposits and neurofibrillary tangles

 ▷ Vascular dementia (VD)

  ▶ Second most common type

  ▶ Formerly called *multi-infarct dementia*

  ▶ Primarily caused by cardiovascular disease and characterized by step-type declines

  ▶ Most common in men with preexisting high blood pressure and cardiovascular risk factors

  ▶ Hallmarks: carotid bruits, fundoscopic abnormalities, and enlarged cardiac chambers

 ▷ Dementia due to HIV disease

  ▶ Classified as a subcortical dementia.

  ▶ Parenchymal abnormalities visualized on magnetic resonance imaging (MRI) scan.

▶ HIV-associated neurocognitive disorder or HIV encephalopathy are less severe forms.

▶ HIV can cause many psychiatric symptoms.

▶ Manifests by progressive cognitive decline, motor abnormalities, and behavioral abnormalities.

▶ Co-occurs with obsessive–compulsive disorder, posttraumatic stress disorder, generalized anxiety disorder, depression, and mania.

▶ Development of dementia in client with HIV is an indicator of poor prognosis; death usually occurs within 6 months.

▶ Psychotic symptoms usually occur in late-stage infection.

▶ Clinical signs of late-stage HIV-related dementia include cognitive, motor, behavioral, and affective impairment:

▷ Global cognitive impairment

▷ Mutism

▷ Seizures

▷ Hallucinations

▷ Delusions

▷ Apathy

▷ Mania

▶ Antiretrovirals and protease inhibitors can interact with psychotropic medications, because many are metabolized by the P450 system or are CYP3A4 inhibitors. Therefore, prescribing psychotropic medications in this client population should be done with caution while monitoring for drug interactions.

▷ Pick's disease

▶ Also known as frontotemporal dementia

▶ Neuronal loss, gliosis, and Pick's bodies present

▶ More common in men

▶ Personality and behavioral changes in early stage

▶ Cognitive changes in later stages

▶ Kluver-Bucy syndrome: hypersexuality, hyperorality, and placidity

▷ Creutzfeldt-Jakob disease

▶ Fatal and rapidly progressive disorder

▶ Occurs mainly in adults in middle age or older

▶ Initially manifests with fatigue, flulike symptoms, and cognitive impairment

▶ Later manifests with aphasia, apraxia, emotional lability, depression, mania, psychosis, marked personality changes, and dementia

▶ Death usually occurs within 6 months.

▷ Huntington's disease

▶ Subcortical type of dementia

> ▶ Characterized mostly by motor abnormalities (e.g., choreoathetoid movements)

> ▶ Psychomotor slowing and difficulty with complex tasks

> ▶ Memory, language, and insight usually intact until late stages

> ▶ High incidence of depression and psychosis

▷ Lewy body disease

> ▶ Caused by Lewy inclusion bodies in the cortex

> ▶ Presents with recurrent visual hallucinations

> ▶ Parkinson features (bradykinesia, cogwheel rigidity, tremor)

> ▶ Adversely react to antipsychotics

Etiology

▶ Multiple theories ranging from psychological to neurobiological

  ▷ Probable multifactorial etiological profile

▶ Primary cause mostly unknown

▶ General medical condition, result of substance use or abuse, reaction to medications or other ingested agents, or combination of some or all of these factors

▶ Diffuse cerebral atrophy and enlarged ventricles in DAT

▶ Decreased acetylcholine (ACh) and norepinephrine in DAT

▶ Genetic loading

  ▷ Genes on chromosomes 1, 14, and 21 have been identified in families with a history of DAT.

  ▷ Autosomal dominant trait.

  ▷ Inherited alleles for apolipoprotein E4 (APOE4) on chromosome 19 are suspected to be related to late-onset dementia.

Incidence and Demographics

▶ Often misdiagnosed or unrecognized, especially in early stages and in young clients

▶ Prevalence of 1.6% for people in the United States ages 65 or older

  ▷ 16% to 25% in people ages 85 or older

▶ DAT the most common

  ▷ Affects an estimated 4 million in the United States

  ▷ Duration of illness averages 8 to 10 years

Risk Factors

▶ Age

▶ Multisystem medical illnesses

▶ Genetic loading

▷ Family history of dementia in first-order relative

▶ History of substance use or abuse

Prevention and Screening

▶ At-risk family education

▶ Community education

▷ Stigma reduction

▷ Signs and symptoms of illness

▷ Treatment potential for control of symptoms

▶ Early recognition, intervention, and initiation of treatment

▷ Allows for ruling out age-related memory changes or unidentified conditions

▷ Cognitive and functional evaluation at least every 3 years for people ages 65 or older

▷ Baseline and regular cognitive evaluation to monitor cognitive decline and treatment response to medications in persons diagnosed with dementia

▶ The U.S. Preventive Services Task Force concluded that there is insufficient evidence to determine if the benefits of routine screening outweigh the harms (U.S. Preventive Services Task Force, 2014).

Assessment

History

▶ Assess for the following:

▷ Detailed history of present illness, including time frame, progression, and associated symptoms

▷ Past medical history of hypertension, strokes, head trauma, and psychiatric illness

▷ Psychiatric history of depression, anxiety, and schizophrenia

▷ Social history, including present living situation; marital status; occupation; education; and alcohol, tobacco, or illicit drug use

▷ Medications, including prescription, over-the-counter, herbals, supplements, and home remedies

▷ Initial and periodic functional history and assessment

▷ Validate history with family or caregiver.

▷ Memory impairment—immediate and intermediate

▶ Most prominent feature of disorder

▶ Usually earliest symptom

▶ Produces multiple deficits in daily functioning

▷ Unable to learn new information

> ▷ Forgets past information
>
> ▷ Loses valuables
>
> ▷ Forgets daily activities such as eating and dressing
>
> ▷ Becomes easily lost
>
> ▷ Has other cognitive deficits such as impaired executive functioning

▷ Instruments for assessing level of impairment

- ▶ Not in public domain
  - ▷ Mini-Mental State Examination (MMSE)
- ▶ In public domain
  - ▷ Montreal Cognitive Assessment (MoCA)
  - ▷ Mini-Cog
  - ▷ St Louis University Mental Status Examination (SLUMS)
- ▶ Remember to always consider visual, sensory, language, and physical disabilities as well as education when administering mental status tests.

Physical Exam Findings

- ▶ *Amaurosis fugax*: Unilateral transient vision loss, described as "curtain over eye"
- ▶ Unilateral focal–motor weakness
- ▶ Asymmetrical reflexes

Mental Status Exam Findings

- ▶ General appearance
  - ▷ Apraxia
  - ▷ Decreased self-care activities of daily living
- ▶ Speech
  - ▷ Deterioration of language skills
  - ▷ Aphasia
  - ▷ Circumlocutory phrases
  - ▷ Indefinite object recognition (such as calling items "things" and being unable to find discrete name)
  - ▷ In advanced stages are
    - ▶ Mutism
    - ▶ Echolalia
- ▶ Affect
  - ▷ Lability
- ▶ Mood
  - ▷ Depressed
  - ▷ Often difficult to elicit from client

- ▶ Thought process
  - ▷ Agnosia
- ▶ Thought content
  - ▷ Difficult to elicit from client
- ▶ Orientation
  - ▷ Disoriented to time and place
  - ▷ Disoriented to person in late stages of disorder
- ▶ Memory
  - ▷ Impaired in many dimensions of memory:
    - ▶ Word registration
    - ▶ Recall
    - ▶ Retention
    - ▶ Recognition
- ▶ Concentration
  - ▷ Distractible
- ▶ Abstraction
  - ▷ Concrete on proverb testing
- ▶ Judgment
  - ▷ Grossly impaired for self- and social judgment

Diagnostic and Laboratory Findings

- ▶ CBC, chemistry profile, thyroid function tests, B_{12} level, and folate level to rule out metabolic causes or unidentified conditions
- ▶ Syphilis drug toxicity screening if indicated by history
- ▶ Alcohol and illicit drug screen if suspected or indicated
- ▶ Urinalysis if urinary tract infection suspected
- ▶ Arterial oxygen or pulse oximetry if hypoxemia suspected
- ▶ Computed tomography (CT) or magnetic resonance imaging (MRI) not routinely used
- ▶ EEG not useful
- ▶ Neuropsychological testing recommended to complete diagnostic assessment

Differential diagnosis

- ▶ Nonpsychiatric
  - ▷ Parkinson's disease
  - ▷ Hearing loss
  - ▷ B_{12} and folate deficiencies
  - ▷ Trauma, especially with history of falls

▷ Hypothyroidism

▷ Infection

▷ Cerebrovascular accident

▷ Polypharmacy

▷ Alcohol intoxication

▶ Psychiatric

▷ Mood disorders (see Chapter 9)

▷ Delirium (see above)

▷ Anxiety disorders (see Chapter 10)

Clinical Management

General Considerations

▶ Rule out or treat any conditions that may contribute to cognitive impairment.

▶ Discontinue unnecessary medications, especially sedatives and hypnotics.

Pharmacological Management

▶ Cognitive symptoms

▷ N-methyl D-aspartate glutamate receptor antagonists

▶ Prevent overexcitation of glutamate receptors and stabilize the neurodegenerative process

▶ Memantine (Namenda; 10 to 20 mg b.i.d.)

▷ Moderate to severe Alzheimer's Dementia

▷ May slow the degenerative process

▷ Promotes synaptic plasticity

▷ May be used in combination with cholinesterase inhibitors.

▷ Memantine/Donepezil (Namzric) combination medication)

▷ Cholinesterase inhibitors

▶ May be initiated for mild to moderate Alzheimer's disease

▶ Can lead to modest clinical improvement in some clients, with studies showing 2- to 3-point improvement in mental state exam (MSE) testing

▶ Treat only symptoms, slow loss of function, and may improve agitated behaviors

▶ Do not prevent pathological progression of disease

▶ Not effective in severe, end-stage disease

▶ Should stop if side effects, usually nausea and vomiting, develop

▶ Commonly used agents:

▷ Donepezil (Aricept; 5 to 10 mg/day; Stahl, 2014)

▶ Approved for mild, moderate, and severe Alzheimer's disease

- ▶ Nausea, diarrhea, vomiting, appetite and weight loss, abnormal dreams, insomnia, dizziness common
  - ▷ Rivastigmine tartrate (Exelon; 1.5 to 6 mg twice a day; increase gradually to avoid nausea)
    - ▶ Indicated for mild to moderate Alzheimer's disease and Parkinson's disease dementia (Stahl, 2014)
    - ▶ Transdermal: 4.5, 9.5, or 13.3 mg / 24 hours
    - ▶ Retitrate if a lapse in treatment occurs
- ▶ Psychosis and agitation
  - ▷ Try nonpharmacological therapies first.
  - ▷ Use antipsychotic agents for agitation or psychotic symptoms regularly.
  - ▷ Use lowest effective dose and attempt to wean periodically.
  - ▷ Antipsychotics may cause many side effects of significance in the older adult:
    - ▶ Extrapyramidal symptoms
    - ▶ Sedation
    - ▶ Postural hypotension
    - ▶ Anticholinergic side effects
  - ▷ Benzodiazepines may be used for treating anxiety or infrequent agitation.
- ▶ Depression
  - ▷ Treat clients with depressive symptoms:
    - ▶ Depressed mood
    - ▶ Insomnia
    - ▶ Fatigue
    - ▶ Irritability
    - ▶ Appetite loss
  - ▷ Use lowest effective dose.
  - ▷ Treat for 6 to 12 months, then attempt to taper; depression may reoccur and need to be treated as a chronic condition.
  - ▷ Clients may have less depression as the dementia progresses and they become less aware of their circumstances.

Nonpharmacological Management

- ▶ Educate client and family about the illness, treatment, and community resources.
- ▶ Assist with long-term planning, including financial, legal, and advanced directives.
- ▶ Assess home and driving safety.
- ▶ Use behavioral therapy to identify causes of problem behaviors and changes to the environment to reduce the behavior.
- ▶ Use recreational therapy, art, and pet therapy to reduce agitation and promote normalized behavior.

▶ Use reminiscence therapy or life review to process through any unresolved issues and recollect the past.

▶ Maintain a simple daily routine for bathing, dressing, eating, toileting, and bedtime.

▶ Integrate cultural beliefs into the management of all clients with dementia.

▶ Psychotherapeutic approaches for HIV-related dementia

▷ Major psychodynamic themes for people with HIV-related dementia are issues of guilt, self-esteem, and fear of dying.

▷ Because the client may not be able to give a complete and accurate history, family or friends should be questioned about any unusual behavior or mental status changes.

▷ Changes in the level of activity, in interest in other people, or in personality are clues to an acute central nervous system disturbance.

▷ Some changes are directly due to brain dysfunction, while other changes are due to psychological distress of a systemic problem—anxiety that the person is dying.

▷ The spectrum of neuropsychiatric and neurological manifestations depends on the severity of immunosuppression.

▷ Psychiatric disorders may preexist or result from HIV.

▷ Even subtle neurocognitive impairment can affect psychological coping.

▷ Neuropsychiatric disorders are much more prevalent in late-stage illness.

Life Span Considerations

▶ Primarily a disease of older adults but can occur in children

▷ Diagnosis based on impaired cognition; diagnoses not applicable until ages 4 to 6 years, when cognition can be fully assessed

▷ Dementia in children usually presents as deterioration in functioning, such as school performance or delay in normal development.

MAJOR OR MINOR NEUROCOGNITIVE DISORDER DUE TO TRAUMATIC BRAIN INJURY

Description

▶ DSM-5 diagnostic criteria are not met for a major or minor neurocognitive disorder.

▶ Evidence of a traumatic brain injury—an impact to the head or other mechanism of rapid movement or displacement of the brain within the skull—with one or more of the following:

▷ Loss of consciousness

▷ Posttraumatic amnesia

▷ Disorientation and confusion

▷ Neurological signs (neuroimaging demonstrating an injury; new onset of seizures; worsening seizure disorder; visual field cuts; hemiparesis; anosmia)

▶ The neurocognitive disorder presents immediately after the occurrence of the traumatic brain injury or immediately after recovery of consciousness and persists past the acute postinjury period.

Etiology

▶ Brain injury resulting when the head is hit or violently shaken, such as from a blast or explosion.

Incidence and Demographics

▶ About 2% of the population and estimated 30% of returning soldiers

Risk Factors

▶ Combat duty exposing personnel to improvised explosive devices (IEDs) used by opposing factions

Prevention and Screening for Military Personnel

▶ Mandatory postdeployment screening for all veterans returning from combat assignment

▶ Traumatic brain injury screening

▷ Exposure to events (such as blasts, vehicle accidents, falls) that may have caused brain injury

▷ Immediate symptoms (such as loss of consciousness, feeling dazed, head injury, amnesia of event)

▷ Onset or worsening of problems (such as with memory, balance, headaches, dizziness, irritability, sensitivity to bright light, sleep problems) that may indicate brain injury

▷ Presence of symptoms in past week

▶ Four factors complicate recovery from combat-related concussions compared with mild TBI acquired in civilian settings.

1. The physically and emotionally traumatic environment in which they occur

2. The potentially repetitive and cumulative nature of concussions sustained over a tour (or multiple tours) of combat duty

3. The high incidence of comorbid mental health conditions

4. The difficulty in following typical recommendations for postconcussion care, such as rest (U.S. Department of Veteran Affairs, 2015)

TABLE 12–1.
SYMPTOMS OF TRAUMATIC BRAIN INJURY

MILD TBI	MODERATE TO SEVERE TBI
Mental status changes:	*Symptoms in first column plus:*
Poor concentration	Chronic, worsening headaches
Memory difficulty	Repeated nausea and vomiting
Intellectual impairment	Seizures
Irritability	Difficult to arouse from sleep
Depression	Slurred speech
Anxiety	Unequal pupils
	Confusion
Physical findings:	Restlessness and agitation
Dizziness	Extreme weakness or numbness
Balance problems	Loss of coordination
Headaches	
Tinnitus (ringing in the ears)	
Numbness and tingling	
Vision changes	
Sensitivity to light	
Sensitivity to sound	
Extreme fatigue	
Sleep problems	
Acute symptoms:	
Dazed and confused	

Assessment

Physical Findings and Mental Status

▶ Symptoms of TBI (see Table 12–1)

▶ Risk for suicide

▷ Factors increasing risk for suicide attempt with TBI:

▶ Males

▶ Ages 18 and 19

▶ Psychiatric disorder

▶ Aggressive behavior

▶ Substance use

Diagnostic and Laboratory Findings

▶ No current diagnostic test can retrospectively diagnose mild TBI or determine that current symptoms or problems are due to a past mild TBI. Conventional structural neuroimaging studies are typically normal in mild TBI.

Differential Diagnosis

▶ Posttraumatic stress disorder (PTSD)

▶ Depression

▶ Anxiety

▶ Other mental health diagnosis

Clinical Management

Pharmacological Management

▶ No specific medications for TBI.

▶ Treat related symptoms according to current evidence-based standards.

▶ Increased sensitivity to side effects of medication (secondary to head injury).

▷ Sedation

▷ Anticholinergic side effects (decrease memory)

▷ Seizures with tricyclic antidepressants (TCAs), buproprion, and amantadine (lower seizure threshold)

▷ Extrapyramidal symptoms, neuroleptic malignant syndrome, tardive dyskinesia

▷ Neuroleptics: decrease neuronal recovery

▷ Benzodiazepines: decrease memory, increase confusion, decrease coordination, abuse potential

▶ Cognitive disorders recommendations:

▷ Methylphenidate: increase attention, processing speed, general cognitive function, learning, and memory

▷ Dextroamphetamine: increase attention, processing speed

▷ Bromocriptine (off label, possibly helpful): increase executive function

▷ Amantadine (off label, possibly helpful): increase general cognitive function, attention, concentration

▶ When using medications, start low and go slow.

Nonpharmacological Management

▶ Treat comorbidities (military personnel with TBI frequently have posttraumatic stress disorder [PTSD], which makes treatment of TBI more difficult).

▶ Safety plan for suicide risk; limit availability of means.

▶ Teach family to identify signs of risk for suicide.

▶ Follow up for 1 year after anyone with TBI makes a suicide attempt.

▶ Treat vestibular dysfunction with physical therapy to reduce dizziness.

▶ Treat traumatic vision syndrome with occupational therapy; scanning and accommodation difficulties lead to headaches, irritability, and fatigue.

▶ Treat memory impairment with occupational therapy to teach memory improvement skills.

▶ Teach about symptoms and implications for relationships, employment, etc.

▶ Avoid alcohol.

▶ Neuropsychological testing.

▶ Psychotherapy

  ▷ Supportive

  ▷ Cognitive behavioral therapy (CBT)

    ▶ Increase understanding of relationships between cognition and emotion

    ▶ Target adjustment or development of new beliefs and assumptions (see Table 12–2)

  ▷ Behavioral therapy

  ▷ Family therapy

    ▶ Behavioral, affective, and personality changes are most difficult for families to adjust to

    ▶ Tips for families:

      ▷ If concentration is an issue, ask the TBI survivor for one thing at a time. Use of white noise machines may reduce distractions. May take longer to complete tasks.

      ▷ If memory is an issue, keep note pads near the phone for messages and in other places throughout the house. Keep a "memory book." Make a calendar and keep in a central location.

      ▷ If anger or irritability is an issue, leave the situation if possible and wait for TBI survivor to calm down. Use a soft, calm voice. Keep your distance and give the TBI survivor space.

      ▷ Resources

        ▶ Defense and Veterans Brain Injury Center: http://www.DVBIC.org

        ▶ Brain Injury Association of America: http://www.biausa.org

        ▶ U.S. Department of Veterans Affairs: www.VA.gov

TABLE 12–2.
COGNITIVE IMPAIRMENT AND ASSOCIATED CORE FEATURES OF COGNITIVE BEHAVIORAL THERAPY

COGNITIVE IMPAIRMENT	CORE FEATURE OF CBT
Impulsivity	"Stop–think–reflect"
Decreased awareness, encoding, and recall	Monitoring problems and successes
Memory	Use of audiotapes of sessions
Executive impairment	Develop independent problem-solving for every day difficulties

- ▶ Tips for the PMHNP for therapy with the client with TBI:
  - ▷ Determine what having a TBI means to the client.
  - ▷ Focus on "real life" difficulties in the here-and-now.
  - ▷ Monitor speed and complexity of comments.
  - ▷ Adjust session length according to level of attention and fatigue.
  - ▷ Reestablish an acceptable sense of self.
  - ▷ Instill hope without making predictions of a successful rehabilitation outcome.

Life Span Considerations

- ▶ Mild TBI
  - ▷ Most clients achieve full recovery within 3 months; if residual symptoms continue, 80% to 85% will clear within 6 months

Follow-up

- ▶ Symptoms may occur immediately but may also appear much later, which underscores the importance of screening for TBI
- ▶ Resource for guidelines, conditions and concerns: Deployment Health Clinical Center http://www.pdhealth.mil/main.asp

CASE STUDY

Mrs. Dean, a 59-year-old homemaker with a positive family history for Alzheimer's disease, has been very worried lately because she believes that she is losing her memory. She has hesitated to go for an evaluation because of her concern and is very upset as she shares her beliefs with the PMHNP. She gives a social history of being happily married for the past 35 years and of having several children and two new grandchildren. She has had no recent stressors and has felt a slow decline in her memory for the past 2 years. She believes no one else has noticed, but recently it is harder to hide her deficit from her family.

She has been employed as a nurse for the past 25 years at the local hospital but has begun to notice a decline in her ability to keep track of all of the information needed to do her job well. She has a history of asthma and periodically uses a rescue inhaler and steroids to manage her asthma. She routinely takes one aspirin a day and uses over-the-counter kava kava when she feels stressed. She has been taking pravastatin (Pravachol) 20 mg/day for her cholesterol level for the past 2 years. She has no significant physical findings but does show mild impairment in short-term memory testing during the MSE. There are many issues to consider in planning care with this client:

1. What is the probable diagnosis at this time?

2. What further assessment is needed?

3. What does the PMHNP need to take into account when considering medication for this client?

4. Would the PMHNP include the family in care planning at this time?

5. Are medications indicated at this time?

ANSWERS TO CASE STUDY DISCUSSION QUESTIONS

1. The correct diagnosis in this case is unspecified neurocognitive disorder.

2. Additional assessment information needed is to refer client for a complete medical examination.

3. Before starting the client on medication the PMHNP needs to understand the correct diagnosis for the client's symptoms and the stage of their illness, and discuss the client's preference for treatment.

4. In this case, yes, family should be involved as early as possible.

5. For this client, medication is not indicated at this time.

REFERENCES AND RESOURCES

American Geriatric Society. (1999). *Geriatric review syllabus.* New York, NY: Kendall/Hunt.

American Psychiatric Association. (2013). *Diagnostic and statistical manual of mental disorders* (5th ed.). Washington, DC: Author.

Bickley, L. S. (2007). *Bates' guide to physical examination and history taking* (9th ed.). Philadelphia, PA: Lippincott Williams & Wilkins.

Borson, S., Scanlan, J., Brush, M., Vitaliano, P., & Dokmak A. (2000). The mini-cog: A cognitive 'vital signs' measure for dementia screening in multilingual elderly. *International Journal of Geriatric Psychiatry, 15,* 1021–1027.

Burke, M., & Laramie, J. A. (2003). *Primary care of older adults* (2nd ed.). St. Louis, MO: Mosby.

Dick, K., & Morency, C. R. (2011). Delirium. In K. Devereaux & S. Crock (Eds.), *Geropsychiatric and mental health nursing* (2nd ed., pp. 255–272). Sudbury, MA: Jones & Bartlett Learning.

Doornbos, M. M. (2002). Family caregivers and the mental health care system: Reality and dreams. *Archives of Psychiatric Nursing, 15*(4), 39–46.

de Lange, E., Verhaak, P. F., & van der Meer, K. (2013). Prevalence, presentation and prognosis of delirium in older people in the population, at home and in long term care: A review. *International Journal of Geriatric Psychiatry, 28*(2), 127–134.

Jacobson, S. (2014). *Clinical manual of geriatric psychopharmacology* (2nd ed.) Arlington, VA: American Psychiatric Publication.

Melillo Devereaux, K., & Houde Crocker, S. (2011). *Geropsychiatric and mental health nursing* (2nd ed.). Sudbury, MA: Jones & Bartlett Learning.

Pfeiffer, E. (1975). A short portable mental status questionnaire for the assessment of organic brain deficit in elderly patients. *Journal of American Geriatric Society, 23,* 433–441.

Sadock, B. J., Sadock, V. A., & Ruiz, P. (2015). *Kaplan and Sadock's synopsis of psychiatry: Behavioral sciences/clinical psychiatry* (11th ed.). New York, NY: Wolters Kluwer.

Stahl, S. (2014). *Essential psychopharmacology prescribers guide* (5th ed.). New York, NY: Cambridge University Press.

Steffens, D., Blazer, D., & Thakur, M. (2015). *The American Psychiatric Publishing textbook of geriatric psychiatry* (5th ed.). Arlington, VA: American Psychiatric Publishing.

U.S. Department of Veterans Affairs. (2015). Polytrauma/TBI system of care. Retrieved from http://www.polytrauma.va.gov/understanding-tbi/

U.S. Preventive Services Task Force. (2014). *Screening for dementia: Recommendations and rationale.* Retrieved from http://www.uspreventiveservicestaskforce.org/Page/Document/UpdateSummaryFinal/cognitive-impairment-in-older-adults-screening?ds=1&s=dementia

CHAPTER 13

SUBSTANCE-RELATED AND ADDICTIVE DISORDERS

One of the most common but least well-addressed classes of disorders is substance use disorders. Psychiatric–mental health nurse practitioners (PMHNPs) who work in primary psychiatric settings or integrated primary care settings commonly treat clients with substance-related disorders. These disorders can stand alone or be part of complex co-occuring illness with either general medical conditions or psychiatric disorders.

Many substances can be used and abused. No matter what the substance, the continuum of use can range from mild to severe. Although the specific substances of abuse will determine many of the physical, behavioral, and cognitive symptoms exhibited by the client, some commonalities exist for all drugs. New to the fifth edition of the *Diagnostic and Statistical Manual of Mental Disorders* (DSM-5; American Psychiatric Association, 2013) is the inclusion of gambling as a behavioral addiction.

This chapter focuses on the PMHNP role in determining the severity of substance use and the available clinical management and treatments. It also emphasizes alcohol use disorders as a primary example. Alcohol is discussed because it is the most commonly abused substance, it is well researched, and PMHNPs will most often encounter people in clinical settings with an alcohol use disorder. Much of what is known about disorders of alcohol use is believed to be transferable to other substances.

SUBSTANCE-RELATED DISORDERS

Description

▶ *Substance use disorders* are a cluster of disorders in which cognitive, behavioral, and physiological symptoms indicate that a person continues using a substance despite significant substance-related problems (American Psychiatric Association, 2013).

▶ Psychiatric symptom clusters may be related to substance use, discontinuation of substance use, or withdrawal from habitual substance use.

▶ Substance use disorders lead to changes in brain circuits and physiological functions that lead to a need for detoxification and a possible need for long-term treatment.

- ▶ The word *substance* can describe a drug of abuse, a medication, or a toxin that produces psychoactivation and alters cognitive, behavioral, and affective perceptions.
- ▶ *Dependence:* repeated use of a substance with or without physical dependence
- ▶ *Abuse:* use that is inconsistent with sociality use patterns
- ▶ *Misuse:* usually applies to a prescribed substance
- ▶ *Intoxication:* reversible syndrome caus ed by a specific substance affecting memory, judgment, behavior, or social or occupational functioning
- ▶ *Withdrawal:* substance-specific symptoms that occur after stopping or reducing use
- ▶ *Tolerance:* needing more of the substance to get the desired effect

Etiology

- ▶ Multiple theories ranging from psychological to neurobiological
- ▶ Probable multifactorial etiological profile
- ▶ Two common types of theories: psychodynamic and biological
  - ▷ Psychodynamic theory
    - ▶ Behaviors of abuse are seated in oral-stage fixation.
    - ▶ A person seeks gratification through oral behaviors.
    - ▶ Maladaptive regressive behaviors can become overlearned, fixed, and reinforced through dysfunctional family patterns.
    - ▶ Sociocultural factors attempt to explain population-based differences in substance abuse rates.
  - ▷ Biological theory
    - ▶ Genetic loading
      - ▷ People with a strong genetic vulnerability to addiction are thought to have defects in the working of the reward center of the brain, which predisposes them to stronger-than-normal positive rewards that draw them to substance use.
      - ▷ Gender differences
      - ▷ Ethnic differences
      - ▷ A person is predisposed to stronger-than-normal negative rewards, making it more difficult to stop abuse once it has begun.
    - ▶ Involves two neurobiological processes:
      1. Reinforcement
         - ▶ Brain-based changes in structure and function can lead to addictive behavior.
         - ▶ The process of positive and negative rewards is physiologically linked to memory function.
         - ▶ Changes appear to occur with any drug of abuse.

▶ Reinforcement results in "feel good" sensations when a drug of abuse is used and in "feel bad" sensations when the drug exits the body.

▶ Positive rewards of reinforcement result in the social rewards commonly associated with drug use, such as disinhibition, euphoric mood, and anxiety reduction.

▷ Mediated by dopamine (DA) pathways

▶ Negative rewards are aversive, such as increased anxiety and dysphoria.

▷ Mediated by the gamma amino butyric acid (GABA) pathways

▶ Reinforcement occurs in the ventral tegmental area and the nucleus accumbens of the brain, collectively called the *reward center*.

▶ DA release within the reward center is enhanced further by the release of natural morphine-like neurotransmitters called *neuropeptides* (enkephalins, beta-endorphins).

▶ Neuropeptides further enhance the reinforcing pleasure experienced by the person.

▶ With repeated drug use, the DA system becomes increasingly sensitized.

▶ Eventually, associated drug use stimuli (e.g., pictures of drug paraphernalia) can cause DA release, leading to reinforcement of use and often to increased drug use.

2. Neuroadaptation

▶ Brain-based changes in structure and function can lead to *tolerance* and *withdrawal*.

▶ Drug-specific alterations in the normal level and function of neurotransmitters occur as the body adapts to the chronic presence of the substance of abuse.

▶ Neuroadaptive processes become very significant when the person stops substance use.

▶ These processes become the basis for withdrawal symptoms, because adaptive responses are unopposed when the substance is no longer present.

▶ Neuroadaptive changes may be more enduring in some persons, possibly lasting for years, thus increasing their potential for relapse.

▶ This concept helps to explain why, after a long period of sobriety, a person who returns to substance abuse often picks up at the same level of tolerance and physical impact as experienced before sobriety.

Incidence and Demographics

▶ Persons age 18 to 24 years of age have high prevalence rates for using most substances.

▶ The United States has higher rates of substance use than any other developed country.

▶ More than 50% of U.S. clients with a psychiatric disorder have a comorbid substance use disorder.

 ▷ Persons with schizophrenia are 4 times more likely to have a substance use comorbidity than the general population.

 ▷ Persons with bipolar affective disorder are 5 times more likely to have a substance use comorbidity than the general population.

▶ More than 2 million admissions annually are made to inpatient substance use treatment facilities.

 ▷ Though now legal in some states, marijuana is the most commonly abused illegal substance.

▶ Alcohol is the most commonly abused legal substance.

 ▷ Rates are higher in men than in women.

  ▶ 90% of men have used alcohol.

  ▶ 70% of women have used alcohol.

  ▶ Rates are highest in African Americans, Hispanic Americans, and Native Americans; rates are lowest in Asian Americans.

   ▷ 55% of fatal driving accidents in the United States occur with a driver under the influence of alcohol.

   ▷ 50% of crimes in the United Stated are committed under the influence of alcohol.

   ▷ The lifetime risk for alcohol use disorder is 15% in the general U.S. population.

Risk Factors

▶ Genetic loading

 ▷ Family history of substance abuse or major depressive disorder (MDD)

▶ Association with peer structure with heavy substance use

▶ Co-occurring psychiatric disorder

▶ Age and gender (younger, males)

▶ Existence of chronic pain

▶ Untreated chronic pathological-level anxiety

Prevention and Screening

► At-risk family education

▷ Stigma reduction

▷ Signs and symptoms of illness

▷ Treatment potential for control of symptoms

► Early recognition, intervention, and initiation of treatment to prevent disease development of complications of disorder

► Implications of alcohol and other drugs of abuse during pregnancy:

▷ Fetal alcohol syndrome (FAS)

► *Prevalence*: one third of all infants born to females with alcohol use disorder

► *Signs*: low birth weight and height, microphthalmia, short palpebral fissure, midface hypoplasia, smooth or short philtrum, thin upper lip

▷ Birth defects

► Acute alcohol intoxication in nontolerant persons such as teenagers:

▷ Coma

▷ Respiratory depression

▷ Death

▷ Administered by asking the client four questions

▷ Each positive answer scored as 1 point; negative answers receive no score

▷ The more positive answers, the greater the likelihood of an alcohol abuse disorder.

▷ Clients scoring 2 or greater are at mild to moderate risk for alcohol dependency, and the score is considered clinically significant

▷ Clients scoring 3 to 4 are considered at high risk for alcohol dependency

► Other screening

▷ AUDIT: Alcohol Use Disorders Identification Test

▷ S-MAST: Short Michigan Alcoholism Screening Test (or Geriatric Version)

▷ CRAFFT: Children and adolescents under 21 years of age

▷ COWS: The Clinical Opiate Withdrawal Scale

CAGE SCREENING TEST IS THE MOST COMMONLY USED SCREENING TOOL FOR ALCOHOL ABUSE (SAMHSA, 2016)

C: Have you ever felt the need to cut down on your drinking?

A: Have people annoyed you by mentioning your drinking?

G: Have you ever felt bad or guilty about your drinking?

E: Have you ever had a drink the first thing in the morning to steady your nerves or get rid of a hangover (eye-opener)?

Assessment

History

▶ Assess for the following:

▷ Detailed history of present illness, including time frame, progression, and associated symptoms

▷ Social history, including present living situation; marital status; occupation; education; and alcohol, tobacco, or illicit drug use

▷ Medication use, including prescription, over-the-counter, alternative, supplements, and home remedies

▷ Initial and periodic functional history and assessment

▷ Validate history with a family member

▷ Identify the category of drug abused by the client

▶ Knowing category allows for anticipation of physical impact of drug and to predict potential symptoms of withdrawal

▶ Clients often abuse drugs from categories with similar pharmacological properties.

▶ Categories of abused agents:

▷ Alcohol

▷ Amphetamines or similar sympathomimetics

▷ Caffeine

▷ Cannabis

▷ Cocaine

▷ Hallucinogens

▷ Inhalants

▷ Nicotine

▷ Opioids

▷ Phencyclidine (PCP) or similar arylcyclohexylamines

▷ Sedatives

▷ Hypnotics

▷ Anxiolytics

▷ Assess for presence of substance abuse

▶ Maladaptive pattern of substance use manifested by recurrent and significant adverse consequences related to repeated use of a substance

▶ Is *not* synonymous with *use, misuse,* or *hazardous use*

▶ Specific criteria needed to identify substance use as abuse:

▷ Maladaptive pattern of use occurring for at least a 12-month period of sustained use

▷ Must be accompanied by repeated failure to fulfill major role obligation

▷ Must be accompanied by use in situation that presents as physically hazardous, such as drinking and driving

▷ Abuse continues despite multiple problems related to substance use patterns, such as legal, interpersonal, or social problems

▷ Assess for presence of substance use disorder

▶ Cluster of cognitive, behavioral, and physiological symptoms indicating that the person continues use of a substance despite significant substance-related problems

▶ Synonymous with *addiction*

▶ Pattern of repeated use that leads to clinically significant impairment or distress with three or more of the following symptoms within a 12-month period:

▷ Tolerance

▷ Withdrawal

▷ Using larger amounts than intended

▷ Persistent craving or unsuccessful attempts to cut down

▷ Large amount of time spent obtaining substance, using substance, or recovering from its effects

▷ Activities decreased or given up because of use

▷ Using despite consequences

▶ Physiological dependence implies tolerance and withdrawal

▶ Degree of tolerance and withdrawal symptoms are substance-specific.

▷ Can be physical, psychological, or both, depending on the substance

▷ Withdrawal symptoms are almost always the opposite of the acute action of the substance.

▷ Categories of abused substances with pronounced, *obvious withdrawal symptoms*:

▶ Alcohol

▶ Opioids

▶ Sedatives

▶ Hypnotics

▶ Anxiolytics

▷ Categories of abused substances with less pronounced, *less obvious withdrawal symptoms*:

▶ Stimulants

▶ Nicotine

▶ Cannabis

▷ Categories of abused substances with *little to no* pronounced, obvious withdrawal symptoms:

▶ Hallucinogens

▶ PCP

▷ Assess for the presence of substance withdrawal or intoxication

▶ Clients abusing substances present for assessment either under the influence of the drug (intoxication) or experiencing problems related to cessation of substance use (withdrawal)

▷ *Intoxication:* Reversible substance-specific syndrome caused by recent ingestion of a psychoactivating substance

▷ *Withdrawal:* Potentially nonreversible substance-specific syndrome caused by cessation or significant reduction in heavy, prolonged use of a substance

▶ Blood alcohol levels determine presence of alcohol in the body

▷ Tolerant persons often have higher blood levels with less impairment than nontolerant persons

▷ Must interpret blood alcohol levels of a client based on his or her degree of tolerance

▶ Diagnostic criteria for substance withdrawal:

▷ Cessation or reduction in substance use that has been heavy or prolonged

▷ Two or more of the following symptoms within several hours or days of reduction or cessation of the substance:

▶ Hand tremor

▶ Insomnia

▶ Autonomic hyperactivity (sweating, increased heart rate, and increased blood pressure)

▶ Nausea or vomiting

▶ Hallucinations or illusions

▶ Psychomotor agitation

▶ Anxiety

▶ Seizures

▶ Structured interview allows for assessment of the use patterns and consequences of a person's substance use

▷ Assess for all dimensions of the impact of substance abuse or dependence in the person.

▶ Current use

▶ Pattern of use

▶ Consequences (interpersonal, occupational, legal)

▶ Physical health consequences

Physical Exam Findings

▶ Substance abuse or dependence produces many physical symptoms.

▷ Usually a result of sequelae of use or abuse rather than findings specific to abuse or dependence

▶ Generally nonspecific when viewed in isolation

▶ Must be considered as a cluster of symptoms that raise an index of suspicion of addiction potential

▷ Abdominal pain and tenderness

▷ Nausea

▷ Weight loss

▷ Gastrointestinal bleeding

▷ Hypertension

▷ Anxiety

▷ First-episode seizure in adult

▶ Physical findings related to alcohol use disorders (Domino, Baldor, Golding, & Stephens, 2015; NIAAA, 2016).

▷ *Brain*: mood changes, behavior changes

▷ *HEENT*: poor oral health

▷ *Cardiovascular*: hypertension, cardiomyopathy, tachycardia

▷ *Gastrointestinal*: liver disease, cirrhosis, peptic ulcer, esophageal malignancies

▷ *Neurologic*: tremor, cognitive deficits, peripheral neuropathy, Wernicke-Korsakoff syndrome

▷ *Metabolic*: hyperlipidemia

Mental Status Exam (MSE) Findings

▶ Nature of findings depends heavily on whether the client is experiencing substance intoxication or withdrawal, or is substance-free at the time of assessment.

▷ Index of suspicion for substance-related disorder should be raised if client presents differently during different periods of assessment (Sadock, Sadock, & Ruiz, 2015).

▶ *Stimulants*: agitation, anxiety, irritability, mood swings, elevated mood

▶ *Opioids*: mood swings, aggression, disinhibition, impaired cognition, slurred speech, psychomotor slowing

▶ *Hallucinogens*: mood swings, hallucinations, paranoia, flashbacks, panic, impaired judgement

▶ *Cannabis*: confusion, paranoia, panic

▶ *Inhalants*: agitation, irritability, confusion, hallucinations

Diagnostic and Laboratory Findings

▶ Complete blood count (CBC), chemistry profile, thyroid function tests, and B_{12} level to rule out metabolic causes or unidentified conditions

▶ Drug toxicity screening, if indicated by history

▶ Alcohol dependence and abuse produce characteristic laboratory findings.

   ▷ Blood alcohol level >100 mg/dL outpatient; >150 mg/dL anytime with sx; >300 mg/dL anytime

   ▷ Aspartate transaminase (AST)/Alanine transaminase (ALT) ration >2.0

   ▷ Elevated: glutamyltransferase, mean corpuscular volume, prothrombin time, uric acid, total cholesterol, and triglycerides

   ▷ Decreased: magnesium, calcium, potassium, blood urea nitrogen, hemoglobin, hematocrit, platelet count and albumin (Domino et al., 2015).

Differential Diagnosis

▶ Endocrine disorders

   ▷ Cushing's disease

▶ Neurological disorders

   ▷ Seizure disorders

▶ Cardiovascular disorders

   ▷ Myocardial infarction

▶ Mood disorders

   ▷ MDD

   ▷ Bipolar (BP) disorder

▶ Anxiety disorders

▶ Personality disorders

▶ Differential diagnostic consideration for acute alcohol withdrawal:

   ▷ Many acute general health conditions can mimic symptoms of alcohol withdrawal.

Clinical Management

▶ Rule out or treat any conditions that may contribute to clinical findings.

▶ *Note:* 80% to 90% of people who require alcohol treatment do not get it.

   ▷ Common reasons for failure to receive needed treatment:

      ▶ Lack of diagnosis

      ▶ Lack of referral

      ▶ Lack of access to services

      ▶ Resistance to treatment

- ▶ The genetics of addiction vulnerability are becoming better known, which allows for preventative and early intervention treatments.
- ▶ The knowledge base of the pathophysiology of dependence has promoted new somatic interventions.
  - ▷ Psychopharmacology offers the promise of a new era in the treatment of addictions.
- ▶ Clinical management differs depending on the substance-related syndrome exhibited by the person.
  - ▷ Acute withdrawal
  - ▷ Acute intoxication
  - ▷ Long-term sobriety maintenance
  - ▷ Relapse prevention
- ▶ Alcohol withdrawal carries a high risk of mortality.
- ▶ Clinical management of alcohol withdrawal is a specialized treatment that requires specific experience in this type of care.
- ▶ Some clinical findings may assist in identification of clients at risk for severe alcohol withdrawal:
  - ▷ Agitation
  - ▷ Decreased short-term memory
  - ▷ Disorientation
  - ▷ Hallucinations
  - ▷ Irregular pulse
  - ▷ Ophthalmoplegia
- ▶ Clinical Institute Withdrawal Assessment for Alcohol
  - ▷ Used to determine likelihood of withdrawal and delirium tremens (DTs), which usually occur within the first 24 to 72 hours after cessation of alcohol.
  - ▷ Assesses 10 common withdrawal symptoms:
    - ▶ Nausea and vomiting
    - ▶ Tremors
    - ▶ Paroxysmal sweats
    - ▶ Anxiety
    - ▶ Agitation
    - ▶ Tactile disturbances
    - ▶ Auditory disturbances
    - ▶ Visual disturbances
    - ▶ Headaches
    - ▶ Altered sensorium

▷ Each symptom is graded on a 0- to 7-point scale with the exception of orientation and sensorium, which are graded on a 0- to 4-point scale. The higher the total score (maximum = 67), the more likely the person will experience severe withdrawal and DTs: 0–9 = absent or very mild withdrawal, 10–15 = mild withdrawal, 16–20 = moderate withdrawal, and 21-67 = severe withdrawal and possible DTs.

Pharmacological Management

▶ Pharmacological treatments are symptom-specific

▶ Clinical management of acute withdrawal

▷ Detoxification (detox) agents replace uncontrolled use of substance with slow tapering of controlled substance to minimize neuroadaptive rebound.

▶ Multiple daily doses of benzodiazepines are used according to a fixed schedule and gradually tapered down over several days.

▶ Examples include:

▷ Lorazepam (Ativan)

▷ Chlordiazepoxide (Librium)

▷ Diazepam (Valium)

▷ Oxazepam (Serax)

▶ Polytherapy is a newer approach that matches drugs required for safe and effective withdrawal with neurotransmitter deficits created by substance use.

▷ Selective serotonin reuptake inhibitors

▷ Opioid antagonists nalmefene hydrochloride (Revex), naltrexone (Revia), or naltrexone for extended-release injectable suspension (Vivitrol)

▷ N-methyl-D-aspartate (NMDA) agonists

▶ Antiseizure medications such as carbamazepine (Tegretol) and valproic acid (Depakene) are sometimes used to decrease the potential for seizures.

▶ Adrenergic medications are sometimes used to decrease blood pressure and pulse rate associated with withdrawal.

▷ Clinical management of craving (see Table 13–1)

▶ Use anticraving medication such as naltrexone (Revia), acamprosate (Campral), ondansetron (Zofran), or buprenorphine (Buprenex).

▶ Use behavior treatment to help client learn substitute behaviors.

▷ Clinical management and maintenance of sobriety (see Table 13–1)

▶ Person may require ongoing treatment for comorbid psychiatric disorder.

▶ May use *aversion treatment* to avoid alcohol in persons with alcohol dependence.

▷ Disulfiram (Antabuse)

▶ Do not administer until the person has been alcohol-free for at least 12 hours.

TABLE 13–1.
PHARMACOLOGICAL AGENTS USEFUL IN TREATING CRAVING AND MAINTAINING (STAHL, 2014)

PHARMACOLOGICAL AGENT	CHEMICAL CATEGORY	ACTION EFFECT
Citalopram (Celexa)	Selective serotonin reuptake inhibitor	Decrease desire
Disulfiram (Antabuse)	Aldehyde dehydrogenase inhibitor	Aversion therapy
Naloxone(Narcan)	Opioid antagonist, antidote	Blocks effects of opioids
Buprenorphine (buprenex)	Opioid partial agonist, opioid antagonist	Agonist and antagonist, decrease cravings
Buprenorphine and naloxone (Suboxone)	Narcotic analgesic	Opioid agonist/antagonist
Methadone (Dolophine)	Narcotic analgesic	Suppresses withdrawal
Nalmefene (Revex)	Opioid antagonist	Increases abstinence
IM (Revia; Vivitrol)	Opioid antagonist	Increases abstinence
Acamprosate (Campral)	Homotaurine	Decreases craving

> ▶ Advise client to refrain from using anything that contains alcohol (e.g., vinegar, aftershave lotion, perfumes, mouthwash, cough medication) while taking disulfiram and up to 2 weeks after discontinuing disulfiram.

> ▶ Disulfiram can elevate liver function tests, so monitor.

> ▶ Antabuse may potentially induce mania in people with BP disorder.

▷ General health maintenance medication to treat vitamin deficiencies in persons with alcohol dependence include thiamine, folic acid, and B-complex vitamins.

Nonpharmacological Management

▶ Multimodality treatment needed.

▶ Lifetime treatment often required.

▶ Inpatient treatment usually needed for safe and effective withdrawal from alcohol.

▶ Indications for inpatient alcohol detoxification include history of severe withdrawal symptoms, seizures, or delirium tremens; multiple past detoxifications; additional medical or psychiatric illness; recent significant alcohol consumption; lack of reliable support system; and pregnancy.

▶ Reduce central nervous system stimulation by maintaining a quiet environment; put client in room close to the nurses' station to facilitate frequent observation and monitoring; minimize abrupt changes in environment; decrease bright light and sharp, sudden noises; decrease room clutter; and do not restrain.

▶ Maintain hydration by monitoring intake and anticholinergic effects of benzodiazepines. Frequently offer fluids.

▶ Before discharge from acute-care setting, have a definite plan for follow-up treatment.

▶ Connect client and family with support groups.

   ▷ 12-step groups in community

   ▷ Concrete plan for first week of support group attendance (may need daily)

▶ Connect client with counseling or psychotherapy.

▶ Identify a primary healthcare provider.

▶ Note medical problems that will require further evaluation and potential treatment:

   ▷ Neurological sequelae of chronic alcohol consumption

   ▷ Nutritional deficiencies

   ▷ Cardiomyopathy, hypertension, arrhythmias, ischemic heart disease

   ▷ Blood dyscrasias

   ▷ Gastrointestinal inflammations

   ▷ Esophageal, liver, nasopharyngeal, and laryngeal cancers

▶ Client care needs:

   ▷ Substance abuse education classes

   ▷ Substance abuse counseling program

   ▷ Continued 12-step program involvement (e.g., Alcoholics Anonymous, Narcotics Anonymous)

   ▷ Halfway housing

   ▷ Cognitive behavioral therapy

▶ Family care needs:

   ▷ Current and understandable information about condition, progress, and treatment plan

   ▷ Connect family to community support groups such as Al-Anon and Alateen

   ▷ Management of feelings such as guilt and anger

   ▷ Referrals to community resources

   ▷ Specific considerations: relationship with treatment team; role strain; financial stresses; social isolation and "code of silence"; family support systems; family violence; marital and family strife; family members' work and school functioning; history of mental disorders, including substance-related disorders

   ▷ Assist family in coping with difficulties incorporating drinking member back into routines; encourage further counseling to resolve these difficulties

   ▷ Refer for further treatment if family members report symptom clusters from anxiety and mood disorders, eating disorders, and addiction

Life Span Considerations

▶ Children and adolescents

   ▷ Most common period for starting drug use

   ▷ Significant impact of peer pressure on substance use patterns

   ▷ 30% to 40% of adolescents report drinking frequently

- ▷ 15% report binge-drinking patterns
- ▷ Approximately 50% of high school–age students report at least a one-time use of illicit drugs
- ▶ Older adults
  - ▷ Referral to specialized treatment program that emphasizes interventions to deal with losses
  - ▷ Large-print psychoeducation materials
  - ▷ Transportation to service locations
  - ▷ Treatment with same-age peer group
  - ▷ Adaptations to home environment to cope with physical disabilities
  - ▷ Close collaboration with primary-care physician for follow-up

CASE STUDY

Mrs. Day is a 61-year-old widow who has multiple health problems. She had been diagnosed with essential hypertension and chronic bronchitis and has non-insulin-dependent diabetes. She has been coming to your primary care clinic for 6 months, and before that she had been receiving her care from multiple other providers in the community. She receives Social Security Disability Insurance.

Mrs. Day's chief complaint for the past few months has been stasis ulcers on her lower left leg, which have not healed well despite multiple approaches to care. She also complains of problems with her "nerves." She currently is taking

- ▶ multivitamin daily
- ▶ ranitidine (Zantac) 150 mg q 12 hrs
- ▶ alprazolam (Xanax) 1 mg b.i.d.
- ▶ glipizide (Glucotrol) 20 mg b.i.d.

Mrs. Day is in today, and this is the first time you see her. On initial approach, she is hostile and difficult to get information from, stating, "You should know all this; you have my chart right there in your hand." She states that today she wants a refill of all of her prescriptions, and she wants you to write a letter to her landlord to "stop harassing me." She reports that her landlord is insisting that she place her garbage in the containers in the parking lot of the complex. She feels that is too far for her to walk, and she wants a letter supporting her current practice of leaving her garbage bags in the hallway outside her apartment door.

She also is reporting that her nerves are worse, and the pain in her legs is worse as well. She also believes that she has had a return of "chronic bronchitis," and she is requesting an antibiotic. She is requesting that you increase her alprazolam and add codeine or morphine or "any other thing like that" for her "constant pain." She states, "Just do this and get me out of here. I know what I need."

Mental Status Exam

- ▶ *Appearance:* moderately obese, well-dressed with appropriate hygiene, poor eye contact
- ▶ *Motor:* mild psychomotor restlessness, slightly ataxic gait, tremulous
- ▶ *Speech:* loud and pressured
- ▶ *Affect:* angry
- ▶ *Mood:* self-described as "cranky"; assessed as irritable
- ▶ *Thought processes:* goal-directed and organized without evidence of psychotic processing but does show some mild thought-blocking and tangentiality
- ▶ *Thought content:* thematic for mistrust of health providers and for fear of pain continuing
- ▶ *Memory:* one-third of objects after 15 minutes
- ▶ *Concentration:* refuses to do numbers testing, stating "I was never good with book work or numbers"
- ▶ *Abstraction:* is abstract on proverbs; asks, "You got any more dumb questions?"

▶ *Judgment:* intact for self-welfare

▶ *Education:* completed 12th grade and went to 2-year secretarial business school

▶ *Employment history:* was a medical claims clerk for 32 years at the VA Medical Center

▶ *Social history:* no children; lives by herself; history of 2-pack-a-day smoker and "I drink a six-pack or so at night to relax myself—wouldn't you?"

Her physical exam is overall unremarkable. Her vital signs are within her documented baseline, with BP 132/88, P 96, RR 26, Temp 98.5° F, Weight 209 lbs. Her lungs are overall clear. On her left leg she has a stasis ulcer, which is circular and approximately 6 cm in circumference. It is open and oozing white–yellow liquid drainage, with redness around the borders. She reports it is painful to touch and increasingly painful when weight-bearing. She was ordered silver sulfadiazine treatments with cling wrap and hot soaks q 6 hours. She refuses to cover it because "it hurts when I remove the bandage" and is not very clear about whether or not she is doing the hot soaks. Recent labs are all within normal limits, including thyroid-stimulating hormone, electrolytes, and CBC.

1. What is the primary healthcare concern of this client?

2. What method of interviewing would be useful for Mrs. Day?

3. What further laboratory testing should be considered?

4. If the client is unwilling to participate in further assessment, how will you deal with her health needs?

ANSWERS TO CASE STUDY DISCUSSION QUESTIONS

1. Given her laboratory values are within normal limits and she has no physical signs of a respiratory infection, the main concern is current or risk for addiction.

2. The method of interviewing Mrs. Day would be using the SBIRT technique.

3. Additional laboratory assessments should be obtained, which include liver function tests, including ALT, AST, GGT, albumin, and possibly uric acid level.

4. If Mrs. Day is unwilling to engage in a further assessment, the use of motivational interviewing techniques, building rapport, and keeping the client engaged would be indicated.

REFERENCES AND RESOURCES

American Psychiatric Association. (2013). *Diagnostic and statistical manual of mental disorders* (5th ed.). Washington, DC: Author.

Barbosa, C., Cowell, A., Bray, J., & Aldridge, A. (2015). The cost effectiveness of alcohol screening, brief intervention, and referral to treatment (SBIRT) in emergency and outpatient medical settings. *Journal of Substance Abuse Treatment, 53*, 1–8.

DiClemente, C., Bellino, L., & Neavins, T. (1999). Motivation for change and alcoholism treatment. *Alcohol Research and Health, 23*(2), 86–92.

Domino, F. J., Baldor, R. A., Golding, J., & Stephens, M. B. (2015). *The 5-minute clinical consult standard* (24th ed.). Philadelphia, PA: Wolters Kluwer.

Dunn, K., Saulsgiver, K., Miller, M., Nuzzo, P., & Sigmon, S. (2015). Characterizing opioid withdrawal during double blind buprenorphine detoxification. *Drug and Alcohol Dependence, 151*(1), 47–55.

Graham, A. W., & Schultz, T. K. (2007). *Principles of addiction medicine* (3rd ed.). Baltimore, MD: American Society of Addiction Medicine.

Mayfield, D., McLeod, G., & Hall, P. (1974). The CAGE questionnaire: Validation of a new alcoholism instrument. *American Journal of Psychiatry, 131*, 1121–1123.

Miller, N., Gold, M., & Smith, D. (1997). *Manual of therapeutics for addictions.* New York, NY: Wiley-Liss.

National Institute on Alcohol Abuse and Alcoholism. (1997). *Alcohol and health* (DHHS Publication No. 97-4017). Rockville, MD: Author.

National Institute on Alcohol Abuse and Alcoholism. (2016). Alcohol's Effects on the body. http://www.niaaa.nih.gov/alcohol-health/alcohols-effects-body

National Institute on Drug Abuse. (2012). *Medical consequences of drug abuse: Mental health effects.* Bethesda, MD: National Institutes of Health. Retrieved from http://www.drugabuse.gov/publications/medical-consequences-drug-abuse/mental-health-effects

Perese, E. F. (2012). *Psychiatric advanced practice nursing: A biopsychosocial foundation for practice.* Philadelphia, PA: F. A. Davis.

Sadock, B., Sadock, V. A., & Ruiz, P. (2015). *Kaplan and Sadock's synopsis of psychiatry: Behavioral sciences/clinical psychiatry* (11th ed.). New York, NY: Wolters Kluwer.

Stahl, S. (2014). *Essential psychopharmacology prescribers guide* (5th ed.). New York, NY: Cambridge University Press.

Substance Abuse and Mental Health Services Administration (SAMHSA). (2016). Screening tools. http://www.integration.samhsa.gov/clinical-practice/screening-tools#drugs

Wheeler, K. (2014). *Psychotherapy for the advanced practice psychiatric nurse* (2nd ed.). New York, NY: Springer Publishing Company.

CHAPTER 14

PERSONALITY DISORDERS

This chapter reviews a category of illnesses called personality disorders, common disorders that can affect the quality of the general health care that a person receives. Although these disorders can create great difficulty for the given person, he or she remains able to perform routine daily functions. Often the person does not recognize a problem or seek treatment.

This chapter briefly reviews the concept of *personality* and then its disorders. Assessment and clinical management features of personality disorders are discussed.

PERSONALITY

Description

▶ *Personality* is the sum total of all emotional, cognitive, and behavioral attributes of a person.

▶ Personality involves an enduring pattern of perceiving, relating to, and thinking about the environment and one's self that are exhibited in a wide array of social and personal contexts.

▶ When healthy, personality structures allow for realistic, happy, and satisfying self-perceptions and interpersonal interactions.

▶ Characteristics

    ▷ Personality is organized early in life and is dynamic and deeply ingrained; however, it can be altered.

    ▷ Patterns of behavior based on personality can be perceived by the person as comfortable (*ego-syntonic*) or uncomfortable (*ego-dystonic*):

        ▶ Ego-syntonic

            ▷ Behavior consistent with personality

            ▷ Causes little concern to the person

            ▷ Person generally fails to recognize problem

            ▷ Person does not seek treatment

▶ Ego-dystonic

▷ Behavior inconsistent with personality

▷ Causes discomfort and concern to the person

▷ Person generally recognizes problem

▷ Person often seeks treatment

▷ Personality is reflected in behavioral traits habitually displayed by the person:

▶ Coping

▷ Interpersonal or interactive style

▷ Perceptions

▷ Cognitive beliefs about events, people, and situations

PERSONALITY DISORDERS

Description

▶ Personality disorders are chronically maladaptive patterns of behavior that cause functional impairment in work, school, or relationships.

▶ These disorders manifest as maladaptive patterns in four areas of functionality:

▷ Maladaptive *affective* traits, such as overly affectual patterns of response

▷ Maladaptive *behavioral* traits, such as poor impulse control patterns of response

▷ Maladaptive *cognitive* traits, such as unrealistic perceptual patterns of response

▷ Maladaptive *social* traits, such as maladaptive unsatisfying interpersonal patterns of response

▶ These disorders can cause *subjective distress*.

▷ A person is unlikely to recognize the problem or seek help if maladaptive patterns of behavior are ego-syntonic.

▷ A person is more likely to recognize problem and seek help if maladaptive patterns of behavior are ego-dystonic.

▷ Maladaptive patterns are *inflexible* and *pervasive* across most personal and social situations.

▷ These disorders are coded in the DSM-5 (see Table 14–1).

▷ Clients seldom fit neatly into one personality disorder diagnosis; rather, they often exhibit features of several similar disorders.

▷ For this reason, personality disorders often are referred to by the category of commonly manifesting symptom clusters (A, B, or C).

Etiology

▶ Multiple theories ranging from psychological to neurobiological

▶ Probable multifactorial etiological profile

TABLE 14–1.
CATEGORIES OF PERSONALITY DISORDERS

CATEGORY	CHARACTERISTIC BEHAVIOR	DISORDERS
Cluster A	Odd, unusual, eccentric, asocial	Paranoid personality disorder
		Schizoid personality disorder
		Schizotypal personality disorder
Cluster B	Dramatic, affective instability	Antisocial personality disorder
		Borderline personality disorder
		Histrionic personality disorder
		Narcissistic personality disorder
Cluster C	Anxious	Avoidant personality disorder
		Dependent personality disorder
		Obsessive–compulsive personality disorder

▶ Less empirical data available on neurobiological etiological factors

▶ Borderline personality disorder is the most well researched.

▶ Two common types of theories of personality disorders:

1. Psychodynamic theory (primarily borderline personality disorder)—based on two etiological factors:

   ▶ Early separation problems

      ▷ Object relations theory

         ▶ Internalized intrapsychic experiences of interpersonal relationships

         ▶ Mental representation of the self in relation to others

         ▶ Stability and depth of a person's relationships

         ▶ During development, child must accomplish two tasks: *separation* and *individuation.*

            ▷ *Separation:* Develop intrapsychic self-representation distinct and separate from mother

            ▷ *Individuation:* Form distinct identity with characteristics unique to the person.

      ▷ Failure in separation–individuation is etiologically linked to development of personality disorders.

      ▷ Different personality disorders linked to problems with different stages of the separation–individuation process.

         ▶ Disturbed parental interaction

         ▶ Family background assumed to be dysfunctional:

            ▷ Enmeshed family patterns

            ▷ Role-reversal patterns of child–parent interaction

            ▷ Restricted involvement of family with the rest of the environment

▷ Social isolation

▷ Confusion of parental authority and nurturing roles

▷ Blurred family boundaries

▶ Dysfunctional family patterns block separation–individuation processes; family rejection occurs if person attempts individuation.

2. Biological theory

▶ Genetic factors

▷ Familial tendency

▷ Genetic overlap between loading for some Axis I disorders and personality disorders

▶ Structural abnormalities

▷ Reduced gray-matter volume in prefrontal cortex

▷ Limbic system deregulation

▶ Neurotransmitter dysfunction

▷ Decreased levels of serotonin

▷ Elevated levels of norepinephrine

▷ Dysregulation of dopamine receptors

▶ Neurobiological impact of trauma

▷ Most studied in borderline personality disorder

▷ Assumes early childhood trauma alters basic brain patterns of response

▷ In genetically susceptible people, may function as the environmental vulnerability that causes expression of genetic load

Incidence and Demographics

▶ Difficult to estimate, because people with personality disorders are rarely hospitalized and often receive no treatment

▶ Incidence varies with disorder

▶ Generally assumed to be 0.5% to 5.4% in the general U.S. population

Risk Factors

▶ Genetic loading

▶ Dysfunctional family of origin

Prevention and Screening

▶ At-risk family education

▶ Community education

▷ Stigma reduction

> ▷ Signs and symptoms of illness

> ▷ Treatment potential for control of symptoms

>> ▶ Early recognition, intervention, and initiation of treatment

>> ▶ Preventative work with young children in identified dysfunctional family settings

Assessment

▶ Symptoms of personality disorder are enduring maladaptive patterns of behavior, generally seen as problems with living.

▶ Often several interviews are needed to clarify the diagnostic picture.

History

▶ Assess for the following:

> ▷ Detailed history of present illness, including time frame, progression, and associated symptoms

> ▷ Social history, including present living situation; marital status; occupation; education; and alcohol, tobacco, and illicit drug use

> ▷ Medication use, including prescription, over-the-counter, alternative, supplements, and home remedies

> ▷ Initial and periodic functional history and assessment

> ▷ Validate history with family member

▶ Long-term patterns of functioning

> ▷ Stability of traits over time and across situations

▶ Cultural issues versus maladaptive personality traits

> ▷ Issues of acculturation in new immigrants

> ▷ Cultural expression of habitual behavior

> ▷ Custom or religious practices

Assessment for Cluster A Disorders

▶ Patterns of pervasive distrust and suspiciousness, with odd and unusual behavior

> ▷ Present in a variety of contexts, even without supportive evidence

▶ Distrust usually not at psychotic level but can display brief psychotic episodes under stress

▶ Significant history includes the following:

> ▷ Limited social network

> ▷ Poor interpersonal relationships

> ▷ Limited disclosure or revealing of self to others, often refusing to answer personal questions

> ▷ Compliments often misinterpreted

▷ Pathological jealousy common

▷ Difficult to get along with

▷ Appearing cold and lacking in feelings

▷ High control needs

▷ Rigid and critical of others

▷ Often highly litigious

▷ Negatively perceive others; often biased and prone to stereotypes

▶ Differences in Cluster A disorders are in degree of suspiciousness and mistrust and in behavioral manifestations of those traits (see Table 14–2).

Assessment for Cluster B Disorders

▶ Patterns of pervasive affective and interpersonal disruption

▷ Present in a variety of contexts, even without supportive evidence

▶ Disturbance usually not at psychotic level but can display brief psychotic episodes under stress

▶ Of all clusters, disorders of Cluster B type may require hospitalization during period of active symptom expression and when client is under significant levels of stress

▶ Significant history includes the following:

▷ Fluctuating emotional states

▷ Dramatic qualities to how the person lives his or her life

TABLE 14–2.
CHARACTERISTICS OF CLUSTER A PERSONALITY DISORDERS

DISORDER	CHARACTERISTIC
Schizoid personality disorder	Neither desires nor enjoys close relationships
	Chooses solitary activities
	Shows little to no interest in sexual activity with another person
	Derives no pleasure in social activities
	Lacks close friends or social supports
	Is indifferent of opinion of others
	Appears cold and detached
	Exhibits affective flattening
Schizotypal personality disorder	Ideas of reference
	Odd beliefs
	Magical thinking
	Unusual perceptual experiences
	Paranoid ideation
	Inappropriate or constricted affect
	Behavior overtly odd, eccentric, or peculiar
	Few or no close friends
	Excessive social anxiety

▶ Antisocial personality disorder

▷ Usually diagnosed by age 18

▷ More common in men

▷ High substance abuse comorbidity

▷ High impulsivity

▷ Often diagnosed with conduct disorder as children

▶ Borderline personality disorder

▷ Predominantly in women

▷ Often with positive history of significant childhood physical abuse, sexual abuse, neglect, or early parental separation or loss

▶ Differences in Cluster B disorders are in degree of affective instability, type of interpersonal disruption, and behavioral manifestations of those traits (see Table 14–3).

Assessment for Cluster C Disorders

▶ Patterns of pervasive anxiety and fear

▷ Present in a variety of contexts, even without supportive evidence

▶ Disturbance usually not at psychotic level but can display brief psychotic episodes under stress

▶ Significant history includes the following:

▷ Avoidant behavior

▷ Procrastination

▷ Difficulty in following through

▷ Fearful of rejection and criticism

▷ Difficulty relaxing

▶ Avoidant personality disorder

▷ Must consider cultural variable when looking at avoidant behavior

▷ Disorder equal for both genders

▶ Dependent personality disorder

▷ Most frequently diagnosed personality disorder

▷ Rates higher in women than in men

▷ Commonly diagnosed in people with history of chronic physical illnesses

▶ Obsessive–compulsive personality disorder

▷ Predominantly in men

▷ Symptoms similar to but less severe than obsessive–compulsive disorder

▶ Differences in Cluster C disorders are in the degree of anxiety and fear and in behavioral manifestations of those traits (see Table 14–4).

Physical Exam Findings

▶ Nonspecific

TABLE 14–3.
CHARACTERISTICS OF CLUSTER B PERSONALITY DISORDERS

DISORDER	CHARACTERISTIC
Antisocial personality disorder	Failure to conform to social norms
	Repeated acts that are grounds for arrest
	Deceitfulness, lying, and use of aliases for profit or pleasure
	Impulsivity and failure of future planning
	Reckless disregard for the welfare of others
	Consistent irresponsibility
	Lack of remorse; indifference to the feelings of others
Borderline personality disorder	Frantic efforts to avoid real or imagined abandonment
	Pattern of unstable, intense interpersonal relationships
	Identity disturbances
	Impulsivity, often with self-damaging behavior
	Recurrent suicidal behavior
	Chronic feelings of emptiness
	Inappropriate, intensified affective anger responses
	Transient psychotic symptoms of paranoia and dissociation
Histrionic personality disorder	Uncomfortable in situations in which he or she is not center of attention
	Interactions with others characterized by inappropriate seductive or sexualized or provocative behavior, rapid shifting, and shallow emotional responses
	Consistent use of physical appearance to draw attention to self
	Speech excessively impressionistic and lacking in detail
	Suggestible and easily influenced
	Relationships considered more intimate than they are
Narcissistic personality disorder	Grandiose sense of self-importance
	Preoccupation with fantasies of power, success, brilliance, and beauty
	Belief of self-importance and being special and unique
	Excessive admiration required
	Unreasonable expectations or sense of entitlement
	Interpersonally exploitative
	Empathy lacking
	Envy of others and belief that others envy him or her
	Arrogant and haughty behaviors

Diagnostic and Laboratory Findings

▶ Complete blood count (CBC), chemistry profile, and thyroid function tests to rule out metabolic causes or unidentified conditions

▶ Drug toxicity screening if indicated by history

TABLE 14–4.
CHARACTERISTICS OF CLUSTER C PERSONALITY DISORDERS

DISORDER	CHARACTERISTIC
Avoidant personality disorder	Avoidance of activities involving significant interpersonal contact
	Fear of criticism, disapproval, or rejection
	Unwillingness to be involved with people unless sure of being liked
	Restraint in intimate relationships for fear of being shamed
	Preoccupation with being criticized or rejected in social settings
	View of self as socially inept, personally unappealing, or inferior
	Unusual reluctance to take personal risks or engage in new activities
Dependent personality disorder	Difficulty making everyday decisions without excessive advice
	Needing others to assume responsibility for most areas of life
	Difficulty expressing disagreement
	Difficulty initiating projects by himself or herself
	Going to excessive lengths to obtain nurturing and support from others
	Urgent seeking of another relationship if a close relationship ends
	Unrealistic preoccupation with fears of being left alone
Obsessive–compulsive personality disorder	Preoccupation with details, rules, order, and organization
	Perfectionism that interferes with task completion
	Excessive devotion to work and productivity
	Overly conscientious, scrupulous, and inflexible on issues of morality
	Inability to discard worn-out or worthless objects
	Reluctance to delegate tasks or work with others
	Adoption of a miserly spending style toward self and others
	Rigidity and stubbornness

Differential Diagnosis

▶ Comorbidity is common

▶ Mood disorders (see Chapter 9)

▷ Affective instability of borderline personality disorder often mistaken for bipolar affective disorder

▶ Substance-induced disorders (see Chapter 13)

Clinical Management

▶ Rule out or treat any conditions that may contribute to cognitive impairment.

▶ Personality disorders are generally managed in a community setting.

▶ In some cases, hospitalization may be required.

Pharmacological Management

- ▶ No specific class of pharmacological agents used to treat personality disorders
- ▶ Individualized symptom control
  - ▷ Impulsivity
    - ▶ Selective serotonin reuptake inhibitors (SSRIs)
    - ▶ Anticonvulsant mood stabilizers
  - ▷ Affective instability
    - ▶ SSRIs
    - ▶ Anticonvulsant mood stabilizers
  - ▷ Anxiety
    - ▶ Non-benzodiazepine anxiolytics
    - ▶ SSRIs
    - ▶ Benzodiazepines are used with extreme caution

Nonpharmacological Management

- ▶ Most common form of treatment for personality disorders
- ▶ Focus on issues of limit-setting, protection from self-harm, improved coping, and enhanced interpersonal functioning
- ▶ Multiple therapeutic interventions may be used, such as
  - ▷ Case management
  - ▷ Psychotherapy
    - ▶ Focus on the person gaining control
    - ▶ Improvement of interpersonal skill level
    - ▶ Enhanced coping
    - ▶ Alteration of problematic patterns of behavior
    - ▶ Forms of therapy:
      - ▷ Dialectical behavioral therapy
      - ▷ Psychodynamic therapy
      - ▷ Interpersonal therapy
      - ▷ Behavioral therapy
      - ▷ Cognitive behavioral therapy (CBT)
      - ▷ Milieu therapy
- ▶ Assist with realistic expectation formation
- ▶ Structure environment
- ▶ Improve realistic self-appraisal ability

Life Span Considerations

▶ Children

▷ Before diagnosis is determined, sufficient life experiences must occur so that chronicity of maladaptive patterns can be observed.

▷ Features of personality disorder usually become apparent during adolescence to early adulthood.

▷ It is unusual for someone to be given personality disorder diagnosis before ages 16 to 18 (an exception is antisocial personality disorder, which often is observable by onset of puberty; however, diagnosis of antisocial personality disorder is not made until age 18).

▷ Separation anxiety and chronic physical illness often precede and predict onset of dependent personality disorder.

Follow-up

▶ These are chronic disorders, and clients may be resistant to change.

▶ Relapse is common and frequent.

▶ How long to treat and success rates vary with client characteristics and motivation.

▶ Prognosis is poor without treatment.

▶ Prognosis improves if treatment is started as early in life as possible.

CASE STUDY

Mr. Jevers is 42-year-old new client who seeks health care for a general physical exam. The family nurse practitioner who examines Mr. Jevers asks the psychiatric–mental health nurse practitioner (PMHNP) to speak with him because of his odd presentation. The client discusses with the PMHNP an unusual, recurrent experience he has been having.

Mr. Jevers lives in an apartment building downtown and works as a bartender in the late evening. He tells the PMHNP that every night as he walks home from work he watches to see if the wind "blows north to south or south to north." He relates that, on the occasions that wind goes north to south, he takes that as a sign that a woman will visit him. He tells of a woman who rides a bicycle down the road and, as she passes him, he receives a blessing from her that protects him from those who wish him harm. He believes the woman is a "spirit from the other side" and that no one but he can see the woman.

As Mr. Jevers tells his story, his affect is inappropriate, his mood pleasant and happy, and he exhibits some paranoid ideation as he worries that others will try to take away the spirit. His mental status examination (MSE) shows ideas of reference and some magical thinking as he shares his "blessing" with customers in the bar, and he describes odd, eccentric, and peculiar behaviors. Mr. Jevers is not at all bothered by his unusual experience and seems to enjoy telling it to others. He considers himself lucky to have "special powers" and to see and understand things that other do not. Mr. Jevers denies the presence of any typical manifestations of hallucinations or delusions, any mood disturbance or anxiety, and alcohol or other drug use. He reports having several close friends, a strong support network, and is in general good health but does experience significant social anxiety. He does not believe his unusual experience is a symptom of an illness and wishes no intervention or assistance at this time.

1.   What is the most probable diagnosis for this client?

2.   What further assessment should occur?

3.   If the client desires no treatment, should the PMHNP attempt to follow up with him?

4.   What treatment should be suggested at this time?

ANSWERS TO CASE STUDY DISCUSSION QUESTIONS

1. The most likely diagnosis for this client is schizotypal personality disorder.

2. Medical work-up including drug screen is indicated to complete a thorough assessment.

3. If the client is unwilling to engage in treatment, the PMHNP should try to follow up with the client at regular intervals and continue to build a therapeutic alliance.

4. If the client is willing to engage in treatment, treatment indicated is using a CBT approach would be helpful for the client to find "evidence" for his unusual thoughts and beliefs.

REFERENCES AND RESOURCES

American Psychiatric Association. (2013). *Diagnostic and statistical manual of mental disorders* (5th ed.). Washington, DC: Author.

Linehan, M., … Lindenboim, N. (2006). Two-year randomized controlled trial and follow-up of dialectical behavior therapy vs therapy by experts for suicidal behaviors and borderline personality disorder. *JAMA, 63*(7), 757–766.

Neacsiu, A., Lungu, A., Harned, M., Rizvi, S., & Linehan, M. (2014). Impact of dialectical behavioral therapy versus community treatment by experts on emotional experience, expression, and acceptance in borderline personality disorder. *Behaviour Research and Therapy, 53*, 47–54.

Nelson, K., Zagoloff, A., Quinn, S., Swanson, H., Garber, C., & Schulz, C. (2014). Borderline personality disorder: Treatment approaches and perspectives. *Clinical Practice, 11*(3), 341–349.

Perese, E. F. (2012). *Psychiatric advanced practice nursing: A biopsychosocial foundation for practice.* Philadelphia, PA: F. A. Davis.

Rees, C., & Prichard, R. (2015). Brief cognitive therapy for avoidant personality disorder. *Psychotherapy, 52*(1), 45–55.

Reichborn-Kjennerud, T., Czajkowski, N., Ystrom, E., Orstavik, R., Aggen, S., & Kendler, K. (2015) A longitudinal twin study of borderline and antisocial disorder traits in early to middle adulthood. *Psychological Medicine, 45*(14), 3121–1331.

Sadock, B. J., Sadock, V. A., & Ruiz, P. (2015). *Kaplan and Sadock's synopsis of psychiatry: Behavioral sciences/clinical psychiatry* (11th ed.). New York, NY: Wolters Kluwer.

Schmahl, C. G., McGlashan, T., & Bremner, J. D. (2002). Neurobiological correlates of borderline personality disorder. *Psychopharmacology Bulletin, 36*(2), 69–78.

Tusaie, K., & Fitzpatrick, J. (2013). *Advanced practice psychiatric nursing integrating psychotherapy, psychopharmacology, and complementary and alternative approached.* New York, NY: Springer Publishing Company.

Wheeler, K. (2014). *Psychotherapy for the advanced practice psychiatric nurse* (2nd ed.). New York, NY: Springer Publishing Company.

CHAPTER 15

DISORDERS OF CHILDHOOD AND ADOLESCENCE

Disorders first diagnosed in infancy, childhood, or adolescence, such as conduct disorder, oppositional defiant disorder, attention-deficit hyperactivity disorder, Rett syndrome, autism spectrum disorder, eating disorders, and intellectual disabilities, are considered brain-based illnesses and have many similarities to disorders diagnosed more commonly in adulthood. In addition, these disorders often are missed during childhood and adolescent years and are therefore not identified until early adulthood.

The disorders diagnosed during childhood or in adolescent differ in presentation based on developmental context of the person, age of onset, and gender. Assessment, treatment planning, and therapeutic interventions for these disorders must always occur within the context of the family and assume a multimodal, systems-oriented approach to care. In addition, assessment of children is different from assessment of adults. Prior to making a psychiatric diagnosis, all possible medical causes of the symptoms must be ruled out. Therefore, psychiatric–mental health nurse practitioners (PMHNPs) must apply principles of child assessment to care and have a good understanding of normal growth and development to detect what is disordered. Effective assessment, diagnosis, and treatment is completed in the context of the family system, however family is defined for the client.

ASSESSMENT AND CARE PLANNING FOR CHILDREN AND ADOLESCENTS

- ▶ Requires alteration in assessment process
  - ▷ Generally takes more time.
  - ▷ PMHNP must develop trusting relationship with the child to put him or her at ease.
  - ▷ Interview the child and parent separately: child can provide information on internal symptoms and family or care providers on external signs (Hamrin & Gray Deering, 2012).
  - ▷ Must attend to developmental needs and interests of the child.
  - ▷ Must attend to the cognitive and language abilities of the child.

▶ Mental status examination (Sadock, Sadock, & Ruiz, 2015).

▷ Modified to reflect developmental and other age-related issues in children

▷ Often requires establishment of a play environment to open communication with the child

▷ Appearance

▶ Conclusions must consider age and developmental processes (e.g., physical appearance and dress for weather and age group).

▶ Gait and motor skills are assessed on expected normative behaviors for age.

▶ Parent–child interaction

▷ Observe interaction in waiting room

▷ Examine way parent and child talk with one another and emotional overtones

▷ Separation and reunion

▶ Examine how child reacts to separation and reunion with parent

▶ Speech and language

▷ Assessed on expected normative and appropriate language use for age

▷ Comprehension, word selection, and range of vocabulary

▷ Rate, rhythm, latency, intonation, spontaneity

▶ Mood and affect

▷ *Mood*: Verbal admission of feelings or assessment based on themes, play, and fantasy

▷ *Affect*: Range of emotions expressed, appropriateness of affect to thought content

▶ Thought process and content

▷ *Thought process*: Looseness of associations, magical thinking, preservation, echolalia, ability to distinguish fantasy from reality (by age 4 children have some understanding of what is real or made up), flight of ideas

▷ *Thought content*: Suicidal or homicidal ideation, perceptual disturbances (hallucinations)

▶ Social relatedness

▷ Child's response to interviewer

▶ Motor behavior

▷ Coordination, activity level, involuntary movements, tremors, tics, unusual asymmetries

▶ Cognition

▷ Intellectual functioning and problem-solving abilities

▶ Memory

▷ Test recall after 5 minutes (school-age children should be able to remember three objects after 5 minutes)

▶ Abstraction

▷ Assessed on expected normative behaviors for age

▷ Children ages 12 or younger not expected to have abstractive thought abilities (young children have concrete thinking)

▷ Proverb testing and similarity testing require prior exposure to concept, word choices, and ability to think abstractly

▶ Judgement and insight

▷ Child's view of problem

▷ Child's understanding of what he or she can do to help the problem

▶ Therapeutic care planning

▷ Variety of effective treatments commonly used with children and adolescents:

▶ Play therapy

▶ Art therapy

▶ Bibliotherapy

▶ Orative therapy (such as storytelling, family narrative therapy)

▶ Behavioral therapy

▶ Interpersonal therapy

▶ Cognitive therapy

▶ Milieu therapy

▶ Pharmacotherapy

OPPOSITIONAL DEFIANT DISORDER (ODD)

Description

▶ *Oppositional defiant disorder (ODD)* is an enduring pattern of angry or irritable mood and argumentative, defiant, or vindictive behavior lasting at least 6 months with at least four of the associated symptoms:

▷ Loses temper

▷ Touchy or easily annoyed

▷ Angry or resentful

▷ Argues with authority

▷ Actively defies or refuses to comply with request or rules from authority figures

▷ Blames others

▷ Deliberately annoys others

▷ Spiteful or vindictive

Etiology

▶ Temperament

▶ Parents who model extreme ways of expressing emotions

▶ Trauma

▶ Unresolved conflicts

Prevalence and Demographics

▶ ODD is more common in children of parents with a history of ODD, conduct disorder, attention-deficit hyperactivity disorder (ADHD), antisocial personality disorder, mood disorders, or substance abuse disorder.

▶ It affects 1% to 11% of the general U.S. population, with an average of 3.3%.

▶ More common in males (1.4:1).

▶ About 30% of children with ODD develop conduct disorder.

Risk Factors

▶ Genetic and physiological

▶ Temperamental

▶ Environmental

Prevention and Screening

▶ At-risk family education

▶ Community education

▷ Stigma reduction

▷ Signs and symptoms of illness

▷ Treatment potential for control of symptoms

▶ Well-child visit mental health screening

▶ Early recognition, intervention, and initiation of treatment

▷ Secondary prevention important in younger clients

Assessment

History

▶ Assess for the following:

▷ Detailed history of present illness, including time frame, progression, and associated symptoms

▷ Social history, including present living situation; education; and alcohol, tobacco, or illicit drug use

▷ Medication use, including prescription, over-the-counter, alternative, supplements, and home remedies

▷ Initial and periodic functional history and assessment

▷ Validate history with a family member

▷ Substance or alcohol use

Physical Exam Findings

▶ Nonspecific

Mental Status Exam Findings

▶ Mood

▷ *Lability:* Low frustration tolerance, angry, argue and lose temper

▶ Concentration

▷ Impaired

▶ Thought content

▷ Often blame others for mistakes

Diagnostic and Laboratory Findings

▶ No specific laboratory tests

▶ Complete blood count (CBC), chemistry profile, thyroid function tests, and B_{12} level to rule out metabolic causes or unidentified conditions

▶ Drug toxicity screening, if indicated by history

▷ Lead toxicity

▷ Toxicology screen to rule out a substance abuse disorder

Differential Diagnosis

▶ ADHD (see below)

▶ Mood disorders (see Chapter 9)

▶ Substance abuse disorders (see Chapter 13)

▶ Intellectual disability (see below)

▶ Conduct disorder (see below)

▶ Psychotic disorders (see Chapter 11)

Clinical Management

▶ Rule out or treat any conditions that may contribute to current symptom manifestation.

Pharmacological Management

▶ Nonspecific: not first-line treatment

▶ Target symptoms: mood or aggression

Nonpharmacological Management

▶ Therapy is mainstay:

▷ Individual therapy

▷ Family therapy, with emphasis on child management skills

▷ Evidence-based treatment: child and parent problem-solving skills training (American Academy of Child and Adolescent Psychiatry [AACAP], 2007b).

▶ Incredible Years (group intervention)

▶ Parent–child interactional therapy (individual or family intervention)

▶ Adolescent Transitions Program (ATP; individual or family and group intervention)

CONDUCT DISORDER

Description

▶ *Conduct disorder* is a repetitive and persistent pattern of behavior in which the rights of others or societal norms or rules are violated. The presence of at least three of the following criteria must be present in the past 12 months, with one in the past 6 months:

▷ Aggression toward people or animals—bullies, threatens, intimidates, initiates physical fights, uses a weapon to cause physical harm to others, physically cruel to people or animals, stealing while confronting a victim, forced sexual activity on someone

▷ Destruction of property—engaged in fire-setting, destroyed others' property

▷ Deceit or theft—broke into house, building, or car; lies, steals items

▷ Serious violation of rules—stays out late before age 13, runs away from home, truant before age 13

▷ Child onset before age 10 or adolescent onset after age 10

Etiology

▶ No single factor accounts for presentation.

▶ Etiology is largely unknown.

▶ Many biopsychosocial factors contribute to the development.

Prevalence

▶ Conduct disorder is more common in children of parents with antisocial personality disorder, alcohol dependence, mood disorders, or schizophrenia than in the general population.

Incidence and Demographics

▶ Affects 2% to 10% of general U.S. population, 6% to 16% of boys and 2% to 9% of girls

▶ Onset is earlier for boys (10 to 12 years) than for girls (16 years)

Risk Factors

▶ Genetic loading

▶ Temperamental: Lower than average IQ

▶ Environmental: Family rejection and neglect, unsupervised, physical or sexual abuse, substance use

Prevention and Screening

▶ At-risk family education

▶ Community education

▷ Stigma reduction

▷ Signs and symptoms of illness

▷ Treatment potential for control of symptoms

▶ Early recognition, intervention, and initiation of treatment

▷ Secondary prevention is important in younger clients

Assessment

History

▶ Assess for the following:

▷ Detailed history of present illness, including time frame, progression, and associated symptoms

▷ Social history, including present living situation; education; and alcohol, tobacco, or illicit drug use

▷ Medication use, including prescription, over-the-counter, alternative, supplements, and home remedies

▷ Initial and periodic functional history and assessment

▷ Developmental history

▷ Validate history with a family member

Physical Exam Findings

▶ Nonspecific

Mental Status Exam Findings

- ▶ Affect
  - ▷ Irritable
  - ▷ Angry
  - ▷ Uncooperative
- ▶ Mood
  - ▷ Anger
- ▶ Thought content
  - ▷ Lack of empathy or concern for others
- ▶ Concentration
  - ▷ Distractible
- ▶ Insight
  - ▷ Poor

Diagnostic and Laboratory Findings

- ▶ No specific laboratory tests
- ▶ Drug screening to rule out possible substance abuse
- ▶ CBC, chemistry profile, thyroid function tests, and B_{12} level to rule out metabolic causes or unidentified conditions

Differential Diagnosis

- ▶ Attention-deficit hyperactivity disorder (ADHD; see below)
- ▶ Oppositional defiant disorder (ODD; see above)
- ▶ Mood disorders (see Chapter 9)
- ▶ Posttraumatic stress disorder (see Chapter 10)
- ▶ Substance abuse disorders (see Chapter 11)
- ▶ Developmental disorders (see below)

Clinical Management

- ▶ Rule out or treat any conditions that may contribute to current symptom manifestation.

Pharmacological Management

- ▶ No specific pharmacological interventions
- ▶ Aggression and agitation treated with antipsychotics, mood stabilizers, selective serotonin reuptake inhibitors (SSRIs), and alpha agonists

Nonpharmacological Management

▶ Multimodality treatment programs that use all available family and community resources

▶ Behavioral therapy is mainstay:
  ▷ Individual therapy
  ▷ Family therapy

Life Span Considerations

▶ May be diagnosed in clients ages 18 years or older if criteria for antisocial personality disorder are not met.

ATTENTION-DEFICIT HYPERACTIVITY DISORDER (ADHD)

Description

▶ *Attention-deficit hyperactivity disorder (ADHD)* is a persistent pattern of inattention or hyperactivity, impulsivity, or both, that interferes with functioning and development.

  ▷ Inattention, six or more of the following:
    ▶ Fails to give attention to details
    ▶ Difficulty sustaining attention
    ▶ Does not listen when spoken to
    ▶ Does not follow through on instructions
    ▶ Disorganized
    ▶ Avoids or dislikes tasks requiring sustained mental effort
    ▶ Loses things
    ▶ Distracted
    ▶ Forgetful

  ▷ Hyperactive and impulsive, six or more of the following:
    ▶ Fidgets
    ▶ Leaves seat
    ▶ Runs or climbs
    ▶ Unable to engage in quiet activities
    ▶ "On the go"
    ▶ Talks excessively
    ▶ Blurts out information
    ▶ Difficulty waiting turn
    ▶ Interrupts others

- ▶ Several symptoms were present prior to age 12
    - ▷ Subtypes:
        - ▶ ADHD, inattentive type
            - ▷ Inattentive symptoms dominate
            - ▷ Lack of criterion symptoms for hyperactivity or impulsivity
        - ▶ ADHD, hyperactive type
            - ▷ Hyperactivity or impulsivity symptoms dominate
            - ▷ Lack of criterion symptoms for inattention
        - ▶ ADHD, combined type
            - ▷ Criterion symptoms met for inattention and hyperactivity or impulsivity

Etiology

- ▶ Many biopsychosocial factors contribute to the development of ADHD.
- ▶ Polygenic neurobiological deficits are associated with ADHD.
    - ▷ Problems with executive functioning
    - ▷ Abnormalities of fronto–subcortical pathways
        - ▶ Frontal cortex
        - ▶ Basal ganglia
    - ▷ Abnormalities of reticular activating system
    - ▷ Structural abnormalities producing neurotransmitter abnormalities
        - ▶ Dopamine dysfunction
        - ▶ Norepinephrine dysfunction

Incidence and Demographics

- ▶ 5% of children and 2.5% of adults in the United States have ADHD.
- ▶ Boys are more likely to be diagnosed (13.2%) than girls (5.6%; CDC, 2010).
- ▶ Average age of onset is 3 years; mean age of diagnosis is 9 years.
- ▶ Approximately 60% of clients have symptoms persisting into adulthood.
    - ▷ Inattention symptoms are more persistent than hyperactivity and impulsivity symptoms.

Risk Factors

- ▶ Genetic loading
    - ▷ Pregnancy and perinatal complications
    - ▷ Family conflict

▶ Environmental

▷ Low birth weight

▷ Neglect, foster placement

▷ Alcohol exposure in utero

▶ Temperamental

▷ Reduced behavioral inhibition

Prevention and Screening

▶ At-risk family education

▶ Community education

▷ Stigma reduction

▷ Signs and symptoms of illness

▷ Treatment potential for control of symptoms

▶ Early recognition, intervention, and initiation of treatment

▷ Secondary prevention is important in young clients.

Assessment

Physical Exam Findings

▶ Nonspecific

▶ Minor physical anomalies at higher rates in people with ADHD than in general population:

▷ Hypertelorism

▷ Highly arched palate

▷ Low-set ears

▶ Higher-than-average accidental injury rates

Mental Status Exam Findings

▶ Restlessness

▶ Inattention

▶ Distractible speech patterns

▶ Overproductive speech patterns

▶ Affective lability

▶ Poor memory

▶ Poor concentration

Diagnostic and Laboratory Findings

▶ Nonspecific

Differential Diagnosis

▶ Understimulated home environment

▶ Substance abuse

▶ Major depressive disorder (MDD)

▶ Bipolar (BP) disorder

▶ Stereotypic movement disorder

Clinical Management

Pharmacological Management

▶ Most commonly used agents (see Table 15–1) are stimulants (Schedule II)—controlled substances that carry risk for abuse.

▷ Monitor for side effects and adverse effects of stimulants:

▶ Gastrointestinal (GI) upset

▶ Cramps

▶ Anorexia

TABLE 15–1.
MOST COMMONLY USED AGENTS FOR ADHD

DRUG	DOSAGE
Ritalin (methylphenidate hydrochloride), Schedule II	5–40 mg/day
Ritalin LA/Ritalin SR (methylphenidate hydrochloride), Schedule II	10–60 mg/day
Metadate CD (methylphenidate hydrochloride), Schedule II	10–60 mg/day
Metadate ER (methylphenidate hydrochloride), Schedule II	10–60 mg/day
Concerta (methylphenidate hydrochloride), Schedule II	18–72 mg/day
Methylin (methylphenidate hydrochloride), Schedule II	5–60 mg/day
Methylin ER (methylphenidate hydrochloride), Schedule II	10–60 mg/day
Daytrana (methylphenidate transdermal patch), Schedule II	10 mg–30 mg/day (9 hours)
Dexedrine (dextroamphetamine), Schedule II	2.5–20 mg/day
Adderall (amphetamine, dextroamphetamine), Schedule II	5–40 mg/day
Adderall XR (amphetamine, dextroamphetamine), Schedule II	5–60 mg/day
Focalin/Focalin XR (dexmethylphenidate), Schedule II	2.5–20 mg/day
Vyvanse (lisdexamfetamine dimesylate), Schedule II	30–70 mg/day
Strattera (atomoxetine hydrochloride), not a controlled substance	10–100 mg/day
Intuniv (guanfacine), alpha agonist; not a controlled substance; FDA-approved for ages 6–17	1–4 mg/day
Catapres (clonidine), alpha agonist; not a controlled substance; not FDA-approved	0.1–0.4 mg/day
Wellbutrin SR/XL (bupropion), norepinephrine dopamine reuptake inhibitor; not FDA-approved	100–450 mg/day

- ▶ Weight loss
- ▶ Blood pressure changes
- ▶ Increased pulse rate
- ▶ Growth suppression (rare)
- ▶ Headache, dizziness
- ▶ Irritability
- ▶ Psychosis (rare)

Nonpharmacological Management

- ▶ Behavioral therapy
- ▶ Patient and parent cognitive behavioral training program
- ▶ Psychoeducation
- ▶ Treatment of learning disorders
- ▶ Family therapy and education
  - ▷ Parents of children with ADHD have many difficult emotions:
    - ▶ Stress
    - ▶ Self-blame
    - ▶ Social isolation
    - ▶ Embarrassment
    - ▶ Depressive reaction
    - ▶ Marital discord
  - ▷ Typical family concerns:
    - ▶ Stigma
    - ▶ Anger
    - ▶ Concerns over treatment options
    - ▶ Presence of controversial information in media
      - ▷ Claims of dietary causes of disorder
      - ▷ Belief in family etiological factors
  - ▷ Family educational needs:
    - ▶ Environmental structuring
    - ▶ Psychiatric comorbidities
    - ▶ School issues and concerns
    - ▶ Peer relationship-building
    - ▶ Smoking and substance abuse rates
    - ▶ Stress management
- ▶ Common comorbidities
  - ▷ Major depressive disorder (see Chapter 9)

    ▷   Bipolar disorder (see Chapter 9)

    ▷   Anxiety disorders (see Chapter 10)

    ▷   Oppositional defiant disorder (see above)

    ▷   Substance abuse disorders (see Chapter 13)

    ▷   Tic disorder

    ▷   Learning disorders

Follow-up

▶ Monitor clinical progress over time.

▶ Use standardized rating scales such as:

    ▷   Conners' Parent and Teacher Rating Scales (copyrighted)

    ▷   Vanderbilt ADHD Diagnostic Parent and Teacher Rating Scales (public domain)

▶ Monitor attainment of growth and development milestones.

▶ Symptoms may persist into adulthood.

    ▷   Plan for long-term needs.

AUTISM SPECTRUM DISORDER

Description

▶ Persistent deficits in social communication and social interaction across multiple settings associated with deficits in:

    ▷   Social reciprocity

    ▷   Nonverbal communication

    ▷   Developing, maintaining, and understanding relationships.

▶ Restricted repetitive behavior:

    ▷   Stereotyped or repetitive motor movements

    ▷   Insistence on sameness

    ▷   Highly restricted with fixed interests

    ▷   Hyper- or hyposensory input

Etiology

▶ No single factor can account for presentation.

▶ Etiology is largely unknown.

▶ Many biopsychosocial factors contribute to the development.

Prevalence

▶ The disorder appears to be more common in families in which other members have autism spectrum disorder (ASD).

▶ Affects about 1% of U.S population, but the disorder is more common in boys.

▶ Imbalances of glutamate, serotonin, and gamma-aminobutyric acid (GABA) are thought to be implicated in causation.

▶ Brain imaging studies of children with autism revealed microscopic and macroscopic abnormalities of the amygdala, hippocampus, and cerebellum.

▶ Decreased numbers of Purkinje cells in the cerebellum are thought to play a role in the development.

Incidence and Demographics

▶ ASD is more common in children with a family history of pervasive developmental disorders.

▶ The concordant rate for an identical twin with autism is 60%.

▶ The incidence is 2 to 5 cases per 10,000 in the United States.

▶ The male-to-female ratio is 4:1.

▶ Onset of symptoms is before age 3 years.

▶ About 10% of people with autism also have a genetic or chromosomal condition such as Down syndrome or fragile X syndrome (CDC, 2015).

Risk Factors

▶ Male

▶ Intellectual disability

▶ Genetic loading

Prevention and Screening

▶ At-risk family education

▶ Community education

   ▷ Stigma reduction

   ▷ Signs and symptoms of illness

   ▷ Treatment potential for control of symptoms

▶ Early recognition, intervention, and initiation of treatment

   ▷ Secondary prevention is important in young clients.

Assessment

History

▶ Assess for the following:

▷ Impairment with social interaction, communications, and behavior

▶ Impaired social interactions such as abnormal gaze, posture, and expression in social interactions

▷ Lack of peer relationships, emotional reciprocity, and spontaneous seeking of enjoyment

▷ Impaired communication, such as a delay or lack in the development of spoken language, impaired ability to initiate and sustain conversations, repetitive and stereotyped use of language, and inability to play with others

▷ Restricted repetitive and stereotyped patterns of behavior, interests, and activities, such as inflexible adherence to specific nonfunctional routines and repetitive, stereotyped motor mannerisms (e.g., hand or finger flapping, rocking, swaying)

▷ Parents may report any of the following symptoms:

▶ No cooing by age 1 year, no single words by age 16 months, no two-word phrases by age 24 months

▶ Loss of language skills at any time

▶ No imaginary play

▶ Little interest in playing with other children

▶ Extremely short attention span

▶ No response when called by name

▶ Little or no eye contact

▶ Intense tantrums

▶ Fixations on single objects

▶ Unusually strong resistance to changes in routines

▶ Oversensitivity to certain sounds, textures, or smells

▶ Appetite or sleep–rest disturbance, or both

▶ Self-injurious behavior

Physical Exam Findings

▶ Nonspecific

Mental Status Exam Findings

▶ Little or no eye contact

▶ Flat or blunted affect

▶ Lack of emotional reciprocity

▶ Stereotyped or repetitive motor mannerisms

▷ Expressive- and receptive-language impairment

Screening

▶ Screened for developmental delays at well-child visit (CDC, 2015).

▷ Modified Checklist for Autism in Toddlers (M-CHAT)

▷ Autism Diagnostic Observation Schedule–Generic (ADOS-G)

▷ Ages and Stages Questionnaires (ASQ)

Diagnostic and Laboratory Findings

▶ No specific laboratory tests

Differential Diagnosis

▶ Rett syndrome (see below)

▶ Asperger syndrome

▶ Childhood disintegrative disorder

▶ Intellectual disability (see below)

▶ Hearing impairment

▶ Developmental language and speech disorders

▶ Tic disorders

▶ Stereotypic movement disorder

▶ Schizophrenia (see Chapter 11)

▶ Cluster A personality disorders (see Chapter 14)

Clinical Management

Pharmacological Management

▶ No specific pharmacological interventions

▶ Antipsychotics effective for symptoms such as tantrums; aggressive behavior; self-injurious behavior; hyperactivity; and repetitive, stereotyped behaviors

▶ Antidepressants, naltrexone, clonidine, and stimulants to diminish self-injurious and hyperactive and obsessive behaviors

Nonpharmacological Management

▶ Behavioral therapy to improve cognitive functioning and reduce inappropriate behavior

▶ Occupational therapy to improve sensory integration and motor skills

▶ Speech therapy to address communication and language barriers

▶ Pivotal response training

▶ Appropriate school placement with a highly structured approach

RETT SYNDROME

Description

▶ *Rett syndrome* is the development of specific deficits following a period of normal functioning after birth.

Etiology

▶ Etiology is unknown.

▶ There is a known, progressive, and deteriorating course after an initial period without apparent disability.

▶ It is compatible with probable metabolic disorder.

▶ Genetic mutation is suspected.

Incidence and Demographics

▶ The disorder occurs primarily in girls.

▶ It is usually associated with an intellectual disability (see below).

Risk Factors

▶ Seizure disorder

Prevention and Screening

▶ At-risk family education

▶ Community education

  ▷ Stigma reduction

  ▷ Signs and symptoms of illness

  ▷ Treatment potential for control of symptoms

▶ Early recognition, intervention, and initiation of treatment

  ▷ Secondary prevention is important in young clients

Assessment

▶ Detailed history of present illness, including time frame, progression, and associated symptoms

▶ Social history, including present living situation and education

▶ Medication use, including prescription, over-the-counter, alternative, supplements, and home remedies

▶ Initial and periodic functional history and assessment

▶ Validate all physical health findings with a family member.

History

▶ Assess for the following:

▷ Normal prenatal and perinatal development

▷ Normal psychomotor development through the first 5 months after birth

▷ Normal head circumference at birth

▷ Onset of all of the following after the period of normal development:

▶ Deceleration of head growth between the ages 5 to 48 months

▶ Loss of previously acquired purposeful hand skills between ages 5 to 30 months, with the subsequent development of stereotyped hand movements

▶ Early loss of social engagement

▶ Appearance of poorly coordinated gait or trunk movements

▶ Severely impaired expressive- and receptive-language development with severe psychomotor retardation.

Physical Exam Findings

▶ Associated features:

▷ Seizures

▷ Irregular respirations

▷ Scoliosis

▷ Loss of purposeful hand skills

▷ Stereotypic hand movements

Mental Status Exam Findings

▶ Appearance

▷ Stereotypic hand movements

▶ Speech

▷ Expressive- and receptive-language impairment

▶ Affect

▷ Flat or blunted affect

▷ Diagnostic and laboratory findings

▷ No specific laboratory or diagnostic findings

▷ CBC, chemistry profile, thyroid function tests, and B_{12} level to rule out metabolic causes or unidentified conditions

▷ Drug toxicity screening, if indicated by history

▷ Electroencephalogram (EEG) and nonspecific abnormalities on brain imaging

Differential Diagnosis

▶ Intellectual disability (see below)

▶ Autism spectrum disorder (see above).

Clinical Management

▶ Rule out or treat any conditions that may contribute to current symptom manifestation.

Pharmacological Management

▶ Nonspecific

Nonpharmacological Management

▶ Multimodality treatment

▶ Treatment aimed at symptomatic intervention

EATING DISORDERS

Description

▶ *Eating disorders* are characterized by disordered patterns of eating, accompanied by distress, disparagement, preoccupation, and a distorted perception of one's body shape.

▶ Common forms of eating disorders:

▷ Anorexia nervosa

▶ Clients refuse to maintain a normal body weight.

▶ Involves restricted caloric intake.

▶ Clients have an intense fear of gaining weight because of a distorted body image.

▷ Bulimia nervosa

▶ Clients engage in binge eating, combined with inappropriate ways of stopping weight gain

▶ Associated with efforts made to lose weight

▶ Usually normal or slightly overweight

▷ Binge eating disorder

▶ Recurrent episodes of binge eating with lack of control

▶ Bingeing occurs at least 2 days weekly for 6 months

▶ Not regularly associated with compensatory behaviors

Etiology

▶ Etiology is multifactorial, with biological, social, and psychological factors implicated in causation.

▶ Neurobiological factors include decreased hypothalamic norepinephrine activation, dysfunction of lateral hypothalamus, and decreased serotonin.

Incidence and Demographics

▶ Incidence is more common in girls, with 85% to 95% of occurrences.

▶ Anorexia nervosa affects approximately 0.28% of the general U.S. population.

▶ Bulimia nervosa affects approximately 1.0% of the general U.S. population.

▶ Onset is typically between ages 14 and 18 years.

Risk Factors

▶ Genetic loading

▶ Increased risk of eating disorders among first-degree biological relatives of people with certain other psychiatric disorders:

▷ Eating disorders

▷ Mood disorders

▷ Substance abuse disorders

Prevention and Screening

▶ At-risk family education

▶ Community education

▷ Stigma reduction

▷ Signs and symptoms of illness

▷ Treatment potential for control of symptoms

▶ Early recognition, intervention, and initiation of treatment

▷ Secondary prevention is important in young clients.

Assessment

▶ Detailed history of present illness, including time frame, progression, and associated symptoms

▶ Social history, including present living situation; marital status; occupation; education; and alcohol, tobacco, or illicit drug use

▶ Medication use, including prescription, over-the-counter, alternative, supplements, and home remedies

▶ Initial and periodic functional history and assessment

▶ Validate history with a family member.

History

▶ Assess for the following:

▷ Anorexia nervosa

    ▶ Refusal to maintain a minimally normal body weight

    ▶ Weight less than 85% of expected weight

    ▶ Fear of gaining weight or becoming fat

    ▶ Distorted body image

        ▷ *Restricting type:* During the current episode, the person has not regularly engaged in binge eating or purging behavior.

        ▷ *Binge eating or purging type:* During the current episode, the person has regularly engaged in binge eating or purging behavior.

▷ Bulimia nervosa

    ▶ Recurrent, episodic binge eating

    ▶ Both binge eating and inappropriate compensatory behaviors occur at least twice weekly for 3 months

    ▶ Recurrent, inappropriate compensatory behaviors to prevent weight gain:

        ▷ Self-induced vomiting

        ▷ Laxatives

        ▷ Enemas

        ▷ Diuretics

        ▷ Stimulants

        ▷ Abuse of diet pills

        ▷ Fasting

        ▷ Excessive exercise

    ▶ Self-evaluation unduly influenced by body shape and weight

        ▷ *Purging type:* During the current episode, the person regularly has engaged in purging or the misuse of laxatives, enemas, or diuretics.

        ▷ *Nonpurging type:* During the current episode, the person has used other inappropriate compensatory behaviors, such as fasting or excessive exercise, but has not regularly engaged in purging or misuse of laxatives, enemas, or diuretics.

Physical Exam Findings

▶ Anorexia nervosa:

    ▷ Low body mass index

    ▷ Amenorrhea

    ▷ Emaciation

    ▷ Bradycardia

    ▷ Hypotension

▷ Electrocardiogram (ECG) changes

  ▶ Inversion of T-waves

  ▶ ST segment depression

  ▶ Prolonged QT interval

▷ Hypothermia

▷ Yellow skin secondary to carotenemia

▷ Dry skin

▷ Brittle hair and nails

▷ Lanugo growth on face, extremities, and trunk

▷ Peripheral edema

▷ Hypertrophy of the salivary glands

▷ Erosion of dental enamel

▷ Russell's sign—scarring or calluses on the dorsum of the hand, secondary to self-induced vomiting

▶ Bulimia nervosa:

  ▷ Weight usually within normal range

  ▷ Erosion of dental enamel

  ▷ Russell's sign

  ▷ Hypertrophy of salivary glands

  ▷ Rectal prolapse

Mental Status Exam Findings

▶ Appearance

  ▷ Emaciated appearance with anorexia nervosa

▶ Affect

  ▷ Lability

  ▷ Anxiety

  ▷ Constricted and sad

▶ Mood

  ▷ Dysphoric mood

▶ Thought content

  ▷ Preoccupation with food and body weight

  ▷ Suicidal ideation

  ▷ Low self-esteem

▶ Concentration

  ▷ Decreased concentration

- ▶ Judgment
  - ▷ Impaired for self-welfare
- ▶ Insight
  - ▷ Impaired

Diagnostic and Laboratory Findings

- ▶ CBC, chemistry profile, thyroid function tests, and B_{12} level to rule out metabolic causes or unidentified conditions
- ▶ Drug toxicity screening, if indicated by history
- ▶ Anorexia nervosa
  - ▷ No definitive laboratory test for diagnosis
  - ▷ Laboratory changes:
    - ▶ Normochromic, normocytic anemia
    - ▶ Leukopenia
    - ▶ Neutropenia
    - ▶ Anemia
    - ▶ Thrombocytopenia
    - ▶ Hypokalemia
    - ▶ Hypomagnesemia
    - ▶ Hypoglycemia
    - ▶ Decreased LH and FSH
- ▶ Bulimia nervosa
  - ▷ No definitive laboratory tests
  - ▷ Laboratory changes:
    - ▶ Hypotension
    - ▶ Bradycardia
    - ▶ Hypokalemia
    - ▶ Hyponatremia
    - ▶ Hypochloremia
    - ▶ Hypomagnesemia
    - ▶ Metabolic acidosis or alkalosis
    - ▶ Elevated serum amylase

Differential Diagnosis

- ▶ General medical condition
- ▶ Mood disorders (see Chapter 9)
- ▶ Cluster B personality disorders (see Chapter 14)

▶ Obsessive–compulsive disorder (OCD; see Chapter 10)

▶ Schizophrenia (see Chapter 11)

Clinical Management

▶ Rule out or treat any conditions that may contribute to current symptom manifestation.

Pharmacological Management

▶ Medication management as adjunctive therapy to psychotherapy

▶ No specific medication therapy for anorexia nervosa

▶ Fluoxetine is FDA-approved for bulimia nervosa.

▶ SSRIs and tricyclic antidepressants (TCAs) effective in reducing the frequency of bingeing and purging

▶ Treat associated symptoms, such as depression and anxiety, with appropriate pharmacological therapy.

Nonpharmacological Management

▶ Multimodal treatment

  ▷ Medical and nutritional stabilization

    ▶ Weight restoration

    ▶ Correction of electrolyte disturbance

    ▶ Vitamin supplementation

    ▶ Nutrition counseling

  ▷ Dental care

  ▷ Psychotherapeutic interventions

    ▶ Individual psychotherapy

    ▶ Behavioral therapy

    ▶ Cognitive behavioral therapy

    ▶ Family therapy

    ▶ Group therapy

  ▷ Community resources

    ▶ Eating disorder support groups

    ▶ 12-step programs

Follow-up

▶ Regular follow up with a multidisciplinary team is necessary

INTELLECTUAL DISABILITY

Description

▶ *Intellectual disability has an onset during the developmental period and includes low intellect and adaptive functioning.*

▶ Onset must occur before age 18 years.

▶ Mild, moderate, severe, or profound.

  ▷ Based on adaptive functioning and *not* IQ scores

  ▷ IQ scores are less valid on the lower end of IQ range

Etiology

▶ Heredity accounts for 5% of cases:

  ▷ Inborn errors of metabolism (e.g., Tay-Sachs disease)

  ▷ Single-gene abnormalities (e.g., tuberous sclerosis)

  ▷ Chromosomal aberrations (e.g., translocation of chromosome 21 [Down syndrome] and X-linked gene of FMR-1 [fragile X syndrome]).

▶ Early alterations of embryonic development account for 30% of cases.

  ▷ Prenatal exposure to toxins (e.g., maternal alcohol consumption, infections)

▶ Pregnancy and perinatal problems account for 10% of cases.

  ▷ Fetal malnutrition

  ▷ Premature birth

  ▷ Fetal hypoxia

  ▷ Birth trauma

▶ General medical conditions acquired during infancy or childhood contribute to approximately 5% of cases.

  ▷ Infections

  ▷ Brain trauma

  ▷ Exposure to toxins (e.g., lead poisoning)

▶ No clear etiology can be found in 30% to 50% of cases.

▶ The most preventable cause of intellectual disability is fetal alcohol syndrome.

  ▷ Characteristics of fetal alcohol syndrome include:

    ▶ Epicanthal skin folds

    ▶ Low nasal bridge

    ▶ Short nose

    ▶ Indistinct philtrum

    ▶ Small head circumference

    ▶ Small eye openings

▶ Wide-set eyes

▶ Thin upper lip

Prevalence

▶ 1% of the general population

Demographics

▶ Highest rates are reported in school-age children (10–14 years of age).

▶ 1.5 percent more males than females

Risk Factors

▶ Genetic loading

▶ Adverse birth events

Prevention and Screening

▶ At well-baby examinations

▶ School screenings

Assessment

Physical Exam Findings

▶ Oblique eye folds

▶ Small, flattened skull

▶ Large tongue

▶ Broad hands with stumpy fingers

▶ Single transverse palm crease

▶ High cheekbones

▶ Small height

▶ Brushfield spots on iris

▶ Abnormal finger and toe prints

▶ Cryptorchidism

▶ Congenital cardiac defects

▶ Early dementia

▶ Hypothyroidism

Mental Status Exam Findings

▶ Communication deficits

▶ Dependency

▶ Passivity

▶ Poor self-esteem

▶ Low frustration tolerance

▶ Aggressiveness

▶ Stereotyped, repetitive motor movement

▶ Self-injurious behavior

Diagnostic and Laboratory Findings

▶ No specific laboratory findings

▶ Some laboratory findings associated with a variety of causes of intellectual disability (e.g., metabolic disturbances)

Differential Diagnosis

▶ Borderline intellectual functioning

▶ Learning and communication disorders

▶ Pervasive developmental disorder (PDD)

▷ 75% of people with a PDD have comorbid intellectual disability.

▶ ADHD (see above)

▶ Stereotypic movement disorder

▶ General medical condition

Clinical Management

Pharmacological Management

▶ Pharmacological treatment is symptom-specific.

▷ Treat concomitant psychopathology (e.g., ADHD, depressive disorder, anxiety disorder, schizophrenia).

▷ Aggressive or self-injurious behavior may be controlled with antipsychotics and mood stabilizers.

Nonpharmacological Management

▶ Therapy

▷ Behavioral therapy

▷ Group therapy

▷ Family therapy

▶ Community resources

  ▷ Day care settings

  ▷ Sheltered workshops

  ▷ Group homes

Separation Anxiety Disorder (refer to Chapter 10)

DISRUPTIVE MOOD DYSREGULATION DISORDER

Description

▶ Childhood depressive disorder that is diagnosed in children older than age 6 but younger than age 18.

▶ The features of this disorder are

  ▷ chronic dysregulated mood,

  ▷ frequent temper outbursts, and

  ▷ severe irritability.

Etiology

▶ Cause is unknown

Prevalence and Demographics

▶ Affects about 2% to 5% of children and adolescents

▶ Higher incidence in boys and school-age children than girls and adolescents

Risk Factors

▶ Complicated psychiatric history including comorbid ADD and ADHD.

Prevention and Screening

▶ Children and adolescents should be screened for a personal and family history of bipolar disorder as symptoms of disruptive mood dysregulation disorder can be similar to bipolar disorder.

Assessment

▶ Assess for comorbid conditions such as:

  ▷ Bipolar disorder

  ▷ ODD

  ▷ ADHD

▷ Depressive and anxiety disorders

▷ Autism spectrum disorder

Clinical Management

Pharmacologic Management

▶ Medications can be used to treat the target symptoms of the disorder.

▶ Selective serotonin reuptake inhibitors, mood stabilizers, and atypical antipsychotics can be helpful.

Nonpharmacologic Management

▶ Individual, group, and family therapy are helpful.

Follow-Up

▶ Regular follow-up is necessary, as is ongoing assessment for comorbid conditions

CASE STUDY

The parents of a 14-year-old with attention-deficit hyperactivity disorder (ADHD) ask to speak to you privately after you complete your assessment of their child. They tell you they have several questions that they want answered, and they want to ask you to keep the answers to yourself and not tell their son what they ask. Their first question is about diet. They have read that ADHD can be managed by dietary therapy instead of medications, and they want your opinion about trying this strategy with their child. They also want to know how likely it is that he will "outgrow" the disorder. You have many issues to consider before answering the parents' questions.

1. What is the most accepted theory of etiology regarding ADHD?

2. What is the empirical database for dietary treatment in ADHD clients?

3. What is the natural course of this illness? Is it likely that the son's symptoms will improve as he ages?

4. What are the other issues to consider regarding the parents' request to keep confidential the concerns that they are expressing?

ANSWERS TO CASE STUDY DISCUSSION QUESTIONS

1. The accepted theory is that ADHD is a neurobiological disorder

2. The best-studied treatment for ADHD is stimulant medication. Elimination of food allergens, sugar, and aspartame can be helpful to decrease hyperactivity. Limited evidence exists about the use of herbal remedies; however, it is always best to meet the client and parents where they are and if nonpharmacological treatments or dietary alterations are requested, the PMHNP should provide evidence for treatment of ADHD so the family can make an informed decision.

3. ADHD is a lifespan disorder; however, as children progress into adulthood, symptoms of inattention usually remain with a decrease in impulsive and hyperactive symptoms.

4. Other issues of concern in a child with ADHD include a lack of involvement of the child in treatment might lead to nonadherence by the child. Working in family therapy would be beneficial.

REFERENCES AND RESOURCES

American Academy of Child and Adolescent Psychiatry. (1997). Practice parameter for the treatment of children and adolescents with conduct disorder. *Journal of the American Academy of Child and Adolescent Psychiatry, 36*(10), 122S–139S.

American Academy of Child and Adolescent Psychiatry. (2007a). Practice parameter for the assessment and treatment of children and adolescents with attention-deficit/hyperactivity disorder. *Journal of the American Academy of Child and Adolescent Psychiatry, 46*(7), 894–921.

American Academy of Child and Adolescent Psychiatry. (2007b). Practice parameter for the assessment and treatment of children and adolescents with oppositional defiant disorder. *Journal of the American Academy of Child and Adolescent Psychiatry, 46*(1), 126–141.

American Psychiatric Association. (2001). Practice parameters for the assessment and treatment of children and adolescents with suicidal behavior. *Journal of the American Academy of Child and Adolescent Psychiatry, 4*(Suppl. 7), 245–478.

American Psychiatric Association. (2009). Practice parameters on the use of psychotropic medication in children and adolescents. *Journal of the American Academy of Child and Adolescent Psychiatry, 48*(9), 961–973.

American Psychiatric Association. (2013). *Diagnostic and statistical manual of mental disorders* (5th ed.). Washington, DC: Author.

Centers for Disease Control and Prevention. (2010). Morbidity and mortality weekly report: Increasing prevalence of parent reported attention-deficit/hyperactivity disorder among children – United States, 2003 and 2007. *Morbidity and Mortality Weekly Report, 59*(44), 1–40.

Centers for Disease Control and Prevention. (2015). *Facts about ASD*. Retrieved from http://www.cdc.gov/ncbddd/autism/facts.html

Hamrin, V., & Gray Deering, C. (2012). Mental health assessment of children and adolescents. In M. Boyd (Ed.), *Psychiatric nursing contemporary practice* (5th ed., pp. 661–678). Philadelphia, PA: Lippincott Williams & Wilkins.

Lock, J., LaVia, M., & The American Academy of Child and Adolescent Psychiatry Committee on Quality Issues. (2015). Practice parameter for the assessment and treatment of children and adolescents with eating disorders. *Journal of the American Academy of Child and Adolescent Psychiatry, 54*(5), 412–425.

Murphy, T., Lewin, A., Storch, E., Stock, S., & The American Academy of Child and Adolescent Psychiatry Committee on Quality Issues. (2013). Practice parameter for the assessment and treatment of children and adolescents with tic disorders. *Journal of the American Academy of Child and Adolescent Psychiatry, 52*(12), 1341–1359.

Nolan, E., Gadow, K., & Sprafkin, J. (2001). Teacher reports of DSM-IV ADHD, ODD, and CD symptoms in school children. *Journal of the American Academy of Child and Adolescent Psychiatry, 40,* 241–249.

Sadock, B. J., Sadock, A. V., & Ruiz, P. (2015). *Kaplan & Sadock's synopsis of psychiatry: Behavioral sciences/clinical psychiatry* (11th ed.). Baltimore, MD: Wolters Kluwer.

U. S. Department of Health and Human Services. (2000). *Mental health: A report of the Surgeon General.* Washington, DC: Author.

Volkmar, F., Siegel, M., Woodbury-Smith, M., King, B., McCracken, J., & The American Academy of Child and Adolescent Psychiatry Committee on Quality Issues. (2014). Practice parameter for the assessment and treatment of children and adolescents with autism spectrum disorder. *Journal of the American Academy of Child and Adolescent Psychiatry, 53*(2), 237–257.

CHAPTER 16

SLEEP

This chapter addresses sleep issues and disorders commonly encountered by the psychiatric–mental health nurse practitioner (PMHNP). These conditions and clinical problems may co-occur with the disorders already discussed or may present in clients with no other identifiable psychiatric or mental health problems. They also may be frequent findings in primary care settings while working with clients with general medical conditions.

GENERAL CONSIDERATIONS

- ▶ Must be systematically assessed
- ▶ Comparison of present level of sleep to historical baseline
- ▶ Can be measured by polysomnography
- ▶ Rapid eye movement (REM) alternating with four distinct nonrapid eye movement stages (NREM).
  - ▷ *Stage I*
    - ▶ NREM
    - ▶ Transitional stage from wakefulness to sleep
    - ▶ 5% of total normal sleep cycle
  - ▷ *Stage II*
    - ▶ NREM
    - ▶ Specific electroencephalogram (EEG) waveforms
    - ▶ 50% of total sleep cycle
  - ▷ *Stages III and IV*
    - ▶ NREM
    - ▶ Slow-wave sleep period
    - ▶ Deepest level of sleep
    - ▶ 20% to 25% of total sleep cycle

    ▷   Sleep stages are organized and sequential during sleep period.

        ▶   Stages III and IV tend to occur in first one-third to one-half of sleep period

        ▶   REM occurs cyclically throughout the night, alternating with NREM on average every 80 to 100 minutes.

        ▶   REM increases in duration toward morning.

    ▷   Sleep patterns vary with age.

        ▶   Children and adolescents have large amounts of slow-wave sleep.

        ▶   Sleep continuity and depth decrease with age.

        ▶   Consider age when assessing for sleep–rest problems.

    ▷   Sleep patterns vary with medication use.

        ▶   Many medications and agents of abuse affect sleep cycle.

        ▶   Assess recent changes in medication or drug use in a person presenting with sleep pattern disturbances.

INSOMNIA

▶   Insomnia is the inability to get the amount of sleep needed to function efficiently during the day.

▶   Situational or acute insomnia lasts from days to weeks.

▶   Insomnia disorder is characterized by a significant inability to initiate or maintain sleep, or early morning awakening with inability to return to sleep and. Occurs at least 3 nights per week and is present for at least 1 month (episodic insomnia disorder) and may persist for greater than 3 months (persistent insomnia disorder).

▶   Insomnia disorder is associated with increased mortality, poor career performance, overeating, and increased hospitalization.

▶   Insomnia disorder is not better explained by or occurring exclusively during the course of another sleep disorder, and is not attributable to the effects of a substance.

Etiology

▶   Dysfunction in sleep–wake circuits of the brainstem

▶   Neurochemical imbalances impinging on these circuits

▶   May be stress-related in brief episodic insomnia

Incidence and Demographics

▶   33% of Americans have difficulty sleeping.

▶   Up to 10% meet criteria for insomnia disorder.

▶   Insomnia is highly comorbid with other psychiatric disorders.

Risk Factors

▶ Female gender and advancing age

▶ Past history of insomnia

▶ Significant stress

▶ Forced pattern changes

  ▷ Working alternating shifts

  ▷ Swing-shift work patterns

  ▷ Travel across time zones

  ▷ Genetic (obstructive sleep apnea)

▶ High-use patterns of medications, drugs, or substances known to affect sleep cycles

  ▷ Caffeine, other stimulants

  ▷ Alcohol

  ▷ Benzodiazepines (BNZs)

Prevention and Screening

▶ At-risk family education for children and adolescents

▶ Limits on shift work

▶ Avoidance of medications known to affect sleep patterns

▶ Good sleep hygiene patterns

▶ Avoidance of stimulants late in the day

▶ Early recognition, intervention, and initiation of treatment

  ▷ Routine screening at all healthcare settings

Assessment

▶ Detailed history of present insomnia, including time frame, progression, and associated symptoms

▶ Social history, including present living situation; marital status; occupation; education; and alcohol, tobacco, or illicit drug use

▶ Medication use, including prescription, over-the-counter, alternative, supplements, and home remedies

▶ Initial and periodic functional history and assessment

▶ Number of hours in usual sleep pattern

▶ Initial- or middle-phase insomnia; early morning awakening

▶ Use of sleep aids

▶ Bed position, use of pillows

▶ Environment: temperature, sound, light

Hypersomnolence Disorder

▶ Self-reported excessive sleepiness despite adequate main sleep period

▶ Difficulty being fully awake—"groggy" after abrupt awakening

▶ Occurs at least 3 times per week and lasts for several months

▶ Causes significant distress or impairment

▶ Not better explained by another sleep disorder, viral infection, or physiologic affect of a substance

▶ May occur within 18 months of experiencing a head trauma

▶ Comorbidity includes various depressive disorders (e.g., major depression with atypical features, seasonal affective disorder [SAD], bipolar disorder depressed state)

Obstructive Sleep Apnea (OSA)

▶ Hallmark of disorder is snoring and repeated apnea during sleep

▶ Daytime sleepiness or sense of feeling unrefreshed despite adequate sleep period is prominent.

▶ Headache upon awakening is common.

▶ Consequences include panic attacks (waking up "gasping"), attention-deficit hyperactivity disorder, depression, hypertension, and motor vehicle and workplace accidents

▶ Affects up to 2% of children, up to 15% to 20% of adults

▶ Etiology due to abnormally small nasopharynx, tonsillar tissue in children; obesity

Polysomnography to Make Definitive Diagnosis

Physical Exam Findings

▶ Nonspecific

▶ Sleep disturbance often a manifestation of an underlying disorder

▶ Clients in whom a sleep disorder is suspected should have full exam

Mental Status Exam Findings

▶ May have preoccupation or excessive worry about "not getting enough sleep"

▶ Depending on duration of sleep deprivation, many areas of mental status exam (MSE) may be affected

Diagnostic and Laboratory Findings

▶ Complete blood count (CBC), chemistry profile, thyroid function tests, ferritin level (if restless legs), and B_{12} level to rule out metabolic causes or unidentified conditions

▶ Drug toxicity screening, if indicated by history

Differential Diagnosis

▶ More than 50% of insomnia cases are related to primary psychiatric disorder.

▷ Mood disorders (see Chapter 9)

▷ Anxiety disorders (see Chapter 10)

▷ Substance-related disorders (see Chapter 13).

▷ Attention-deficit hyperactivity disorder (ADHD; see Chapter 15)

▷ Early-morning wakefulness a possible sign of depression

▷ Sudden, dramatic decrease in sleep a sign of possible mania or schizophrenia

▷ Poor sleep a sign of possible obsessive–compulsive disorder (see Chapter 10)

▷ Panic and anxiety episodes during sleep a sign of possible panic disorder

▷ Alcohol may cause numerous awakenings during the night

▷ Cardiac illnesses

▷ Parasomnias

▷ Gastrointestinal disorders

▷ Chronic obstructive pulmonary disease

▷ Medication side effects

▷ Sleep apnea

▷ Restless leg syndrome

▷ Chronic pain

▷ Stress reaction

▷ Active substance abuse

▷ Drug use

   ▶ Caffeine

   ▶ Stimulants

Clinical Management

▶ Rule out or treat any conditions that may contribute to current symptom manifestation.

▶ Weight loss and avoiding supine sleep position may alleviate sleep apnea

▶ Positive airway pressure, continuous(CPAP) or bilevel (BPAP) for OSA

Pharmacological Management

▶ Melatonin is particularly useful to correct sleep onset issues and may be helpful for the person with ADHD.

▶ Benzodiazepine (BNZ) or hypnotics (should not be used in OSA)

▶ Flurazepam (Dalmane)

▷ Long-lasting agent

- ▷ May cause excess drowsiness
- ▷ Avoid in older adults
- ▶ Temazepam (Restoril)
  - ▷ Intermediate acting agent
- ▶ Triazolam (Halcion)
  - ▷ Short-acting agent
  - ▷ Little to no excess sedation
  - ▷ Common side effects:
    - ▶ Impaired memory
    - ▶ Efficacy decreases over time
    - ▶ Should not be used on a long-term basis
- ▶ Nonbenzodiazepine hypnotics
  - ▷ Zaleplon (Sonata)
    - ▶ Ultra-short half-life makes this drug particularly useful for initial or middle-phase insomnia
  - ▷ Zolpidem (Ambien, Ambien CR)
    - ▶ Short half-life drugs, but may affect person the next morning; must allow for 8 hours before planned awakening
    - ▶ Give on empty stomach
  - ▷ Eszopiclone (Lunesta)
    - ▶ Intermediate-acting agent
  - ▷ Rozerem
    - ▶ Melatonin receptor agonist
  - ▷ Suvorexant (Belsomra)
  - ▷ Orexin antagonist, suppresses wakefulness
    - ▶ Must consider long half-life
- ▶ Antidepressants
  - ▷ Used for sedating properties
  - ▷ Amitriptyline (Elavil), doxepin (Sinequan, Silenor); generally avoid use in older adults
  - ▷ Mirtazapine (Remeron)
  - ▷ Trazadone
- ▶ Wake-promoting drugs
  - ▷ Armodafinil (Nuvigil) indicated for daytime sleepiness associated with OSA

Nonpharmacological Management

- ▶ Sleep hygiene practices
  - ▷ Establish a bedtime routine.

▷ Have a regular time to sleep and wake.

▷ Avoid computer and other electronic device use 1 hour before bedtime.

▷ Never lie in bed for more than 15 minutes if not able to sleep.

▷ Reduce stress.

▷ Do stress reduction activities before bedtime.

▷ Avoid late-in-the-day exercise intensive.

▷ Avoid late-in-the-day stimulant use, such as caffeine.

▷ Use bed/bedroom for sleep or sex only.

▷ Consider moving phone and other devices away from sleeping area; restrict phone and computer use to 1 or more hours before bed time.

▷ Psychotherapy.

▷ Cognitive therapy for insomnia.

▶ Relaxation and other therapies

▷ Abdominal breathing

▷ Progressive muscle relaxation

▷ Meditation

▷ Imaging

▷ Hypnosis

▷ Biofeedback

▷ Stimulus control

▷ Sleep curtailment

▷ Light therapy

▶ Somatic and other therapies

▷ Exercise (during the day)

▷ Warm bath

▷ Warm milk

▷ Change bedroom environment

Life Span Considerations

▷ *Insomnia in children*

▶ Most commonly related to stress

▶ Children with insomnia often have been poor sleepers since birth.

▶ Pharmacological treatment is not recommended for most children.

▷ *Insomnia in older adults*

▶ If first presentation is in older years, insomnia often is the result of changes in chronobiological rhythms. Older adults often become sleepier early in the evening and wake up early.

▶ Sleep latency, decreased REM sleep, and increased sleep fragmentation are common.

▶ Insomnia may be related to underlying psychiatric disorders:

▷ Mood disorders

▷ Anxiety disorders

▷ Attention-deficit hyperactivity disorder

▷ Alzheimer's disease

▶ Older adults often manifest confusion and restlessness as aspects of insomnia.

▶ A careful, complete assessment is necessary when pharmacological interventions are planned.

CASE STUDY 1

Ms. Jones, a 43-year-old receptionist, presents at the PMHNP's clinic with a primary complaint of insomnia. She reports lifelong problems with sleeping that "comes and goes" depending on her stress level and general health. She has been experiencing a 4- to 5-day period of poor sleeping, reporting only 3 to 4 hours of sleep and early morning awakening. She has tried over-the-counter medication and has received no relief. She reports that her health is generally good but states that she is a 2-pack-a-day smoker and has increased her recreational use of alcohol to 1 to 2 drinks a night in the past few weeks in order to get to sleep. Her insomnia is now beginning to impair her daily functioning and her interest in social activities. She reports an irritable mood since her sleep has been difficult and problems with memory and concentration in the morning after she has slept poorly. She denies depression or any other mood problem and currently is taking no routine medication. Her physical exam is unremarkable, and routine lab studies, including thyroid-stimulating hormone (TSH), CBC, and electrolytes, are all normal.

1. What is the most likely diagnosis for this client at this time?
2. What further assessment should the PMHNP make?
3. What treatment should the PMHNP consider?
4. Is medication warranted at this time to induce sleep?

CASE STUDY 2

Mr. Smith is a 40-year-old married man who presents to the PMHNP with a chief complaint of "I can't fall asleep. I've tried everything. Nothing works! That medicine the doctor gave me made me feel worse. It made me feel really anxious. I'm exhausted! I can't function. I'm going to lose my job." Mr. Smith states his primary care provider has prescribed various sleeping medications, "Ambien, Lunesta, and Ativan," which have all caused a worsening of his insomnia. His physical exam and routine labs performed by his primary care provider have all been within normal limits.

1. What further assessment should the PMHNP make at this time?
2. What treatment should the PMHNP consider?
3. Why might a person report feeling more anxious and have more trouble sleeping in response to a hypnotic or anxiolytic medication?
4. Mr. Smith begins psychotherapy with the PMHNP and he begins to discuss growing up in an alcoholic family in which his parents fought at night after the children went to bed. In addition to continuing psychotherapy, should medication be considered?

CASE STUDY 3

Ms. Johnson, a 39-year-old single, obese woman is self-referred to the PMHNP for assessment and treatment of "depression and exhaustion." Ms. Johnson states "I sleep just fine, but I'm always tired. My doctor did some blood work and said that everything was normal. I can't concentrate. I'm dragging at work. The other day I had to go out to my car and take a nap. I can't take this any more! This is really getting me down. Do you think an antidepressant would help?" Ms. Johnson has had a CBC, comprehensive metabolic panel, serum iron, B_{12}, folate levels, and thyroid function tests which were all within normal limits.

1. What further assessment should be completed?
2. Should Ms. Johnson be started on medication?

ANSWERS TO CASE STUDY DISCUSSION QUESTIONS

Case Study 1

1. Ms. Jones is suffering from transient insomnia.

2. The PMHNP should identify life stressors, complete a full psychiatric assessment, and identify any other mental health needs.

3. The PMHNP should assist Ms. Jones in managing her sleep by using effective sleep hygiene strategies, encouraging diet changes, reducing smoking, and omitting the use of alcohol for sleep induction.

4. Short-term use of sleep induction medications such as a low-dose sedating antidepressant would provide relief with little risk to this client and may help her reduce current reliance on alcohol.

Case Study 2

1. The PMHNP should complete a comprehensive psychiatric evaluation exploring for signs and symptoms of a mood or anxiety disorder. The history should include a thorough evaluation of past sleep patterns and issues with insomnia. The PMHNP should carefully assess for issues such as childhood or more recent trauma, alcohol, or other related violence exposure. Clients who have experienced significant trauma directed at them, or who have been raised in an environment of violence, may have fear related to falling asleep.

2. The PMHNP should consider psychotherapy, which should include psychoeducation about insomnia, the impact of anxiety on sleep, and sleep hygiene measures.

3. Children raised in traumatic environments commonly have difficulty falling and staying asleep. Many children become hypervigilant. These patterns can persist into adulthood. Adults may not be cognizant of the connection between current sleep issues and childhood trauma. Any medication that prevents a person from being hypervigilant could be experienced as a lack of control, thus causing an increase in anxiety and insomnia.

4. The PMHNP should discuss the possibility of using a selective serotonin reuptake inhibitor (SSRI) or perhaps another sedating antidepressant to address Mr. Smith's heightened arousal and insomnia.

Case Study 3

1. The PMHNP should complete a comprehensive psychiatric evaluation to rule out a mood, anxiety, or substance abuse disorder. A careful sleep and energy history should be taken and the PMHNP should screen for evidence of snoring or apnea. Further assessment should be done by a sleep specialist to rule out obstructive sleep apnea (OSA) or other sleep disorder.

2. The PMHNP should consider that medications may be indicated. If Ms. Johnson does have OSA, she will be treated with a continuous or bilevel airway pressure device (CPAP or BPAP). Wake-promoting medication such as armodafinil may also be helpful in reducing Ms. Johnson's excessive daytime sleepiness.

REFERENCES AND RESOURCES

American Psychiatric Association. (2013). *Diagnostic and statistical manual of mental disorders* (5th ed., text rev.). Washington, DC: Author.

Buysse, D. (2013). Insomnia. *The Journal of the American Medical Association, 309*(7), 706-716.

Redeker, N., & McEnany, G. P. (2011). *Sleep disorders and sleep promotion in nursing practice.* New York, NY: Springer Publishing.

Rajput, V., & Johnson, R. (1999). Chronic insomnia: A practical review. *American Family Practice, 11,* 1–6.

Stahl, S. M. (2013). *Stahl's essential psychopharmacology* (4th ed.). New York, NY: Cambridge University Press.

CHAPTER 17

VIOLENCE

This chapter deals with the psychiatric–mental health nurse practitioner's (PMHNP's) role in identifying and treating clients who are impacted by intimate partner violence (IPV), sexual assault, homicide, and suicide. Assessment of lethality will also be reviewed. These issues may co-occur with the disorders already discussed or may present in clients with no other identifiable psychiatric or mental health problems. They also may be frequent findings in primary care settings while working with clients with general medical conditions.

INTIMATE PARTNER VIOLENCE (IPV)

Description

- ▶ *IPV* is physical, emotional, economic, or sexual pain and injury that is intentionally inflicted by a person's intimate partner.
- ▶ The goal of the abuser is to:
  - ▷ Establish power
  - ▷ Manipulate the other person
  - ▷ Intimidate the other person
  - ▷ Control the other person

Etiology

- ▶ *Characteristics of abusers*:
  - ▷ Personality disorders
    - ▶ Antisocial personality disorder
    - ▶ Narcissistic personality disorder
    - ▶ Borderline personality disorder

▷ Environmental stressors

▶ Financial difficulties

▶ Ending of a relationship

▶ Unemployment

Incidence and Demographics

▶ IPV occurs among heterosexual and homosexual couples.

▶ IPV is the leading cause of injury to women ages 15–44.

▶ It is the leading cause of death among African-American women between the ages of 15 and 24.

▶ 1 in 10 female high school students in the United States have reported violence from their dating partners.

▶ 15% to 25% of pregnant women are physically abused.

▶ 22% to 35% of all women seen in emergency rooms experienced injuries as a result of IPV.

▶ 1 in 3 women and 1 in 4 men are victims of IPV.

▶ 50% of homeless women experience IPV.

▶ 63% of men incarcerated for murder between the ages of 11 and 20 have murdered their mother's abuser.

▶ 33% of male abusers are well educated and include men in professional jobs. (National Coalition Against Domestic Violence, 2015)

Risk Factors

▶ *For abusers:*

▷ Exposure to violence at an early developmental age

▷ Low self-esteem

▷ Social isolation

▷ Lack of support

▷ Cognitive impairment

▷ Physical or financial dependency

Prevention and Screening

▶ Public education and awareness beginning in high school

▶ Social programs

▶ At-risk family education

▶ Community education

▷ Stigma reduction to allow victims to come forward

▷ Signs and symptoms of being the victim of abuse

▷ Prevention programs

▷ Early recognition, intervention, and initiation of treatment for victims

▷ Routine screening for victimization at all healthcare settings

Assessment

▶ Interview the person who has experienced the violence alone.

▶ Determine primary caregivers, living arrangements, legal custodian

History

▶ Assess for the following:

▷ Determine recurrent history of medical treatment consistent with abuse:

▶ Accidents

▶ Suspicious or repeated fractures

▶ Physical injuries

▶ Traumas

▶ Refusal of ongoing treatment or follow-up

▶ Missed medical appointments

▷ Determine environmental, psychosocial, and financial stressors

Physical Exam Findings

▶ Monitor nutritional status for dehydration and malnutrition.

▶ Look for lacerations, bruises, wounds, burns, or fractures.

▶ Look for poor skin and personal hygiene.

Mental Status Exam Findings

▶ Findings of traits and behaviors suggestive of experiencing abuse:

▷ Fearful

▷ Evasive

▷ Guarded

▷ Depressed

▷ Passive

▷ Dependent

Diagnostic and Laboratory Findings

▶ None specific to abuse

▶ Determine general health and nutritional status

Differential Diagnosis

▶ Accidental injuries

▶ Mood disorders (see Chapter 9)

▶ Anxiety disorders (see Chapter 10)

▶ Substance use disorders (see Chapter 13)

Clinical Management

▶ Most state laws mandate reporting of suspected abuse and neglect of vulnerable populations:

▷ Older adults

▷ People with disabilities

▷ Children

Pharmacological Management

▶ None specific to condition

Nonpharmacological Management

▶ The safety and medical well-being of the person experiencing the abuse is most important.

▶ Refer the person to a domestic abuse shelter when feasible.

▶ Help the person develop a safety plan.

▷ Assist client in developing a "code word" for family or other support system as an attempt to inform them that the person is in need of help.

▷ Advise client to tell one person in his or her support system about the situation.

▷ Advise client to pack an "emergency bag" and hide it in case of need to leave quickly.

▷ Advise client to keep the IPV hotline and other telephone numbers (e.g., police department, counselor, shelter) in a secure place.

▷ Monitor medical status as symptomology presents.

▷ Monitor nutritional status and vital signs.

▷ Suggest psychotherapy to assist in gaining insight and in developing new coping skills.

▷ Suggest hospitalization when in the best interest of the client.

SEXUAL ASSAULT AND ABUSE

Description

▶ *Sexual assault or abuse* is any sexual act or penetration committed through coercion or physical force.

▷ This includes rape, incest, sodomy, oral and anal acts, and use of a foreign object.

▷ It is an act of violence and humiliation expressed through sexual means.

▷ It is used to express power or anger.

Etiology

▶ *For abusers:*

▷ Character disorders

▷ Behavioral act of violence is reinforcing

▶ Once done, likely to repeat

▷ Social exposure to violence in culture, media, and home

Incidence and Demographics

▶ Women have a greater incidence of being assaulted than men.

▶ Sexual assault is the most common form of abuse.

▶ Perpetrators are more frequently men than women.

▷ Sexual assaults are often committed by fathers and stepfathers, uncles, older siblings, other family members, and men that women are dating.

▶ Alcohol is involved in 34% of all rapes.

▶ Only 1 in 4 rapes is reported.

Factors that Increase Incidence of Abusing

▶ Substance abuse disorders

▶ Psychiatric disorders

▶ Divorce

▶ Family or personal history of physical or sexual abuse

▶ Long-term exposure to violence

▶ Social isolation and lack of support systems

▶ Environmental stressors such as unwanted pregnancy in an intimate partner, unemployment, or financial difficulty

Prevention and Screening of Victims

▶ Public education and awareness campaigns

▶ Community resources and support

▶ Community emergency shelters, help lines, and safe houses

▶ Assertiveness training and self-defense

▶ Early recognition, intervention, and initiation of treatment

▷ Routine screening at all healthcare settings

Assessment

▶ Interview persons who have experienced the assault alone when possible.

▶ Establish a safe, trusting relationship to promote sharing.

▷ Routine inclusion of questions concerning sexual assault in medical history.

▷ Interview alone and not in presence of family, friend, or partner.

▷ Interview for social history, including history of living arrangements and relationships.

Physical Exam Findings

▶ Nonspecific

▶ Presentation of traits and behaviors consistent with potential for having suffered sexual assault or other abuse:

▷ Withdrawn

▷ Frightened appearance

▷ Hyperreactive to touch

▶ Associated findings:

▷ Unexplained bruises, abrasions, cuts, laceration, burns, soft-tissue swellings, and hematomas

▷ Sexually transmitted diseases

▷ Genital rash or discharge

▷ Rectal tissue swelling or discharge

▷ Physical signs that are strongly suggestive of sexual abuse in children:

▶ Lacerations, ecchymosis, and newly healed scars of the hymen or posterior fourchette

▶ No hymenal tissue in 3- to 9-o'clock area

▶ Healed hymenal transactions, especially in the above area

▶ Perianal lacerations

Remember that any child presenting with concerning physical signs should be evaluated by a sexual abuse expert. A complete history and a sexual abuse examination need to take place.

Mental Status Exam Findings

▶ Withdrawn

▶ Frightened

▶ Anxious

▶ Scattered appearance

▶ Hyperreactive to touch

▶ Dissociative

Diagnostic and Laboratory Findings

- ▶ Nonspecific
- ▶ Assessment and documentation labs
  - ▷ Forensic specimens
  - ▷ Pregnancy tests
  - ▷ Rectal, throat, and vaginal cultures
  - ▷ Screening for sexually transmitted diseases: Syphilis, HIV, hepatitis B, herpes simplex, human papillomavirus, trichomonas vaginalis

Differential Diagnosis

- ▶ Accidental injuries
- ▶ Consensual sexual activity
- ▶ Lichen sclerosis
- ▶ Posttraumatic stress disorder
- ▶ Anxiety disorder (see Chapter 10)

Clinical Management

- ▶ Use sensitivity and respectful care.
- ▶ Be aware of legal reporting requirements.
- ▶ Use available community resources.

Nonpharmacological Management

- ▶ Ensure safety and well-being.
- ▶ Ensure confidentiality.
- ▶ Complete accurate documentation.
- ▶ Assess for potential suicidal ideation if the person is showing any depressive symptoms.
- ▶ Suggest cognitive behavioral therapy (CBT).
- ▶ Offer support groups and community resources.
- ▶ Assist with access to criminal and legal supports.

LETHALITY ASSESSMENT

- ▶ *Lethality assessment*: evaluation, screening, or testing.
- ▶ *Lethality* refers to the likelihood that a person will commit suicide or homicide— focused violence at the extreme.
- ▶ *Violence:* the behavioral expression of anger, rage, and hostility that is demonstrated by the use of physical force directed toward persons (in case of suicide, toward self) or property.

VIOLENCE IN SCHOOL

▶ Serious physical fighting with peers or family members

▶ Severe destruction of property

▶ Severe rage for seemingly minor reasons

▶ Detailed threats of lethal violence

▶ Possession, use, or both of firearms or other weapons

▶ Self-injurious behaviors or threats of suicide

▶ Bullying or being bullied

▶ When warning signs indicate that danger is imminent, safety must always be the first and foremost consideration. Action must be taken immediately. Immediate intervention by school authorities and possibly law enforcement officers is needed when a child:

  ▷ Has presented a detailed plan (time, place, method) to harm or kill others, particularly if the child has a history of aggression or has attempted to carry out threats in the past

  ▷ Is carrying a weapon, particularly a firearm, and has threatened to use it

SUICIDE ASSESSMENT

Risk Factors

▶ Depression

▶ All antidepressants have black box warnings about increased risk of suicide in children, adolescents, and young adults under the age of 24.

▶ Prior suicide attempt

▶ Family history of mental disorder or substance abuse

▶ Family history of suicide

▶ Family violence

▶ Firearms in the home

▶ Incarceration

▶ Males are 5 times more likely than females to commit suicide

▶ White males over age 85 have highest rate of suicide

Signs of Imminent Danger

▶ Threatening to hurt or kill oneself

▶ Looking for ways to kill oneself (weapons, pills, or other means)

▶ Talking or writing about death, dying, or suicide

▶ Plans or preparations for a potentially serious attempt

▶ Alcohol use increases the risk of suicide attempts in persons with ideation

HOMICIDE: EARLY WARNING SIGNS

▶ Prior history of threatening or violent behavior

▶ Paranoia or easily panicked behavior

▶ A fascination or preoccupation with weapons, particularly weapons or explosives that could be used for mass destruction, such as semi-automatic guns

▶ Extreme stress from personal problems or a life crisis

▶ Identifying with incidents of workplace violence reported in the media and either condoning or sympathizing with the actions of the persons committing violence

▶ Being a loner with little or no involvement with other employees

▶ Engaging in frequent disputes with supervisors or coworkers

▶ Persistent violation of company policy

▶ Obsessive involvement with one's job, particularly where it occurs with no apparent outside interests

▶ Volatile or violent home or other personal situation that has the potential to bring violence into the workplace

THREATS OF VIOLENCE

▶ Throwing objects

▶ Making a verbal threat to harm another person or destroy property

▶ Making menacing gestures or physical posturing without actually touching the person

▶ Displaying an intense or obsessive romantic interest that exceeds the normal bounds of interpersonal interest

▶ Attempting to intimidate or harass other persons

▶ Behavior indicating that the person is significantly out of touch with reality and that he or she may pose a danger to himself or herself or to others

▶ Volatile or violent personal situations such as found in some custody battles

▶ Alcohol use increases the risk for violence

Safety is the number one priority and any threatening behavior must be taken seriously.

CASE STUDY

Ms. Smith, a 24-year-old single Caucasian female is referred to the PMHNP for persistent insomnia and depression after being treated in the emergency department of her local hospital for headaches, stomach pain, and various other physical complaints five times in the past 6 months. The PMHNP suspects that Ms. Smith is a victim of IPV.

1. What should the PMHNP's assessment include?

2. How should the PMHNP approach suspicions of IPV with Ms. Smith?

3. Should anyone beside Ms. Smith be interviewed?

4. If the PMHNP concludes that Ms. Smith meets criteria for major depression, should medication be included as part of the treatment plan?

Assume Ms. Smith is an immigrant.

5. What other considerations must be included in the assessment?

6. How should the PMHNP approach the client with her suspicions of IPV?

7. What other considerations must be included in this woman's treatment plan?

Assume Ms. Smith is an 80-year-old widowed woman.

8. What other considerations must be included in the assessment?

9. Who should be included in the assessment findings?

10. What other considerations must be included in the treatment plan for any person suspected of being the victim of IPV?

ANSWERS TO CASE STUDY DISCUSSION QUESTIONS

1. Ms. Smith should undergo a complete physical assessment, labs as indicated (likely working in conjunction with primary care providers) and a comprehensive psychiatric evaluation. The PMHNP should also inquire about sexual partner(s), sexual behaviors, birth control, and possibility of sexually transmitted infection.

2. The PMHNP should approach Ms. Smith privately (1:1). Questions should be posed in a matter-of-fact manner, using language that is not stigmatizing, such as "Has _____ ever threatened you or made you feel afraid?" or "Does _____'s temper ever make you feel scared?"

3. Generally no one else besides the victim should be interviewed. Women often feel reluctant to discuss being abused because they think if their partner finds out, things will get worse. Women may feel embarrassed or judged if anyone else were to know what is going on.

4. Possibly. Treating significant depression will allow Ms. Smith to be in a better position to make decisions and take action.

5. The PMHNP must make sure the interview is done in the woman's native language. Interpreters must not be a family member or friend.

6. The PMHNP must consider that different cultures may have different perceptions of IPV. The PMHNP must use culturally sensitive language. The PMHNP will need to consider the woman's concerns about legal issues related to immigration status.

7. The availability of culturally sensitive and relevant resources for therapy and medication management.

8. The client's living situation and her ability to care for her own needs. Whether or not she has caregivers, and whether or not her family member or other caregiver is possibly abusing her.

9. All states have mandatory reporting for suspected elder abuse.

10. A safety plan should be first and foremost. The victim should know where and how to get help. Resources should include 24-hour hotlines, shelters, support groups, and the like. The victim should have an escape plan that includes having some clothing and money packed and ready, in case she decides to leave.

REFERENCES AND RESOURCES

American Nurses Association, American Psychiatric Nurses Association, & International Society of Psychiatric-Mental Health Nurses. (2014). *Psychiatric–mental health nursing: Scope and standards of practice* (2nd ed.). Silver Spring, MD: Nursesbooks.org

Davidson, J. R. (2000). Trauma: The impact of post-traumatic stress disorder. *Journal of Psychopharmacology, 14*(Suppl. 1), 5–12.

Blunt, E., & Reinisch, C. (2013) *The family nurse practitioner review manual* (4th ed). Washington, DC: American Nurses Credentialing Center.

National Coalition Against Domestic Violence. (2015). National statistics. Retrieved from http://www.ncadv.org/learn/statistics

Sadock, B. J., Sadock, V. A., & Ruiz, P. (2015). *Kaplan and Sadock's synopsis of psychiatry: Behavioral sciences/clinical psychiatry* (11th ed.). Philadelphia, PA: Walters Kluwer.

Tusaie, K., & Fitzpatrick, J. (2013). Advanced practice psychiatric nursing: integrating psychotherapy, psychopharmacology and complementary and alternative approaches. New York, NY: Springer.

U. S. Department of Health and Human Services. (2000). *Mental health: A report of the Surgeon General*. Washington, DC: Author.

APPENDIX A

REVIEW QUESTIONS

1. The purpose of the American Nurses Association's *Psychiatric–Mental Health Nursing: Scope and Standards of Practice* is to

   a. Define the role and actions for the NP
   b. Establish the legal authority for the prescription of psychotropic medications
   c. Define the legal statutes of the role of the PMHNP
   d. Define the differences between the physician role and the NP role

2. Primary prevention care practices are an essential aspect of the PMHNP role. Which of the following is the best example of a primary prevention care strategy for community behavioral health?

   a. Aftercare program for chronically mentally ill clients recently discharged from the hospital
   b. Court-ordered counseling for abusive parents
   c. 24-hour crisis hotlines
   d. Parenting skills classes for pregnant adolescents

3. The trend in legal rulings on cases involving mental illness over the past 25 years has been to

   a. Encourage juries to find defendants not guilty by reason of insanity
   b. Protect the person's freedoms or rights when he or she is committed to a mental hospital
   c. Place increasing trust in mental health professionals to make good and ethical decisions
   d. Decrease the "red tape" associated with commitments so that commitments are faster and easier

4. Mr. Smithers, an involuntarily hospitalized patient experiencing psychotic symptoms, refuses to take any of his ordered medication because he believes "Jesus Christ told me I am the prophet and must fast for a year." Your actions should be based on your knowledge of which of the following?

   a. Psychiatric clients cannot refuse treatment
   b. Psychiatric clients do not always know what is good for them
   c. Psychiatric clients can refuse treatment
   d. Psychiatric clients cannot be trusted to make good healthcare decisions and, therefore, the nurse's best clinical judgment should guide actions

5. Which of the following statements best reflects the difference between the nurse–client (N–C) relationship and a social relationship?

   a. In the N–C relationship, the primary focus is on the client and the client's needs.
   b. Goals in the N–C relationship are deliberately left vague and unspoken so that the client can work on any issue.
   c. In the N–C relationship, the nurse is solely responsible for making the relationship work.
   d. In the N–C relationship, there is no place for social interaction.

6. A community has an unusually high incidence of depression and drug use among the teenage population. The public health nurses decide to address this problem, in part, by modifying the environment and strengthening the capacities of families to prevent the development of new cases of depression and drug use. What is this is an example of?

    a. Primary prevention
    b. Secondary prevention
    c. Tertiary prevention
    d. Protective factorial prevention

7. Mrs. Kemp is voluntarily admitted to the hospital. After 24 hours, she states she wishes to leave because "this place can't help me." The best nursing action that reflects the legal right of this client is

    a. Discharge the client
    b. Explain that the client cannot leave until you can complete further assessment
    c. Allow the client to leave but have her sign forms stating she is leaving against medical advice
    d. Immediately start the paperwork to commit the client and to allow you to treat her against her wishes

8. In forming a therapeutic relationship with clients, the PMHNP must consider developing many characteristics that are known to be helpful in relationship-building. Which of the following is an essential part of building a therapeutic relationship?

    a. Collecting a family history
    b. Like-mindedness
    c. Authenticity
    d. Accuracy in assessment

9. According to the DSM-5, which of the following is true? (Ch. 3)

    a. A mental disorder is equivalent to the need for treatment.
    b. Diagnostic criteria are used to inform clinical judgment.
    c. Socially deviant behavior is considered a mental disorder.
    d. A culturally expected response to a stressor is not a mental disorder.

10. Mrs. French has been in individual therapy for 3 months. She has shown much growth and improvement in her functioning and insight and is to discontinue services within the next few weeks. In the next session, after you discuss service termination, she suddenly begins to demonstrate the original symptoms that had brought her to treatment initially. She is now hesitant to discharge, wants to continue services, and is displaying an increase in regressive defense mechanisms. What is the best explanation for Ms. French's behavior?

    a. An exacerbation of her symptoms related to stress
    b. The normal cyclic nature of chronic mental health symptoms
    c. A sign of normal resistance to termination seen in the termination phase of therapy
    d. A sign of pathological attachment to the therapist that must be addressed

11. A client is displaying low self-esteem, poor self-control, self-doubt, and a high level of dependency. These behaviors indicate developmental failure of which of the following stages of development:

    a. Infancy
    b. Early childhood
    c. Late childhood
    d. School age

12. Mr. Thompson has been forgetful lately, for example, forgetting where he has placed his keys or what time appointments are scheduled, and he has stated that he thinks these are just random behaviors that have no particular meaning. Which Freudian-based psychodynamic principle assumes that all behavior and actions are purposeful?

    a. Pleasure principle
    b. Psychic determinism principle
    c. Reality principle
    d. Unconsciousness principle

13. An example of a mature, healthy defense mechanism is

    a. Denial
    b. Rationalization
    c. Repression
    d. Suppression

14. Mr. Johnson is a 54-year-old client you have been seeing for several weeks in therapy. While discussing his current concerns of marital stress, he lies on the floor and assumes the fetal position. This is most likely an example of

    a. Immature regressive defense mechanism
    b. Denial of reality
    c. Immature fantasy defense mechanism
    d. Repressive behavior

15. Defense mechanisms are best viewed as a function of the ego

    a. To alert us to harm and danger
    b. To alert us to problems
    c. Used to resolve a conflict
    d. Used to protect the id

16. One of the health care changes that has occurred as a result of the affordable care act (ACA) is that doctors/hospitals/clinic groups or health systems are coming together and assuming the responsibility for quality care to large groups of individuals insured by Medicare. The

health care clinics/systems doctors or hospitals that join together are called which of the following?

a. Health Maintenance Organization (HMO)

b. Preferred Provider Network (PPO)

c. Accountable Care Organization (ACO)

d. Individual Health Plan (IHP)

17. Health care economics is concerned with making decisions so the benefits outweigh the cost of resource utilization. What are two concepts that healthcare economics is concerned with in regard to fair distribution of resources and allocation?

a. Equity and efficiency

b. Cost and benefits

c. Opportunity and waste

d. Affordable and quality

18. What four elements need to be present for a malpractice lawsuit to be filed?

a. Beneficence, Non-Maleficence, Truthfulness, and Justice

b. Duty of care, Breach of standard of care, Injury, and Injury must be related to breach of the standard of care

c. Abandonment, Breach of care, Violation of ethics, and Reimbursement for poor care

d. Breach of standard of care, Injury, Deceit, and Malpractice

19. Mary is a Psychiatric–Mental Health Nurse Practitioner (PMHNP) who is working in a hospitalist role. Mary has encountered over five incidences in which attending psychiatrists and medical residents have been demeaning to nursing staff and not answering calls in the middle of the night or telling the nursing staff to write orders and the MD would sign off in the a.m. Mary is concerned about errors and wants to improve quality, reduce errors to promote safety. What concept is Mary employing?

a. Bullying

b. Abuse

c. Civil Disobedience

d. Just Culture

20. The role of neurotransmitters in the central nervous system is to function as

a. A communication medium

b. A gatekeeper for transmissions

c. A building block for amino acids

d. An agent to break down enzymes

21. Serotonin is produced in which of the following locations:

a. Locus ceruleus

b. Nucleus basalis

c. Raphe nuclei
d. Substantia nigra

22. Dopamine is produced in which of the following locations:

    a. Locus ceruleus
    b. Nucleus basalis
    c. Raphe nuclei
    d. Substantia nigra

23. A client presents with complaints of changes in appetite, feeling fatigued, problems with sleep–rest cycle, and changes in libido. What is the neuroanatomical area of the brain that is responsible for the normal regulation of these functions?

    a. Thalamus
    b. Hypothalamus
    c. Limbic system
    d. Hippocampus

24. In considering whether to order an MRI of the head for a client, which of the following would be a contraindication to this diagnostic test?

    a. Prosthetic limb
    b. History of head trauma
    c. Pacemaker
    d. Pregnancy

25. The primary excitatory neurotransmitter is

    a. GABA
    b. Serotonin
    c. Dopamine
    d. Glutamate

26. A client who is experiencing difficulties with working memory, planning and prioritizing, insight into his problems, and impulse control presents for assessment. In planning his care, the PMHNP should apply his or her knowledge that these symptoms represent problems with the

    a. Frontal lobe
    b. Temporal lobe
    c. Parietal lobe
    d. Occipital lobe

27. The concept of target symptom identification is best explained as

    a. Identification of the major clinical presentation of the client
    b. Identification of specific, precise, and individualized symptoms reasonably expected to improve with medication
    c. Identification of the secondary messenger system syndrome
    d. Intentional modulation of synaptic pathways

28. The goal of the psychiatric assessment process performed by the PMHNP is to

    a. Gain an understanding of the life experiences of the client
    b. Correctly diagnose the client
    c. Identify the mental health needs of the client
    d. Be able to communicate with other staff about the client's health needs

29. Mr. Johnson is a client newly admitted to an inpatient psychiatric hospital. The PMHNP on call at the facility plans to perform the initial intake assessment and diagnostic process. Mr. Johnson asks to please talk in his room because, he says, "People make me nervous." His room is at the end of the hallway and is the farthest away from the nursing station. The PMHNP's action should be based on awareness that the best location to do the assessment is

    a. In Mr. Johnson's room, because it is least noisy and most comfortable for him, thus facilitating data collection
    b. In the dayroom, which is full of people, to observe his interactions with other people
    c. In a quiet place, but public enough to get assistance with client care should it be required during the assessment
    d. In the treatment room with the door closed, a neutral location

30. Which communication technique is the PMHNP using in the following situation? Client: "Sorry I was late. I didn't realize what time it was." PMHNP: "This is the third time now that you have been late for our sessions. I am wondering how committed you are to our working on your problems."

    a. Theming
    b. Recognizing
    c. Validating
    d. Sequencing

31. In assessing a client, you ask him the meaning of the proverb "People who live in glass houses shouldn't throw stones." He replies, "Because it will break the windows." The correct interpretation of this findings is

    a. Client has a probable mood disorder
    b. Client has a probable anxiety disorder
    c. Client has limited intellectual ability
    d. Unable to interpret the finding without knowing the client's age

32. The PMHNP is planning to work with a client using an individual therapy model of care. During the first session, the client makes the following statement: "This is the third time my son has run away. I've grounded him, taken away his bike, even tried cutting off his allowance and confining him to his room. What should I do now?" The most therapeutic response for the PMHNP to make is

   a. "I wonder if confining him to his room was abusive?"

   b. "Maybe that depends on what you are trying to accomplish."

   c. "Perhaps talking to his friends and teachers would help."

   d. Remain silent

33. A client says to the PMHNP, "Some days life is just not worth it. All my wife and I ever do is fight and scream. Things at home would be calmer and simpler if I just wasn't there anymore." The most therapeutic response for the PMHNP to make is

   a. "Do you mean that you are thinking about leaving your wife and moving out?"

   b. "Tell me what you mean by 'it would be simpler if you just weren't there anymore.'"

   c. "So you are thinking suicide might be an option for you?"

   d. Remain silent

34. Mrs. Shea has come to the mental health center seeking treatment for depression. She has a history of a suicide attempt by overdose 1 month ago. She was started on imipramine (tricyclic antidepressant [TCA]) after that event but stopped taking the medication 1 week later because it "did no good." The PMHNP meets with Mrs. Shea to plan care with her. Which of the following is the most appropriate initial action?

   a. Asking Mrs. Shea how to help her

   b. Providing client teaching about the long time frame for TCAs to work

   c. Contracting with Mrs. Shea for 6 sessions of individual therapy

   d. Providing Mrs. Shea with feedback about how suicide might affect her family

35. In completing the PMHNP assessment for the Mrs. Shea, the most appropriate lab test for the PMHNP to order at this time is

   a. CBC

   b. TSH

   c. Liver function tests

   d. Electrolyte panel

36. A client comes into the clinic with a longstanding history of depression and chronic renal failure. He is on an antidepressant and a diuretic and complains of increased depression, mild confusion, irritability, and overall apathy from being too tired to do anything. The best initial PMHNP action to take at this time is

   a. Increase his dose of antidepressant medication to better capture symptoms

   b. Change him to another antidepressant for better symptom control

   c. Augment his antidepressant with an atypical antipsychotic medication

   d. Order a comprehensive metabolic panel

37. Sarah presents for her initial intake appointment with complaints of depression. She is being treated for hypertension and asthma by her primary care provider. Knowing that certain medications can cause or exacerbate depression, you obtain a complete medication history. Which of the following medications is known to exacerbate or cause depression?

    a.   Omeprazole

    b.   Propranolol

    c.   Levothyroxine

    d.   Clarithromycin

38. When treating older adults, you should keep in mind that they are more sensitive to issues of drug toxicity because of which of the following reasons?

    a.   Decreased body fat

    b.   Increased liver capacity

    c.   Decreased protein binding

    d.   Increased muscle concentration

39. Which known teratogenic effects can be caused by the common psychotropic medications divalproex and lithium?

    a.   Divalproex—Epstein anomaly; lithium—cleft palate

    b.   Divalproex—spina bifida; lithium—Epstein anomaly

    c.   Divalproex—limb malformations; lithium—seizure disorder

    d.   Divalproex—mental retardation; lithium—spina bifida

40. The study of what the body does to drugs is called

    a.   Pharmacodynamics

    b.   Pharmacology

    c.   Pharmacokinetics

    d.   Distribution

41. Your client Sam is being treated for panic disorder with agoraphobia. He currently is being prescribed paroxetine (Paxil CR, 37.5 mg q.d.) and clonazepam (Klonopin, 0.5 mg q.d., p.r.n.). He has been on clonazepam for 2 years and admits to needing 4 pills to achieve the same effect that 1 pill initially produced. This is possibly an example of which process?

    a.   Kindling

    b.   Addiction

    c.   Tolerance

    d.   Potency

42. Why is group therapy beneficial?

    a.   It assists the client to focus on self

    b.   It lacks theoretical frameworks

   c. It enables participants to acquire therapeutic factors

   d. It is always time limited

43. Which of the following is the best rationale for using cognitive behavioral therapy?

   a. Recognize and change his or her automatic thoughts

   b. See reality as you see it

   c. Change his or her reality by changing his or her environment

   d. Recognize and accept that automatic thoughts suggest delusional thinking

44. When working with a dysfunctional family, you find that the father, Jim, worries excessively and is resistant to change. You give Jim a paradoxical directive to worry extremely well for 1 hour per day, knowing that he will likely be noncompliant, and thus change will occur. With this technique, you are using which type of therapy?

   a. Experiential therapy

   b. Structural therapy

   c. Strategic therapy

   d. Solution-focused therapy

45. Which of the following best describes homeostasis in a family system?

   a. Choices a family makes to keep the peace

   b. Balance or stability that the family returns to despite its dysfunction

   c. Need for change and balance in a family

   d. Calm in a family that returns after a crisis

46. In an attempt to bring the client toward the goal he or she is working on, you ask the client, "If a miracle were to happen tonight while you slept, and you awoke in the morning and the problem no longer existed, how would you know, and what would be different?" This technique is used in which type of therapy?

   a. Behavioral therapy

   b. Solution-focused therapy

   c. Adlerian therapy

   d. Existential therapy

47. Ms. Thomas has been diagnosed with major depressive disorder (MDD) and is placed on fluoxetine 20 mg for her depression. For the PMHNP to effectively monitor her use of the medication, which of the following actions should be part of ongoing care?

   a. Use of a standardized rating scale of depression

   b. Monitoring for potential abuse of the medication

   c. Monitoring of labs for renal functioning

   d. Monitoring for potential cardiac side effects

48. Which of the following is the best reason for considering the SSRI among the first-line drug choices for treating major depression?

    a. Need to stair-step initial dosages

    b. Sedating and calming effect of the medication

    c. Safe use in suicidal overdose clients

    d. Ability to obtain therapeutic serum drug levels

49. A 23-year-old woman is brought into the ER after attempting suicide by cutting her wrists. Which nursing action by the PMHNP would be of highest priority initially?

    a. Assess her coping behaviors

    b. Assess her current level of suicidality

    c. Take her vital signs

    d. Assess her health history

50. Which of the following interventions by the PMHNP for a person experiencing *ataque de nervios* demonstrates culturally informed care?

    a. Offering brief supportive psychotherapy

    b. Offering a brief hospitalization

    c. Requesting a family member act as an interpreter

    d. Offering low-dose, short-term anxiolytic medication

51. The PMHNP working at a student mental health clinic has now been working with a freshman student for several weeks. The PMHNP learns that the student considers himself shy. He tells the NP that he has always felt uncomfortable in social situations or when he has to do oral presentations in class. He had few friends up until his senior year of high school when he discovered he could enjoy himself if he "had a couple of drinks before going out." He has continued this pattern in college and now occasionally drinks "2 to 3 beers" on weekends as well. According to the DSM-5, does the student have a mental disorder?

    a. Yes, alcohol use disorder, mild

    b. Yes, generalized anxiety disorder

    c. No, at this point, the student does not meet criteria for a mental disorder.

    d. Yes, adjustment disorder with mixed features

52. Jason misses several appointments. The PMHNP notes she feels resentful toward Jason and is struggling with how to respond to Jason when he finally comes in for his appointment. Which of the following demonstrates a therapeutic response?

    a. "Jason, since you have missed several appointments, we are closing your case."

    b. "Jason, it's pretty clear to me that you don't want to be here."

    c. "Jason, you are ambivalent about seeking treatment."

    d. "Jason, help me understand what's going on so we can figure out how to proceed."

53. Which is true about pharmacologic treatment of anxiety in older adults?

 a. Course of treatment is generally shorter than for younger adults.

 b. Drugs that are highly oxidized are more unpredictable than drugs that are mostly conjugated.

 c. The therapeutic dose of SSRIs is generally lower than for young adults.

 d. Highly lipophilic drugs have a more linear elimination in older adults.

54. A client returns for a follow-up appointment 3 weeks after starting on fluoxetine 20 mg. During this appointment you notice that her speech is a little rapid, in marked contrast to the psychomotor retardation and paucity of spontaneous speech she displayed on her first visit. Instead of looking at the floor, she now makes normal eye contact. Her affect has gone from constricted to expansive. She continues to have difficulty sleeping, but her energy has improved and she states she feels "so much better!" What should you conclude about the shift in the client's presentation?

 a. She is experiencing the activating side effects of fluoxetine.

 b. She is becoming euthymic.

 c. She is becoming hypomanic.

 d. She is in a mixed state.

55. Mr. D. is a 35-year-old, married, high-tech industry executive who is referred to the PMHNP for "insomnia." Mr. D. reports that he falls asleep quickly, but has difficulty staying asleep. He wakes up several times during the night, and believes he tosses and turns even when he is sleeping. He wakes up feeling exhausted and drinks "a pot of coffee" to stay awake and concentrate during his long work day. He drinks 1 glass of wine most evenings. He denies any illicit substance use. He denies any symptoms of a mood or anxiety disorder, but is feeling increasingly frustrated and concerned about his sleep. Which of the following is the most likely contributing factor to Mr. D.'s ongoing middle insomnia?

 a. Obstructive sleep apnea (OSA)

 b. Caffeine dependence

 c. Alcohol withdrawal

 d. Attention-deficit hyperactivity disorder (ADHD)

56. Tina is a 54-year-old single white woman who has been a Psychiatric–Mental Health Nurse Practitioner for over 20 years. She is considering making application to a Doctor of Nursing Practice (DNP) program but states "if a DNP is required to practice I'll get grandfathered in, no need for me to go back to school." Following the 2008 License, Accreditation, Certification, and Education (LACE) Consensus Model for Advanced Practice Registered Nurse Regulation, which statement is correct?

 a. Tina is correct: if the DNP becomes a requirement, she will be grandfathered in and obtain a DNP degree.

 b. The DNP is an academic terminal degree and there will not be an opportunity for Tina to be grandfathered in a DNP.

c. Tina will be grandfathered in and obtain a DNP only if her state requires a DNP to practice as an APRN.

d. The DNP is a certification and Tina will have to take an examination to be grandfathered in to obtain a DNP.

57. Tim is a board-certified Psychiatric–Mental Health Nurse Practitioner (PMHNP) working in a busy community mental health center (CMHC). He is currently seeing a client diagnosed with bipolar I disorder who has comorbid hypertension and diabetes. During the visit, Tim takes the client's blood pressure and her reading is 160/94 mm Hg. The client denies any headaches, nausea, chest pain, or shortness of breath. The client states "I can't afford all these medications so I haven't seen my doctor in 7 months and I am out of all my blood pressure and sugar medications, can you give me some?" What is Tim's most appropriate action?

a. Call the pharmacy to find out what medications the client is taking and refill for 1 month to cover until she can get in to see his primary care provider.

b. Tell the client he cannot refill her medications and inform her to go to the emergency room should she develop any signs or symptoms of an elevated blood pressure or hyperglycemia.

c. Call the client's primary care provider, explain the situation, and coordinate the client getting an appointment and medication refills.

d. Send the client to an urgent care clinic to get refills today.

58. The chief nursing officer of a large behavioral health system approached the PMHNP to discuss the new Healthcare Effectiveness Data and Information Set (HEDIS) behavioral health measures and specifications. The PMHNP is asked to do a retrospective chart review of all hospital discharge clients who received a follow-up visit within 7 days of discharge and within 30 days of discharge. The PMHNP has been asked to engage in which of the following?

a. Needs assessment project

b. Plan, do, study, act project

c. A task that is outside of the PMHNP's scope of practice

d. Quality improvement initiative

59. A PMHNP who is working on the consult liaison service is referred to a patient in the medical intensive care unit by the attending hospitalist. The consult note read "Evaluate the patient for competency to make independent medical decisions and consent for a surgical procedure." Based on the scope of practice of a PMHNP, which response would be most appropriate?

a. Complete the patient assessment and write up the findings in the patient's medical record.

b. Complete a patient assessment, including the mini mental status examination and family collateral data to determine competency.

c. Call the hospitalist and provide education that competency is a legal concept and explain that you can assess the patient for the capacity to make medical decisions.

d. Refuse the consult and inform the hospitalist that this is outside your scope of practice.

60. You are asked by a church organization to work with members within your health system to develop a flu vaccination program. According to public health principles, this is an example of what level of prevention?

    a. Secondary
    b. Preventative
    c. Tertiary
    d. Primary

61. A client with bipolar I disorder presents to your PMHNP office for a follow-up visit. During the visit the client informs you that he no longer wants to be treated with medication, and he does not have bipolar disorder, that was a misdiagnosis. He further informs you he stopped all his medication 2 months ago and is here to thank you for your care and tell you that he no longer needs follow-up appointments. Understanding the ethical conflict, you use which of the following ethical principles in working with this client?

    a. Autonomy
    b. Nonmaleficence
    c. Justice
    d. Beneficence

62. A new client reveals to the PMHNP that her boyfriend screams at her and has repeatedly slapped and pushed her in front of her 3-year-old son. She goes on to say that the boyfriend has thrown things at her and on one occasion threw a glass of water at her that hit her son in the back. Should the PMHNP report this to child protective services (CPS)?

    a. Yes, the client is issuing a cry for help for her son.
    b. Yes, the PMHNP has a duty to report.
    c. No, this does not constitute a reportable offense.
    d. No, a report to CPS will escalate the violence.

63. Which of the following is a function of the psychiatric interview?

    a. Understand the client's psychosocial needs and communicate them to the treatment team
    b. Identify the mental health needs of the client
    c. Review previous medical records
    d. Evaluate a treatment plan

64. A 74-year-old married white woman was referred to you by her primary care provider for a psychiatric evaluation. She had a normal medical and neurological examination in the last 2 months. The client presents with her husband of 45 years who states, "My wife is just not the same anymore, she is irritable and asks the same question several times, even though I've answered it many times." The client responds, "Oh, Henry, you do the same thing, it's just a normal part of getting older, and the kids think everything is fine." During the assessment you compete the mini mental status examination (MMSE) and the client scores 18. As

the PMHNP treating the client, you know the results of her MMSE indicate which level of cognitive impairment?

a. No cognitive impairment

b. Mild cognitive impairment

c. Moderate cognitive impairment

d. Severe cognitive impairment

65. You are the PMHNP treating Tim, a 10-year-old child, for ADHD and social anxiety disorder. His mother presents with Tim for his scheduled individual therapy session. At the end of the session his mother says, "I need to take Tim to see his pediatrician and at the last visit I was told he needed some HPV shot. I don't know, he's a boy, why would he need that? What do you think?" What is the PMHNP's best response to her question?

a. "The Centers for Disease Control and Prevention (CDC) recommends the human papillomavirus (HPV) vaccine for all boys and girls at age 10. HPV can cause cancer in both men and women, and the vaccine is effective in protecting against the virus. Can you tell me your concerns about Tim getting this vaccine?"

b. "While the Centers for Disease Control and Prevention (CDC) recommends the vaccine, every parent has the right to choose and if you do not think Tim needs this vaccine, as his parent you have the right to refuse."

c. "The Centers for Disease Control and Prevention (CDC) recommends the human papillomavirus (HPV) vaccine for older teenagers, starting at age 18, so you have time to research and think about your decision."

d. "My daughters received the vaccine, and I'm like you, I did not let my sons receive the vaccine. They don't need it. I agree, vaccines can be scary, can you tell me your concerns?"

66. As a PMHNP working in a crisis evaluation center, you are aware that the initial focus of a crisis assessment is on which of the following?

a. Client's past diagnosis and medication trials

b. Psychosocial history and supports

c. Safety of the client and others

d. Current living situation and coping skills

67. When conducting a neurological examination on a client, the PMHNP asks the client to hold out her arms and stick out her tongue while assessing for tremors. Which cranial nerve is being assessed?

a. Glossopharyngeal

b. Vagus

c. Trigeminal

d. Hypoglossal

68. A 20-year-old Asian man who was recently diagnosed with schizophrenia comes to your office for a follow-up appointment. During the assessment, he talks about his experience

in the group home, thinking that the television is sending him messages through news anchors during the 10 p.m. evening news. What symptom is the client describing?

a. Paranoia

b. Illusions

c. Ideas of reference

d. Neologisms

69. You are working with a family: mother, father, and two biological children. Sam, the father, is very rigid and controlling, which seems to be out of fear that something might happen to his family. He worries daily and it affects his family relationships. You give Sam a paradoxical directive and instruct him to intensely worry about everything he can think of for 1 hour a day. Using a paradoxical directive is part of which therapy?

a. Experimental

b. Structural

c. Strategic

d. Cognitive

70. As a PMHNP working in an outpatient addiction clinic, you often refer your clients to community AA and NA meetings. Using Yalom's therapeutic factors, you are aware that peer-led groups can inspire and encourage other group participants. Which therapeutic factor is instilled in AA and NA group members?

a. Hope

b. Altruism

c. Catharsis

d. Existential factors

71. Which of the following client statements best describes imitative behavior as a therapeutic factor in group therapy?

a. Group members talk over one another so the loudest person is heard

b. Group members begin to model aspects of other members of the group and group leaders

c. Group members discuss past situations when they were bullied and felt ashamed

d. Group leaders take charge of the group and redirect members when they monopolize the group

72. Dialectical behavioral therapy (DBT) draws on cognitive theory and behavioral theory, along with other theories. Elements of behavioral theory in DBT include which of the following?

a. Skills training and exposure

b. Examination of feelings and relating feelings to visceral sensations

c. Working through the transference with the therapist

d. Cognitive interpretation of past traumatic experiences

73. Dialectical behavioral therapy (DBT) affirms dialectical thinking, which involves examining and discussing opposing ideas to find the truth. This philosophy is a supportive principle of DBT training. The central dialectical pattern emphasized in DBT involves the tension between:

    a. Radical acceptance and change
    b. Cue exposure and block avoidance
    c. Problem avoidance and problem-solving
    d. Crisis survival and acceptance

74. Samantha is a 26-year-old partnered woman who works full time as a teacher. She is in a long-term relationship with Mary and they are getting along well, and doing well financially. They have two children, ages 2 and 6. Samantha is seeing the PMHNP to address her concerns that she is feeling down and sad for no reason and states, "I know my life is going well but I just don't feel happy. I have always worried a lot and have been sad most of my life." As a PMHNP trained in transactional analysis (TA), you understand that personality is multifaceted and wonder if which of the following is affecting her ability to experience happiness:

    a. She had long periods of separation from her primary caregiver as a child and now has a difficult time accepting and receiving love and experiencing happiness
    b. She likely had a traumatic event in her childhood and her thoughts and feelings related to the event are locked together in her brain and cannot be accessed
    c. Her unhappiness is likely related to distorted thoughts and feelings about her relationship
    d. As an adolescent she experienced an event that was processed in an ego state as an older sibling

75. You have been working with a 54-year-old man who has been treated for schizophrenia since age 19. He has limited social interactions, likes to be alone, and has never dated nor had a desire to date. His symptoms are best explained by which of the following?

    a. Antisocial personality disorder
    b. Lack of personal hygiene
    c. Negative symptoms
    d. Positive symptoms

76. Following evidence-based (EB) practice, which laboratory screening tests and assessments should be completed prior to placing a person on a second-generation ("atypical") antipsychotic medication?

    a. Serum glucose, lipid profile, weight, blood pressure, waist circumference, and family history of cardiovascular disease
    b. Comprehensive metabolic panel, body mass index, complete blood count, and thyroid panel

(c.) Serum glucose or hemoglobin A1c, lipid profile, weight, body mass index, blood pressure, waist circumference, and family history of cardiovascular disease

d. Serum glucose, complete blood count, assessment of family history of cardiovascular disease and cancer

77. Which type of hallucination is rare in persons with psychotic illnesses and is often associated with an organic etiology?

a. Auditory hallucinations

(b.) Gustatory hallucinations

c. Visual hallucinations

d. Combination hallucinations

78. What differentiates atypical antipsychotic medications from first-generation or typical antipsychotic medications?

(a.) 5HT2a receptor antagonist properties

b. 5HT2a receptor agonist properties

c. Specific dopamine receptor 3 and 5HT2a blockade

d. Dopamine receptor 2 antagonist properties

79. You are treating a client with schizophrenia who takes clozapine. What laboratory values will indicate the client needs to discontinue treatment?

a. White blood cell count of less than 1,800/mm3 and absolute neutrophil count of less than 1,200/mm3

(b.) Absolute neutrophil count of less than 1,000/uL

c. White blood cell count of less than 1,200/mm3

d. Absolute neutrophil count of less than 2,000/uL

80. Sean is a 47-year-old Gulf War veteran who was in combat during Operation Desert Storm. Sean has been treated by the PMHNP for major depressive disorder and associated anxiety symptoms. During the most recent visit, the PMHNP learns that Sean sustained a traumatic brain injury during his service, which was recently diagnosed at the TBI clinic in the Veterans Affairs clinic. What is the rationale for the PMHNP to taper Sean off clonazepam?

(a.) Benzodiazepines causes memory problems and confusion in clients with a history of a TBI.

b. Benzodiazepines lower the seizure threshold in clients with a history of a TBI.

c. Veterans Affairs has banned benzodiazepines from the medication formulary.

d. Benzodiazepines place clients with a TBI at risk for a second head injury.

81. Alice is a 68-year-old woman who presents to you with concerns about her memory. She explains that her mother and grandmother both experienced dementia and she wants to do what she can to prevent this terrible disease. Alice is treated for hypertension, which is well controlled; other than that she is in good health. She is socially and physically active and participates in a monthly cooking class, volunteers at her church, and plays bridge twice a

week at the senior center. She says, "I understand that I am losing brain cells at my age, but I would still like to keep my mind and body active." Which is the best response to Alice?

a. "You are correct that you cannot form new brain cells at your age but you should continue with your activities because they offer excellent physical and mental health benefits and in turn will lower your risk for dementia."

b. "Although most brain development occurs early in life, we still form some new brain cells in a couple of areas of the brain during adulthood. You should continue with your activities because they offer excellent physical and mental health benefits and are neuroprotective."

c. "Scientists now know that we do continue to form new brain cells throughout the entire brain during adulthood. Continue with your activities because you are producing new brain cells in the frontal lobe and this will decrease your risk of dementia."

d. "You should continue the social activities such as bridge, volunteering, and the book club but should consider the risks and benefits of physical activities such as dancing. If you were to fall and break a hip, this could lead to prolonged hospitalization, loss of independence, and ultimately increase your risk of dementia."

82. What is the best treatment for AIDS dementia complex?

a. Acetylcholinesterase inhibitors

b. Symptom-targeted pharmacologic treatments

c. Nonpharmacologic supportive care

d. Antiretroviral therapy

83. As a PMHNP working on the consult liaison team, you know the importance of preventing delirium due to which of the following?

a. Risk of 1-year mortality rate

b. Risk of harm to the client and staff

c. Risk of unremitting psychosis

d. Risk of aspiration

84. When working with a 26-year-old, Mike, who presents for treatment of cannabis use and gambling, you use motivational interviewing techniques. As a PMHNP, you are familiar with the core counseling skills used in motivational interviewing. Mike made the following statement: "I don't know why I came here in the first place but I thought maybe some medication would help me." You respond by saying, "You're feeling confused about the process" and Mike replies, "I never thought I'd need to come to a place like this." You respond, "You kept your appointment today and I appreciate the courage it took for you to come here." What two motivational interviewing techniques are used in this interaction?

a. Interrupting and reassurance

b. Affirming and reflecting

c. Open-ended questions and summarizing

d. Clarification and data collection

85. You are a PMHNP working in a hospitalist role on an acute inpatient psychiatric unit at a local hospital. As you make rounds, the registered nurse informs you that a 32-year-old client who was admitted for alcohol detox has a score of 17 on the Clinical Institute Withdrawal Assessment for Alcohol. What phase of withdrawal is this client in?

    a. Mild withdrawal
    b. Moderate withdrawal
    c. Severe withdrawal
    d. Delirium tremens

86. A client who has been addicted to opioids has not used in 15 days. During your medication management visit, the client states, "I'm going to die from not having my Opanas. You need to give me something now." The PMHNP's best response is:

    a. "I know you are feeling very uncomfortable and we need to get you to the emergency room immediately to prevent a seizure."
    b. "I know you are feeling very uncomfortable, let's take your vital signs and talk about a trial on Catapres to treat your withdrawal symptoms."
    c. "You have been using Opana for a long time and it is going to take several months for the withdrawal to end. In the meantime, I will see you weekly."
    d. "There is no treatment for opioid withdrawal; you will have to wait it out."

87. Signs and symptoms of cannabis intoxication include:

    a. Increase sensitivity to external stimuli
    b. Enhanced motor skills
    c. Fast passage of time
    d. Lower heart rate

88. Which defense mechanisms are commonly used by persons with obsessive–compulsive personality disorder?

    a. Rationalization, isolation, and intellectualization
    b. Projection, distortion, and hypochondriasis
    c. Regression, somatization, and dissociation
    d. Sexualization, displacement, and reaction formation

89. You have been working with Cody, a 30-year-old single man, in weekly individual psychotherapy for 3 weeks. At the start of session 4 he says, "I noticed when I came in that your usual parking spot has a new car in it with temporary tags, and it's a BMW. Nice car." What is the best response from the PMHNP psychotherapist to Cody?

    a. "Thanks for noticing, it is a nice car."
    b. "How do you know what spot I park in?"
    c. "I noticed you drive a BMW as well, how do you like your car?"
    d. "Sounds like having expensive things is important to you."

90. When working in individual psychotherapy with a client who has a personality disorder, what are the primary treatment goals?

    a.   Change the client's personality structure and make him or her more adaptable in every-day life.

    b.   Reparent the client, following Bowlby's theoretical framework.

    c.   Allow the client to reprocess his or her childhood trauma because all clients with personality disorders have a history of severe abuse.

    (d.)   Assist the client in changing dysfunctional interpersonal relationships and use of immature defense mechanisms.

91. For a client who has paranoid personality disorder, what are the best treatment strategies?

    a.   Confront negative and misinterpreted thoughts and feelings.

    b.   Deflate grandiose thoughts.

    c.   Engage the client in detailed and emotional responses and dialog.

    (d.)   Do not challenge negative views or recollections of events.

92. John, a client with paranoid personality disorder, states the following: "I noticed there is a red light in the upper corner of your door and it has been going on and off during our sessions. Are you recording me?" What is the PMHNP best response?

    a.   "No, it would be illegal for me to record you, and that is not a camera it's just a red light."

    (b.)   "John, thank you for asking the question. The light you see in the upper corner of my door tells me when a client has arrived and is in the waiting room. The client turns on the light, as you do, when they arrive in the waiting room, alerting me their arrival, and I turn off the light when we get into the office using the switch by my desk."

    c.   "Come on John, do you think I would record your sessions? You are not that interesting. I'm just kidding, no John, it is not a recorder or camera."

    d.   "John, it takes courage to ask me the question. Tell me a time in your life when you had a similar experience."

93. As a PMHNP, you understand the genetic factors that contribute to psychiatric and personality disorders. Persons who develop antisocial personality disorder often are raised in families with high rates of which of the following?

    a.   Psychotic disorders

    (b.)   Alcohol use disorders

    c.   Anxiety disorders

    d.   Mood disorders

94. Persons with obsessive–compulsive personality disorder often use isolation as a defense mechanism. Which of the following examples best describes isolation as a defense mechanism?

    a.   Staying in the house for days or weeks to clean

    b.   Declining invites by friends or family to attend social gatherings

    c. Describing information with very little affect variation

    d. Being an introvert in the work setting to prevent talking with coworkers

95. In the *Diagnostic and Statistical Manual of Mental Disorders,* 5th Edition (DSM-5), how should a personality disorder be coded?

    a. Coded with the major psychiatric disorder

    b. Coded on Axis II

    c. Coded on Axis III

    d. Coded on Axis IV

96. When prescribing a selective serotonin reuptake inhibitor (SSRI) for a child or young adult up to age 24, what education must be included?

    a. Black box warning about increased suicidality in this population

    b. Black box warning about increased risk of mania in this population

    c. Risk of sexual side effects on this class of medication

    d. Risk of stomach upset and headaches, to prevent unnecessary primary care visits

97. Tommy is an 8 year-old who presents to the PMHNP for evaluation of attention-deficit hyperactivity disorder. His mother completed the Vanderbilt ADHD rating scale and brought in the Vanderbilt teaching rating scale. Both your clinical interview and the rating scales indicate Tommy has ADHD. What assessment indicator(s) need to be completed prior to starting a stimulant mediation?

    a. Get a copy of the rating scale completed by his grandparents.

    b. Assess for family history of cardiovascular disease and, if positive for conduction problems, order an electrocardiogram before prescribing medication.

    c. Obtain blood pressure, and pulse, and begin the stimulant medication.

    d. Assess for a family history of bipolar disorder.

98. A mother brings in her 7-year-old son for a psychiatric follow-up visit with the PMHNP. This is the fourth visit the PMHNP has had with the client, his mother, and his younger sister, Renee, now 7 months old. You notice that she has a decrease in head growth, along with stereotypic motions of the hands, often licking and slapping. Renee has also lost her language skills. What medical condition do you suspect Renee has developed?

    a. Autism spectrum disorder

    b. Rett syndrome

    c. Selective mutism

    d. Childhood onset diabetes

99. You are treating Timothy, a 16-year-old boy, for an eating disorder. Timothy is of normal weight and socially extroverted, at times appearing to seek attention when in a peer group or class. Timothy's symptoms are most consistent with which eating disorder?

    a. Anorexia nervosa

    b. Bulimia nervosa

    c.   Binge eating disorder

    d.   Anxiety-induced eating disorder

100. You are treating a 14-year-old female for attention-deficit hyperactivity disorder (ADHD) who has a family history of bipolar disorder. As a PMHNP familiar with symptoms of both ADHD and pediatric bipolar disorder, you know the following are overlapping symptoms of both disorders:

    a.   Excessive talking, increased activity, and distractibility

    b.   Irritability, sleep problems, and mood swings

    c.   Excessive talking, irritability, and sleep problems

    d.   Sleep problems, mood swings, and distractibility

APPENDIX B

REVIEW QUESTION ANSWERS

1. Correct Answer: A. The ANA's *Psychiatric–Mental Health Nursing: Scope and Standards of Practice* defines the role and actions of the nurse practitioner.

2. Correct Answer: D. Information reduces incidence of disease.

3. Correct Answer: B. Identifies the trend of ensuring the protection of individual civil liberties for psychiatric clients.

4. Correct Answer: C. As with any client, psychiatric clients can refuse treatment unless a legal process resulting in involuntary commitment or mandatory court order for treatment has been obtained.

5. Correct Answer: A. Social relationships are mutual interpersonal relationships in which the needs of both parties are addressed. The N–C relationship is most concerned with meeting the needs of the client.

6. Correct Answer: A. This action focuses on interventions designed to reduce the incidence of new cases of disease.

7. Correct Answer: B. Almost every state allows for a brief period of detainment to assess a client for dangerousness to self or others before allowing the client to leave a hospital setting, even if the admission was voluntary.

8. Correct Answer: C. Authenticity. Being genuine, honest, and respectful are essential elements in establishing a working relationship with any client. Like-mindedness is not a part of the therapeutic relationship. Although an important aspect of the PMHNP role, collecting a family history and accuracy in assessment does not in and of itself facilitate relationship-building.

9. Correct Answer: D. All DSM-5 disorders need to be made taking a person's culture into account. A cultural expression of a response to grief, loss, or stress is not considered a DSM-5 diagnosis.

10. Correct Answer: C. Clients frequently display resistance and regression at the termination of a meaningful therapeutic process. The PMHNP is responsible for planning an effective termination and monitoring clients during the termination period.

11. Correct Answer: B. These signs indicate developmental failure of early childhood.

12. Correct Answer: B. The psychic determinism principle states that all behavior has purpose and meaning, often unconscious in nature, and that no behaviors occur randomly or by coincidence.

13. Correct Answer: D. Suppression is the only defense mechanism listed in which the client channels conflicting energies into growth-promoting activities.

14. Correct Answer: A. Immature regressive defense mechanism is a return to a behavior common to an earlier stage of development.

15. Correct Answer: C. Defense mechanisms are a function of the ego used to resolve a conflict.

16. Correct Answer: C. ACO's are groups of doctors or other health care providers who voluntarily come together and assume the care provided to Medicare patients.

17. Correct Answer: A. Health care efficiency is making risk and benefit decision about how care resources are allocated and equity is ensuring that there is a fair distribution of the resources.

18. Correct Answer: B. The four elements that must be satisfied for malpractice to have occurred are a duty of care between clinician and patient, breach of standard of care, an injury to the patient, and the patient's injury must be related to the clinician's breach of care.

19. Correct Answer: D. The ANA has a position statement that nurses are responsible for developing health care settings that include just culture initiatives understanding that human error can cause error and harm by creating an open and fair environment.

20. Correct Answer: A. Neurotransmitters in the central nervous system function as a communication medium.

21. Correct Answer: C. Serotonin is produced in the raphe nuclei.

22. Correct Answer: D. Dopamine is produced in the substantia nigra.

23. Correct Answer: B. Appetite, sleep, and libido are regulated by the hypothalamus.

24. Correct Answer: C. A client with a pacemaker should not receive an MRI of the head.

25. Correct Answer: D. Glutamate is the primary excitatory neurotransmitter.

26. Correct Answer: A. Problems with working memory, planning and prioritizing, insight into problems, and impulse control indicate a problem in the frontal lobe.

27. Correct Answer: B. Target symptom identification is the identification of specific, precise, and individualized symptoms reasonably expected to improve with a given medication.

28. Correct Answer: C. Although diagnosis is an important aspect of the assessment process, the assessment ultimately should identify the needs of the client.

29. Correct Answer: C. One PMHNP role is to control the milieu as an aspect of assessment, so the PMHNP should choose a quiet place that is public enough to get assistance with client care should it be required during the assessment.

30. Correct Answer: B. This exchange is an illustration of the technique of recognizing.

31. Correct Answer: D. The answer demonstrates concrete thought processes, which are normal in persons younger than age 12 but are abnormal after age 12. To interpret the finding, the PMHNP must know the age of the client.

32. Correct Answer: B. This response will be the most therapeutic in moving forward with the client.

33. Correct Answer: B. This response is the most therapeutic, allowing the client to further clarify and express feelings.

34. Correct Answer: A. Asking the client how to help is an aspect of assessment—all other answers are aspects of interventions, which are not initial actions of the PMHNP.

35. Correct Answer: C. Client overdosed and then was placed on a medication that affects the liver. The PMHNP needs to assess the client's liver function as an aspect of care planning for her.

36. Correct Answer: D. Client symptoms are consistent with electrolyte imbalance and a physical cause of his symptoms must be ruled out first.

37. Correct Answer: B. Beta blockers can cause or exacerbate depression.

38. Correct Answer: C. Older adults usually have decreased protein levels. Most psychotropic medications are highly protein-bound. It is the unbound (free) concentration of the drug that is active; the bound concentration of the drug is inert. Thus, with decreased protein available for binding, more free (active) drug remains in the body, which then predisposes older adults to toxicity.

39. Correct Answer: B. Divalproex can cause spina bifida and lithium can cause Epstein's anomaly.

40. Correct Answer: C. Pharmacokinetics is the study of what the body does to drugs.

41. Correct Answer: C. Tolerance means needing more to achieve the same effect.

42. Correct Answer: D. Group therapy is beneficial because it increases social skills, is cost-effective, and enables participants to acquire the curative factors.

43. Correct Answer: A. Cognitive behavioral therapy helps clients recognize and change their automatic thoughts.

44. Correct Answer: C. Paradoxical directives are used in strategic therapy.

45. Correct Answer: B. Homeostasis is balance or stability that the family returns to despite its dysfunction.

46. Correct Answer: B. Miracle questions are used in solution-focused therapy.

47. Correct Answer: A. The use of a standardized rating scale will allow the PMHNP to monitor the level of client symptoms and to evaluate the efficacy of the medication.

48. Correct Answer: C. SSRIs are considered among the first-line medications used to treat depression because of safety in suicidal overdose clients.

49. Correct Answer: C. The PMHNP needs to ensure that her suicide attempt has not led to medical instability.

50. Correct Answer: A. The literature suggests that although short-term anxiolytic medication may be offered in an emergency room setting, ataque de nervios is best treated by brief supportive therapy by a Spanish-speaking Latino therapist.

51. Correct Answer: C. The student does not meet criteria for alcohol use or other disorder at this point, but if he does not learn alternative coping skills to deal with his shyness, he is at risk of developing an alcohol use disorder.

52. Correct Answer: D. Although the PMHNP's resentment is in response to actual behavior by Jason (his missing several appointments), clarifying what is going on for him, his expectations for treatment and the PMHNP's (and the clinic's) expectations in a non-judgemental manner will help to develop a therapeutic alliance.

53. Correct Answer: B. Liver enzyme functioning (among other things) diminishes as we age. All of the other statements are false.

54. Correct Answer: C. In this case, you see a shifting set of symptoms, the most important being her expansive mood and statement "so much better" that indicates she has gone beyond euthymia.

55. Correct Answer: A. OSA is the only plausible possibility if the rest of the information given by the client is accurate. OSA causes clients to have frequent awakenings and a sense that they are not sleeping deeply ("tossing and turning") that is caused by apnea. The client should be assessed further for snoring and awareness of apnea. Although the client states he drinks a lot of coffee, this is driven by his sleep issues.

Drinking 1 glass of wine in the evening would not cause the degree of sleep pathology he is exhibiting. Other than diminishing concentration that is consistent with sleep deprivation, there are no other signs and symptoms of ADHD.

56. Correct Answer: B. APRNs are not grandfathered into an academic degree; degrees must be earned from accredited academic institutions.

57. Correct Answer: C. It is not within the scope of practice of a PMHNP to treat hypertension. Coordination of care to ensure the client does not run out of medication is the appropriate course of action.

58. Correct Answer: D. Engaging in a project to assess whether a standard of care was met is a quality improvement project.

59. Correct Answer: C. The legal system makes determination whether a person is competent; practitioners can assess and make a determination about a person's capacity to make medical decisions.

60. Correct Answer: D. Prevention of illness is primary prevention and administration of flu vaccinations in a community is intended to prevent a flu outbreak.

61. Correct Answer: A. Clients who are legally competent have the ability to make medical decisions and maintain individual autonomy.

62. Correct Answer: B. PMHNPs are mandated reporters of child abuse. The 3-year-old is being exposed to violence and although not the target, could have been injured when the boyfriend threw the glass of water.

63. Correct Answer: B. During a psychiatric interview, the PMHNP is responsible to identify symptoms and needs of a client to develop an appropriate treatment plan.

64. Correct Answer: C. Cut points on the MMSE are as follows: total score 30, 25–30 questionable significance, 20–25 mild impairment, 10–20 moderate impairment, and 10 or lower severe impairment.

65. Correct Answer: A. When family members or clients ask questions about illnesses and treatment, it is the PMHNP's responsibility to provide data and then assess understanding and meaning.

66. Correct Answer: C. In a crisis, the first assessment should be safety of the client and those near the client.

67. Correct Answer: D. The tongue is controlled by the hypoglossal cranial nerve.

68. Correct Answer: C. Ideas of reference are misinterpretations of incidents and events that one believes have a direct personal reference to oneself.

69. Correct Answer: C. Paradoxical directives may be used in strategic family therapy.

70. Correct Answer: A. Working in support groups such as AA and NA, hearing stories of others who had similar struggles, instills hope.

71. Correct Answer: B. As group progresses the leader is less active and the members of the group take over and begin to model other members and the leaders.

72. Correct Answer: A. DBT focuses on cognitive and behavioral techniques, mindfulness including meditation, and emotional regulation.

73. Correct Answer: A. DBT emphasis acceptance of the current reality of what is and the ability to engage in personal change.

74. Correct Answer: B. According to TA, when a person is traumatized the thoughts and feelings get tied together and the process of therapy is to unlock the two.

75. Correct Answer: C. Negative symptoms include flat affect, alogia, avolition, poor attention, and anhedonia. In the case study, the symptoms are avolition and anhedonia.

76. Correct Answer: C. EB practice guidelines indicate that all clients should have the following prior to starting antipsychotic medication: fasting glucose or A1c, lipid profile, weight, body mass index, blood pressure, waist circumference, and family history of cardiovascular disease.

77. Correct Answer: B. The most common type of hallucinations in persons with psychotic illnesses are auditory and visual. Tactile and gustatory hallucinations are less common and more likely related to an organic illness.

78. Correct Answer: A. Typical antipsychotic medications block D2 receptors; atypical antipsychotic medications block D2 receptors and have 5HT2a antagonist properties.

79. Correct Answer: B. The recent change in monitoring clozapine clients using the risk evaluation and mitigation strategy (REMS) indicates persons treated on clozapine need to have absolute neutrophil count monitored and, if it drops below 1,000/uL, treatment must be interrupted and can be resumed once the absolute neutrophil count normalizes above 1,000/uL.

80. Correct Answer: A. Benzodiazepines are contraindicated in clients with a TBI due to increase rates of confusion and memory problems.

81. Correct Answer: B. While it was once thought that brain neurons did not regenerate, we now known that while most brain development occurs early in life, we continue to form some new brain cells throughout life. As we age, we need to engage in activities that keep our brains healthy by encouraging this growth. Examples are diet, exercise, socialization, and cognitive stimulation.

82. Correct Answer: D. All persons with AIDS should be treated with antiretroviral therapy. Those who develop dementia complex should have those symptoms treated with appropriate pharmacological or nonpharmacological interventions.

83. Correct Answer: A. Studies have identified high rates of mortality post hospitalization for delirium so the best treatment is prevention.

84. Correct Answer: B. When a person is in contemplation stage, interventions should be affirming and reflecting.

85. Correct Answer: B. CIWA cut off scores are as follows: 0–9, absent or very mild withdrawal; 10–15, mild withdrawal; 16–20, moderate withdrawal; and 21–67, severe withdrawal.

86. Correct Answer: B. Opioid withdrawal symptoms can be treated with central alpha agonists.

87. Correct Answer: A. Persons intoxicated on cannabis exhibit distorted perceptions, increase relaxation and sensitivity, and loss of coordination.

88. Correct Answer: A. Persons with obsessive–compulsive personality disorder use defense mechanisms of rationalization, isolation of affect, and intellectualization to make sense of their behavior.

89. Correct Answer: D. In a therapy relationship, the therapist should try to understand the meaning of a client's statement rather than engage in social conversations.

90. Correct Answer: D. Persons with personality disorders have a pervasive maladaptive pattern of behavior and the goal of therapy is to slowly shift how they relate in the world and begin to use higher-order defenses.

91. Correct Answer: D. Persons with fixed false beliefs should not be challenged.

92. Correct Answer: B. When working with a paranoid client, help the person find proof of meaning and explain any questions in a matter-of-fact manner.

93. Correct Answer: B. Being raised in an alcoholic family increases the likelihood of chaos, unpredictability, and lack of rules and order, leading to higher rates of developing antisocial personality disorder.

94. Correct Answer: C. Isolation is a defense mechanism often used by people with obsessive–compulsive personality disorder.

95. Correct Answer: A. DSM-5 no longer uses the axial system.

96. Correct Answer: A. The SSRIs all carry a black box warning for increased suicidal ideation for this age group.

97. Correct Answer: B. American Academy of Child and Adolescent Psychiatry practice parameters require physical exam, pulse, weight, height, and blood pressure workup prior to the start of stimulant medication. Because his grandfather had a cardiac conduction problem, an electrocardiogram (ECG) should also be obtained prior to the start of medication.

98. Correct Answer: B. Girls with Rett's syndrome develop normally and around the 7th month regress, with a decrease in head size and language loss.

99. Correct Answer: B. Clients with bulimia are often of normal weight or overweight and are outgoing.

100. Correct Answer: A. Clients with ADHD and bipolar disorder often have excessive talking, increased activity, and distractibility.

INDEX

A

Abdomen 85–86
Absorption 111
  of drugs 111
Abuse 294
Access to care 56
Acetylcholine
  explanation of 69
  function of 72
  psychiactric disorders and 70
Acupressure 132–133
Acupuncture 132–133
Addiction. *See* Substance-related disorders
Addictive disorders. *See* Substance-related
    disorders
Adolescent Transitions Program (ATP) 332
Advance directives 23
Affect 328
Affordable Care Act (2010) 57
Aggression-turned-inward theory 140–141
Agonist effect 113
Agoraphobia 210–211. *See also* Anxiety
    disorders
  assessment of 210–211
  clinical management of 211
  comorbidities of 211
  description of 210
  diagnostic and laboratory findings and 211
  history of 210
  mental status exams for 210
  nonpharmacological management of 211
  pharmacological management of 211
  physical exams for 210
Alanine aminotransferase 95
Alcohol use disorders identification test
    (AUDIT) 297
Alzheimer's dementia 283
Amaurosis fugax 281
Amino acids 69
Amygdala 66
Anal stage 42
Analysis of variance (ANOVA) 54
Anhedonia 146
Anorexia nervosa 348
Antagonist effect 113
Antiadrenergic 156
Anticholinergic 156
Anticipatory guidance 98–99
Anticonvulsants 182–183

Antidepressants 158–159, 161
  classes of 152–154
  target symptons of treatment 152
  tricyclic 154
Antihistaminergic 156
Antipsychotics 115
  atypical 244–247
  typical 249–250, 250
Anxiety
  certification examination and 1
  description of 195–196
  levels of 195, 196
  pathological levels of 200
  tips for dealing with 6
Anxiety disorders 196–207, 197
  agoraphobia as 210–211
  assessment of 200–202
  clinical management of 202
  comorbidities of 206
  demographics for 199
  description of 196–197
  diagnostic and laboratory findings 202
  differential diagnosis of 202, 203
  etiology for 197–199
  follow-up for 206–207
  generalized anxiety disorder as 215–218
  health considerations for 206
  history of 200–201
  incidence of 199
  life span considerations for 205
  mental status exams for 201–202
  nonpharmacological management of 205
  obsessive–compulsive disorder as 218–221
  panic disorder as 207–210
  pharmacological management of 203–205,
    205
  physical exams for 201
  posttraumatic stress disorder as 222–225
  prevention of 199–200
  risk factors for 199
  screening for 199–200
  separation anxiety disorder as 218
  social anxiety disorder as 214–215
  specific phobias as 211–214
Anxiolytics 116, 205
Arbitration 52
Aromatherapy 132, 133
Aspartate 69
  aminotransferase 95–96

Assessment
  gender-based 99–101
  health behavior guidelines and 101–103
Assessment components
  abdomen as 85–86
  back as 84–85
  breasts as 85
  coordination and fine-motor skills as 82
  ears as 84
  eyes as 83
  head, skin, and nails as 83
  heart as 85
  indicators of child abuse as 86
  motor functions as 82
  musculoskeletal system as 86
  neck as 84
  neurological exam as 80–86
  neurological soft signs as 82–83
  nose and sinuses as 84
  physical exam as 79–86
  sensory functions as 82
  thorax and lungs as 85
  vital signs as 83
Attention deficit disorder 117
Attention-deficit hyperactivity disorder
      (ADHD) 117, 335–340
  agents for treatment of 338
  assessment of 337
  clinical management of 338–339
  comorbidities of 339–340
  demographics of 336
  description of 335–336
  diagnostic and laboratory findings 337–338
  differential diagnosis of 338
  etiology of 336
  follow-up for 340
  incidence of 336
  mental status exams for 337
  nonpharmacological management
      of 339–340
  pharmacological management of 338–339
  physical exams for 337
  prevention of 337
  risk factors for 336–337
  screening for 337
Autism spectrum disorder 340–343
  assessment of 342
  clinical management of 343–344
  demographics of 341
  description of 340
  diagnostic and laboratory findings 343
  differential diagnosis of 343
  etiology of 340
  history of 342
  incidence of 341
  mental status exams for 342
  nonpharmacological management
      of 343–344
  pharmacological management of 343
  physical exams for 342
  prevalence 341
  prevention of 341
  risk factors for 341
  screening for 341, 343
  symptons of 342
Autonomic nervous system 64
Aversion treatment 304
Axon 64, 68

B
Back 84–85
Bandura, Albert 46
Basal Ganglia 67
Beck, Aaron 125, 141
Beck depression inventory (BDI) 145
Becker, Marshall 46
Behavioral therapy 289
  explanation of 126
Belladonna 135
Benzodiazepines (BNZs) 116, 204
Bereavement. See Grief and bereavement
Berg, Insoo 131
Binge eating 348
Biofeedback 132, 133
Biological
  based therapies 132
  preventative factors 104
  risk factors 103
  theories of personality disorders 316
  theories of substance-related
      disorders 294–296
Biopsychosocial framework of care, recovery
      and 37
Bipolar (BP) disorder 173–184
  anticonvulsants and 182–183
  assessment of 175–177
  clinical management of 179–180
  demographics of 174

Bipolar (BP) disorder (continued)
  description of 173–174
  diagnostic and laboratory findings for 179
  differential diagnosis of 179
  drugs for 182–183
  etiology of 174
  history of 175–177
  incidence of 174
  lithium for treatment of 180
  medications for 179
  mental status exam for 177–178
  pharmacological management of 180–182
  phycial exam for 177
  prevention of 175
  rapid cycling and 177
  risk factors for 175
  screening for 175
  symptoms of 176, 179
  types of 177
Black cohosh 134
Body dysmorphic disorder 226
Body mass index (BMI) 83
Bowen, Murray 130
Brain/brain function
  brainstem and 67–68
  cerebrum and 65–67
  depression and 143
  gray matter and 64
  neuroanatomy and 64–68
  neurophysiology and 68–70
  outermost surface of 64–65
  white matter and 64
Brainstem 67–68
Breasts 85
Brief psychotic disorder 264–265
  assessment of 265
  clinical management of 265
  demographics of 264
  description of 264
  diagnostic and laboratory findings 265
  etiology of 264
  history of 265
  incidence of 264
  mental status exams for 265
  nonpharmacological management of 265
  pharmacological management of 265
  physical exams for 265
  prevention of 264
  risk factors for 264

  screening for 264
Brief therapy 162
Bright Futures 98–99
Bulimia nervosa 348

C
CAGE alcohol screening test 297
Calcium 89–90
Cardiac disorders 150
Caring theory 47
Carrier proteins 113
Case management 22
Catecholamine. *See* Dopamine (DA)
Catnip 135
Cell body and neurons 64, 68
Central nervous system (CNS) 64
Cerebellum 67
Cerebral cortex 66
Cerebrum
  basal ganglia in 67
  brainstem and 67–68
  cerebral cortex in 66
  function of 65
  limbic system in 66
  lobes in 65–66
Certification 15–16
Certification examination 1–10
  anxiety 1
  current knowledge about 2
  depth of knowledge required 3
  expectations for 2
  facts about 8–9
  general content 2
  instituting a study plan for 3–5
  internet resources for 9
  mentally preparing for 2
  physically preparing for 2
  preparing for 1–8
  review courses for 2
  strategies prior to 5–6
  test-taking strategies for 6–8
Chamomile 135
Child abuse 86
Childhood and adolescence
      disorders 327–360
    assessment and care planning for 327–329
    attention-deficit hyperactivity disorder
      (ADHD) 335–340
    autism spectrum disorder 340–342

conduct disorder 332–334
  disruptive mood dysregulation
      disorder 355–356
  eating disorders 346–351
  intellectual disability 352–355
  oppositional defiant disorder
      (ODD) 329–332
  Rett syndrome 344–346
Children and adolescents under 21 years of
      age test (CRAFT) 297
Chloride 92–93
Cholinergics 69
Chronic fatigue syndrome 150
Chronobiological theory 143–144
Circadian rhythms 143
Circular causality 129
Client advocacy 22
Clinical Opiate Withdrawal Scale
      (COWS) 297
Cluster A personality disorders 317–318
  characteristics of 318
Cluster B personality disorders 318–319
  characteristics of 320
Cluster C personality disorders 319
  characteristics of 321
Cognitive behavioral therapy (CBT) 162, 289,
      379
Cognitive disorders 271
  description 271
  etiology 271
Cognitive theory 43–45, 141
Cognitive therapy 125–126
Combined structural and functional
      imaging 73
Commitment, involuntary 21
Competency, elements of 21
Complementary and alternative therapies
      (CATs)
  origins of 132
  types of 132–135
Complete blood count (CBC) 149
Computed tomography (CT) 72
Concrete operations stage 44
Conduct disorder 332–335
  assessment of 333
  clinical management of 334
  demographics of 333
  description of 332
  diagnostic and laboratory findings 334

differential diagnosis of 334
  etiology of 332
  history of 333
  incidence of 333
  life span considerations for 335
  mental status exams for 334
  nonpharmacological management of 335
  pharmacological management of 334
  physical exams for 333
  prevalence of 332
  prevention of 333
  risk factors for 333
  screening for 333
Confidentiality 16
  exceptions to guaranteed 17
Conflict 52
  defense mechanisms and 43
  of interest (COI) 57–58
  resolution 52
Confusion Assessment Method (CAM) 273
Conservation 44
Coordination 82
Corpus striatum 67
Corticotropin-releasing hormone (CRH) 142
Countertransference 38–39
Cranial nerves 80–82
Credentialing 15
Creutzfeldt-Jakob disease 278
Critical thinking 52
Cultural differences and health influences and
      determinants 24
Culturally competent care 23–24
  forensics and corrections and 27–28
  homeless individuals and 24–25
  migrant and seasonal farm workers and 25
  sexual orientation and 26–27
Culture 23
Culture-bound syndromes 23
Cyclothymic disorder 186–187
  assessment of 187–188
  clinical management of 188
  demographics of 186–187
  description of 186–187
  diagnostic and laboratory findings 188
  differential diagnosis of 188
  etiology of 186–187
  follow-up for 188
  history of 187
  indicence of 186–187

Cyclothymic disorder (continued)
  life span considerations for 188
  mental status exams for 187–188
  nonpharmacological management of 188
  pharmacological management of 188
  physical exams for 187
  prevention of 187
  risk factors for 187
  screening for 187
Cytochrome P450
  inhibitors and inducers 112

D

Defense mechanisms 43, 44
Delirium 271–277
  assessment of 273
  clinical management of 275
  demographics of 272
  description of 271
  diagnostic and laboratory findings 275
  differential diagnosis of 275
  etiology of 272
  health considerations for 276
  history of 273
  incidence of 272
  life span considerations for 276–277
  mental status exams for 274
  nonpharmacological management of 276
  pharmacological management of 276
  physical exam for 273
  prevention of 273
  risk factors for 272–273
  screening for 273
  subtypes of 272
Delusional disorder 262–265
  assessment of 262–263
  clinical management of 264
  demographics of 262
  description of 262
  diagnostic and laboratory findings 264
  erotomanic 262–263
  etiology of 262
  grandiose 263
  history of 262–263
  jealous 263
  mental status exam for 263–264
  nonpharmacological management of 264
  persecutory 263
  pharmacological management of 264
  physical exam for 263
  prevalence of 262
  prevention of 262
  risk factors for 262
  screening for 262
  somatic 263
  subtypes 262–263
Dementia 277–285
  assessment of 280–281
  clinical management of 283
  demographics of 279
  description of 277–279
  diagnostic and laboratory findings 282
  differential diagnosis of 282–283
  etiology of 279
  history of 280–281
  incidence of 279
  life span considerations for 285
  mental status exams for 281
  nonpharmacological management of 284
  pharmacological management of 283–284
  physical exams for 281
  prevention of 280
  risk factors for 279
Dendrites 64, 68
Deontological theory 19
Dependence 294
Depolarization 68
Depression. *See also* Cyclothymic disorder;
    See also Persistent depressive disorder
    (Dysthymia); *See also* Premenstrual
    dysphoric disorder; *See also* Stevens
    Johnson syndrome (SJS)
  aggression-turned-inward theory 140–141
  anhedonia during 146
  biological theories of 142–144
  chronobiological theory of 143–144
  circadian rhythms and 143
  cognitive theory 141
  corticotropin-releasing hormone (CRH)
    and 142
  diagnostic and laboratory findings 149
  dysphoria and 142
  endocrine dysfunction and 142–143
  etiology of 140–146
  genetic predisposition to 142
  hypothalamic–pituitary–adrenal axis deregu-
    lation and 142

learned helplessness-hopelessness
    theory 141–142
major depressive disorder (MDD) 140–166
medications that induce 119
menses and 146
mental status exams for 147
mood and 146
neurotransmitter abnormalities and 143
object loss theory 140
physical exams for 147
psychodynamic theories of 140–142
versus sadness 139
sex steroid hormones and 173
sleep disruption and 146
structural brain changes causing 143
weight loss from 146
Descriptive statistics 54
deShazer, Steve 131
Developmental stages 99–101
Developmental theories 40–41
Dexamethasone suppression test (DST) 143
Diagnostic and laboratory testing 86–97
Diagnostic and Statistical Manual of Mental
    Disorders 293
Dialectical behavioral therapy 126
Differential diagnosis
    anxiety disorders and 202, 203
    obsessive–compulsive disorder and 220–221
    panic disorder and 208–209
    posttraumatic stress disorder and 224
    specific phobias and 213
Disclosure
    benefits of 20
    of disability 20
    ethics of provider 19–20
    risk of 20
Discontinuation syndrome 165
    symptoms of 165–166
Disease prevention strategies
    immunization and 97–98
    implementation of 98–99
Disruptive mood dysregulation
    disorder 355–356
    assessment of 355–356
    clinical management of 356
    demographics of 355
    description of 355
    etiology of 355
    follow-up for 356

nonpharmacological management of 356
pharmacological management of 356
prevalence of 355
prevention of 355
risk factors for 355
screening for 355
Dissociative disorders 225–226
    body dysmorphic disorder as 226
    excoriation disorder as 226
    hoarding disorder as 226
    trichotillomania as 226
Distribution 111
    of drugs 111
DNA 74
Donabedian model 55
Dopamine (DA) 295
    explanation of 69
    function of 71
    pathways 248–249
    psychiatric disorders and 70
Double depression 168
Drug Enforcement Administration (DEA) 115
Drug screening and false positives 119
Dysphoria 142
Dysthymia. *See* Persistent depressive disorder
    (Dysthymia)

E

Ears 84
Eating disorders 346–351
    assessment of 347
    clinical management of 351
    description of 346
    diagnostic and laboratory findings 350
    differential diagnosis of 350–351
    etiology of 346–347
    follow-up for 351
    history of 348
    incidence of 347
    mental status exams for 349–350
    nonpharmacological management of 351
    pharmacological management of 351
    physical exams for 348–349
    prevention of 347
    risk factors for 347
    screening for 347
Edinburgh Postnatal Depression Scale
    (EPDS) 145
EEG 73

Ego 43
Electrocardiogram (EKG) 156
Electroconvulsive therapy (ECT) 159
Electrolytes 89
Electronic health records, function of 17
Elimination 112
   of drugs 112
Emancipated minors 18
Endocrine
   disorders 150
   dysfunction 142–143
Enzymatic destruction 70
Epinephrine 69
Erikson, Erik 40
Ethical issues
   in decision-making 19
   disclosure by providers as 19–20
   for nurse practitioners 18–19
   in research 54–55
Evidence-based practice 53
Evoked potentials testing 73
Excitatory response 113
Excoriation disorder 226
Exercise
   benefits of 101
   client teaching regarding 101–102
   monitoring intenstity of 102
   recommendations for 102
Existential therapy 126
Experiential therapy 130–131
External validity 54
Extrapyramidal side effects (EPSE) 249
   medications used to treat 251
   side effects of 252
Eye movement desensitization and reprocess-
      ing (EMDR) 127
Eyes 80, 83

F
Family history, explanation of 73–74
Family homeostasis 129
Family structure 130
Family systems theory 129–130
Family systems therapy 130
Family therapy 162, 289
   family system concepts in 129–130
   types of 130–132
Federal Drug Administration (FDA)
   pregnancy ratings for medications from 118

Fetal alcohol syndrome (FAS) 297, 352–353
Fibromyalgia 150
Fine-motor skills 82
First-pass metabolism 112
Fish oil 134
Fissures in the brain 65
Folie á Deux. *See* Shared psychotic disorder
Forensics
   corrections and 27–28
   knowledge base of 27
Formal operations stage 45
Frankl, Viktor 126
Free thyroxine T4 87
Freud, Sigmund 41, 42, 125, 140–141, 197
Frontal lobe 65
Functional imaging 73

G
GABA
   explanation of 69
   function of 72
   psychiatric disorders and 70
Gamma amino butyric acid (GABA) 295
Gamma glutamyl transpeptidase 96–97
Gender
   based screening 99–101
   dysphoria 26
   identity 26
Generalized anxiety disorder (GAD) 215–218
   assessment of 216–217
   comorbidities of 218
   description of 215–216
   history of 216
   life span considerations for 218
   mental status exams for 217
   nonpharmacological management of 217
   pharmacological management of 217
   physical exams for 216–217
Genes 74–75
Gene therapy 74
Genetic
   counseling 74
   loading 294
   predisposition to depression 142
   terms 74
   testing 75
Genital stage 42
Genomics 73–75
Ginkgo 135

Ginseng 135
Glia 68
Glutamate
  explanation of 69
  function of 72
  psychiatric disorders and 70
Glycine 69
Gray matter 64
Grief and bereavement 150, 169–173
  assessment of 171
  clinical management of 172
  demographics of 170
  description of 169–170
  diagnostic and laboratory findings 172
  differential diagnosis of 172
  etiology of 170
  follow-up for 173
  history of 171
  indidence of 170
  life span considerations for 172
  mental status exams for 171
  nonpharamacological management of 172
  pharamacological management of 172
  physical exams for 171
  prevention of 171
  psychotherapy and 172
  risk factors for 171
  screening for 171
Group therapy 162
  explanation of 127–128
  phases in 128–129
Gyri 65

H

Haley, Jay 131
Half-life 112
Hamilton Depression Rating Scale
  (HAM-D) 145
Health
  behavior guidelines 101–103
  belief model 46
  cultural influences on 24
  delivery systems 56
  policy and nurse practitioners 22–23
  policy development 58
  promotion 103
Health care home 57

Health Information Technology for Economic
    and Clinical Health Act (HITECH) of
    2009 17
Heart 85
Herbal products/supplements 132, 133–135
Hierarchy of needs theory 45–46
HIPAA, privacy protections under 16–17
Hippocampus 66
Hoarding disorder 226
Homelessness 24–25
  strategies for reducing 25
Homicide 381
  early warning signs of 381
Human Genome Project 74
Humanistic therapy 126–127
Huntington's disease 278
Hypercalcemia 90
Hyperkalemia 94
Hypermagnesemia 92
Hypernatremia 91
Hypersomnia. *See* Sleep disorders
Hypersomnolence disorder 364
Hypertensive crisis 157
Hyperthyroidism 88
Hypocalcemia 90
Hypokalemia 94
Hypomagnesemia 92
Hypomania 177
Hyponatremia 91
Hypothalamic–pituitary–adrenal axis 142
Hypothalamus 66
Hypothyroidism 88
Hypovolemic hippocampus 143
Hypovolemic prefrontal cortex 143

I

Id 42
Illness management recovery (IMR) 255
Immunization 97–98
Improvised explosive devices (IEDs) 286
Incredible years 332
Individual therapy 162
Indole. *See* Serotonin
Infectious and inflammatory states 150
Inferential statistics 54
Informed consent 17–18
Inhibitory response 113
Insomnia 362–367. *See also* Sleep disorders
  assessment of 363–364

Insomnia (continued)
  in children 367
  clinical management of 365
  demographics of 362
  diagnostic and laboratory findings 364
  differential diagnosis of 365
  etiology of 362
  hypersomnolence disorder and 364
  incidence of 362
  life span considerations for 367–368
  mental status exams for 364
  nonpharmacological management
      of 366–367
  obstructive sleep apnea (OSA) and 364
  in older adults 367–368
  pharmacological management of 365–366
  physical exams for 364
  polysomnography and diagnosis of 364
  prevention of 363
  risk factors for 363
  screening for 363
Institutional review boards (IRBs) 54–55
Intellectual disability 352–354
  assessment of 353–354
  clinical management of 354
  demographics of 353
  description of 352
  diagnostic and laboratory findings 354
  differential diagnosis of 354
  etiology of 352–353
  and fetal alcohol syndrome 352–353
  mental status exams for 354
  nonpharmacological management
      of 354–355
  pharmacological management of 354
  physical exams for 353–354
  prevalence of 353
  prevention of 353
  risk factors for 353
  screening for 353
Internal validity 54
Interpersonal theory 45, 47, 198
Interpersonal therapy 127
Intimate partner violence (IPV) 373–376
  assessment of 375
  clinical management of 376
  demographics of 374
  description of 373
  diagnostic and laboratory findings 375
  differential diagnosis of 376
  etiology of 373–374
  history of 375
  incidence of 374
  mental status exams for 375
  nonpharmacological management of 376
  pharmacological management of 376
  physical exams for 375
  prevention of 374–375
  risk factors for 374
  screening for 374–375
Intoxication 294, 300
Inverse agonist effect 113
Involuntary admission 21
Involuntary commitment 21

J
Just culture of safety 55–56

K
Kidney disease 113
Kindling 174
Klerman, Gerald L. 127

L
Laboratory testing, diagnostic and 86–97
Latency stage 42
Lazarus, Arnold 126
Leadership, nurse practitioners and 51
Learned helplessness-hopelessness
      theory 141–142
Left hemisphere (of brain) 65
Leininger, Madeline 47
Lethality assessment 379
Lewy body disease 279
Licensure 15
Limbic system 66
Linehan, Marsha 126
Lithium 180
  side effects of 181
  Stevens Johnson syndrome (SJS) and 186
Liver disease 113
Liver function tests (LFTs) 95, 181
Living wills 23
Lungs 85

M
Macrobiotics 135
Magnesium 91–92

Magnetic resonance imaging (MRI) 73–74
Magnetoencephalography (MEG) 73
Major depressive disorder (MDD) 140–166.
          See also Depression
    adults and 163–164
    age and 142
    assessment of 145
    brain damage and 143
    children and 163
    clinical management of 151
    demographics of 144–145
    description of 140
    diagnostic and laboratory findings
          for 149–151
    electroconvulsive therapy (ECT) treatment
          for 159
    etiology of 140–146
    expected course of 166
    follow-up for 164–166
    history of 145–146
    hospitalization for 151
    HPA dysregulation causing 142
    incidence of 144–145
    individual therapy 162
    life span considerations for 163–164
    mental status exams for 147–149
    nonpharmacological management
          of 159–162
    pharmacological management of 151–155
    phototherapy 162
    prevention of 145
    risk factors for 145
    screening for 145
    transcranial magnetic stimulation (TMS)
          treatment for 160
    vagal nerve stimulation (VNS) treatment
          for 160
Malpractice
    insurance 20–21
    negligence as proof of 21
Mania 177
    medications inducing 119
Manipulative and body-based therapies 132
Maslow, Abraham 45
Massage 132, 135
Mean 54
Mediation 52
Medications
    absorption of 111

    antipsychotics 115
    for anxiety disorders 116
    anxiolytics 116
    for attention deficit disorder 117
    for attention deficit hyperactivity
          disorder 117
    benzodiazepines (BNZs) 116
    for bipolar affective disorders 115
    for bipolar (BP) disorder 179, 182–183
    depression inducing 119
    for depressive disorders 116
    distribution in organs 111
    and drug screening results 119
    enzyme inducers and 112
    enzyme inhibitors and 113
    FDA pregnancy ratings for 118
    first-pass metabolism and 112
    half-life of 112
    kidney disease from 113
    liver disease from 113
    mania inducing 119
    median effective dose 114
    median toxic dose 114
    metabolism and 112
    monoamine oxidase inhibitors
          (MAOIs) 113, 116, 152, 156
    mood altered states as side effects 151
    for mood disorders 115, 153
    mood stabilizers 115
    norepinephrine dopamine reuptake inhibi-
          tors (NDRIs) 154
    pharmacodynamics and 113
    pharmacokinetics and 111–113
    potency of 113
    for psychiatric disorders 115
    for psychotic disorders 115
    schedules for controlled substances 118
    for schizophrenia 115
    selective serotonin reuptake inhibitors
          (SSRIs) 113, 116, 152, 156
    serotonin agonist and reuptake inhibitors
          (SARIs) 154
    serotonin norepinephrine reuptake inhibi-
          tors (SNRIs) 152–153, 159
    steady state of 112
    stimulants 117
    tachyphylaxis 114
    teratogenic nature of 118–119
    therapeutic index for 114

Medications (continued)
  tolerance to 114
  tricyclic antidepressants (TCAs) 152, 156
  for unipolar affective disorders 116
Meditation 132, 135
Medulla 67
Melatonin 134
Mental state exam (MSE) 283
Mental status exams
  for agoraphobia 210
  for anxiety disorders 201
  for attention-deficit hyperactivity disorder
      (ADHD) 337
  for autism spectrum disorder 342
  for bipolar (BP) disorder 177–178
  for brief psychotic disorder 265
  for conduct disorder 334
  for cyclothymic disorder 187–188
  for delirium 274
  for delusional disorder 263–264
  for dementia 281
  for depression 147
  for eating disorders 349–350
  for generalized anxiety disorder (GAD) 217
  for grief and bereavement 171
  for insomnia 364
  for intellectual disability 354
  for intimate partner violence (IPV) 375
  for major depressive disorder
      (MDD) 147–149
  for obsessive–compulsive disorder
      (OCD) 220
  for oppositional defiant disorder (ODD) 331
  for panic disorder 208
  for persistent depressive disorder
      (Dysthymia) 168
  for phobias 213
  for posttraumatic stress disorder
      (PTSD) 223
  for Rett syndrome 345
  for schizoaffective disorder 261
  for schizophrenia 241–242
  for schizophreniform disorder 259
  for sexual assault and abuse 378
  for shared psychotic disorder 266
  for social anxiety disorder 215
  for substance-related disorders 301
Mentoring 22
Messenger RNA (mRNA) 74

Metabolism 112
  of drugs 112
Midbrain 67
Migrant workers 25
Mind–body interventions 132
Mini-cog 281
Mini-Mental State Examination (MMSE) 281
Minuchin, Salvador 130
Misuse (of substances) 294
Monoamine oxidase inhibitors (MAOIs) 69,
      113, 116, 152, 155, 156
  hypertensive crisis from 157
  side effects of 158
Montreal Cognitive Assessment (MoCA) 281
Mood 328
  depression and 146
  stabilizers 115
Morphogenesis 130
Morphostasis 130
Motivational interviewing 46
Motor functions 82
Musculoskeletal system 86

N
Neck 84
Negotiation 52
Nervous system
  central 64
  components of 64
  function of 63
  peripheral 64
Neuroadaptation 295
Neuroanatomy 64–68
Neurobiological theory 198–199
  of schizophrenia 235
Neurocognitive disorders 271–292
  cognitive disorders 271
  delirium 271–277
  dementia 277–285
  traumatic brain injuries and 285–290
Neuroimaging 72–74
Neuroleptic malignant syndrome (NMS) 253
Neurological
  disorders 150
  examinations 80–86
  soft signs 82–83
Neurons 63–64, 68
Neuropeptides 70, 70–71
Neurophysiology 68–70

Neurotransmitters 113
  abnormalities of 143
  categories of 68–70
  classification requirements for 69
  function of 68, 71–72
  psychiatric disorders and 70
  recovery and degradation of 70
Nonpharmacological management
  of agoraphobia 211
  of anxiety disorders 205
  of generalized anxiety disorder 217
  of obsessive–compulsive disorder 221
  of panic disorder 209–210
  of personality disorders 322
  of posttraumatic stress disorder 225
  of social anxiety disorder 215
  of specific phobias 214
Nonpharmacological treatment
  complementary and alternative therapies
      as 132–135
  family therapy as 129–132
  group therapy as 127–129
  individual therapy as 125–127
  issues related to 125
Nonrapid eye movement stages (NREM) 361
Norepinephrine
  explanation of 69
  function of 71
  psychiatric disorders and 70
Norepinephrine dopamine reuptake inhibitors
      (NDRIs) 154
Nose 84
Nurse practitioners. See also Psychiatric-
      mental health nurse practitioners
      (PMHNPs)
  admissions criteria and 21
  client advocacy and 22
  commitment process and criteria and 21–22
  competency issues and 21
  core competencies of 11–12
  disclosure issues and 19–20
  ethical behavior for 18–19
  growth of 14
  health policy and 22–23
  historical background of 13–14
  leadership and 51
  legal considerations for 20–21
  mentoring of 22
  public health principles and 103–104

  regulatory dimensions of 14–16
  research utilization and 52–53
  role responsibilities of 16–19
  scholarly activities of 22
  specialty competencies of 12–13
  statutory dimensions of 14–16
Nursing theories 47
Nutritional disorders 150

O
Object loss theory 140
Obsessive–compulsive disorder
      (OCD) 218–221
  assessment of 219–220
  clinical management of 221
  comorbidities of 221
  description of 218
  differential diagnosis of 220–221
  history of 219–220
  life span considerations for 221
  mental status exams for 220
  nonpharmacological management of 221
  pharmacological management of 221
  physical exams for 220
  risk factors for 219
Obstructive sleep apnea (OSA) 364
Occipital lobe 66
O'Hanlon, Bill 131
Omega-3 fatty acids 134
Opioid neuropeptides 70, 72
Oppositional defiant disorder
      (ODD) 329–332
  assessment of 330–331
  clinical management of 331
  demographics of 330
  description of 329–330
  diagnostic and laboratory findings 331
  differential diagnosis of 331
  etiology of 330
  history of 330–331
  mental status exams for 331
  nonpharmacological management of 332
  pharmacological management of 331–332
  physical exams for 331
  prevalence of 330
  prevention of 330
  risk factors for 330
  screening for 330
Oral stage 42

Orem, Dorothy 47
Organization of practices 56

P

Panic disorder 207–210. *See also* Anxiety
disorders
assessment of 207–208
clinical management of 209
comorbidities of 210
description of 207
diagnostic and laboratory findings 208
differential diagnosis of 208–209
history of 207–208
mental status exams for 208
nonpharmacological management
of 209–210
pharmacological management of 209
physical exams for 208
Parasympathetic nervous system 64
Parietal lobe 66
Partial agonist effect 113
Pathways
mesocortical 248
mesolimbic 248
nigrostriatal 249
tuberoinfundbular 249
Patient-centered care model (PCC) 56
Patient Health Questionnaire 9 (PHQ-9) 145
Pearson's r correlation 54
Peplau, Hildegard 47
Peptides 72. *See also* Opioid neuropeptides
Peripheral nervous system (PNS) 64
Persistent depressive disorder
(Dysthymia) 166–194
assessment of 167–168
clinical management of 168–169
comorbities of 168–169
demographics of 166–167
description of 166
diagnostic and laboratory findings for 168
differential diagnosis of 168
double depression and 168–169
etiology of 166
follow-up for 169
history of 167–168
indicence of 166–167
life span considerations for 169
and major depressive disorder
(MDD) 168–169

mental status exams for 168
nonpharmacological management of 168
personality disorders and 169
pharmacological management of 168
physical exams for 168
polysomnographic findings for 168
prevention of 167
risk factors for 167
screening for 167
symptoms of 167–168
Personality 313–314
Personality disorders 314–323. *See
also* Cluster A, B, and C personality
disorders
assessment of 317–320
categories of 315
client history and 317
clinical management of 321
demographics of 316
description of 314
diagnostic and laboratory findings 320
differential diagnosis of 321
etiology of 314–316
follow-up for 323
history of 317
incidence of 316
life span considerations for 323
nonpharmacological management of 322
pharmacological management of 322
physical exams for 319–320
prevention of 316–317
risk factors for 316
screening for 316–317
Person-centered therapy. *See* Humanistic
therapy
Phallic stage 42
Pharmacodynamics 111, 113
agonist effect 113
antagonist effect 113
excitatory response 113
inhibitory response 113
inverse agonist effect 113
monoamine oxidase inhibitors (MAOIs) 113
neurotransmitters and 113
partial agonist effect 113
selective serotonin reuptake inhibitors
(SSRIs) 113
target sites and 113
Pharmacogenomics 75

Pharmacokinetics 111–113
  absorption of 111
  alterations in 112–113
  distribution of 111
  elements of 111–113
  elimination and 112
  explanation of 111
  first-pass metabolism and 112
  half-life of medications 112
  metabolism and 112
  steady state 112
Pharmacological management
  concepts in 111–114
  of agoraphobia 211
  of anxiety disorders 203–205, 205
  of generalized anxiety disorder 217
  of obsessive–compulsive disorder 221
  of panic disorder 209
  of personality disorders 322
  of posttraumatic stress disorder 224–225
  of social anxiety disorder 215
  of specific phobias 214
  psychiatric–mental health nurse practitio-
    ners (PMHNPs) role in 114–120
Pharmacology 111. *See*
    also Psychopharmacology
  considerations related to 118–119
  explanation of 111
Phenotype 74
Phototherapy 162
Physical exams 79–86
  for agoraphobia 210
  for anxiety disorders 201
  for attention-deficit hyperactivity disorder
    (ADHD) 337
  for autism spectrum disorder 342
  for bipolar (BP) disorder 177
  for brief psychotic disorder 265
  for conduct disorder 333
  for cyclothymic disorder 187–188
  for delirium 273
  for delusional disorder 263
  for dementia 281
  for depression 147
  for eating disorders 348–349
  for generalized anxiety disorder (GAD) 217
  for grief and bereavement 171
  for insomnia 364
  for intellectual disability 353–354

  for intimate partner violence (IPV) 375
  for major depressive disorder (MDD) 147
  for obsessive–compulsive disorder
    (OCD) 220
  for oppositional defiant disorder (ODD) 331
  for panic disorder 208
  for persistent depressive disorder
    (Dysthymia) 168
  for personality disorders 319–320
  for phobias 213
  for posttraumatic stress disorder
    (PTSD) 223
  for Rett syndrome 345
  for schizoaffective disorder 261
  for schizophrenia 240–241
  for schizophreniform disorder 259
  for sexual assault and abuse 378
  for shared psychotic disorder 266
  for social anxiety disorder 215
  for substance-related disorders 301
Piaget, Jean 43
Pick's disease 278
PICO method 53
Polygenic single nucleotide polymorphism
    (SNP) disorder 142
Polysomnography 364
Pons (of brainstem) 67
Population genetics 75–76
Positron emission tomography (PET) 73
Posttraumatic stress disorder (PTSD) 222–225
  assessment of 222–224
  clinical management of 224
  comorbidities of 225
  description of 222
  diagnostic and laboratory findings 223–224
  differential diagnosis of 224
  history of 222
  life span considerations for 225
  mental status exams for 223
  nonpharmacological management of 225
  pharmacological management of 224–225
  physical exams for 223
  risk factors for 222
Potassium 93–94
Potency 113
Premenstrual dysphoric disorder 173
  description of 173
  symptoms of 173
Preoperational stage 44

Preventative factors 104
Primary prevention of mental disorders 103
Probability 54
Professional civility 52
Psychiatric
  nursing 11
  research in psychotropic medications 111
Psychiatric disorders 151
  age of onset for 41
  among incarcerated individuals 27–28
  classification of 38
  neurotransmitters and 70
  schizophreniform 258–260
Psychiatric–mental health nurse practi-
      tioners (PMHNPs). *See also* Nurse
      practitioners
  assessment of childhood and adolescent
      disorders 327–329
  bipolar disorders treatment of and 139–194
  and childhood disorders 327–360
  culturally competent care and 23–24
  depressive disorders treatment of
      and 139–194
  foundational theories supporting role
      of 41–47
  and grief and bereavement 170
  health policy of 22–23
  major depressive disorder (MDD) follow-up
      care practices from 164
  nursing theories and 47
  origins of 11
  pharmacological management role
      of 114–120
  psychopharmacology and 111–124
  research utilization by 52–53
  roles of 22
  specialized content for 12–13
Psychiatry 19
Psychic determinism 41
Psychoanalytic
  theory 41
  therapy 125
Psychodynamic theories
  anxiety disorders and 197–198
  explanation of 41–43
  of personality disorders 315–316
  of substance-related disorders 294
  psychotherapy 162
Psychological preventative factors 104

Psychological risk factors 104
Psychopharmacology 111–124
  management concepts 111–112
  pharmacological considerations in 118–119
  principles of 111
Psychosexual stages of development 42
Psychosis, symtoms of 234
Psychotic 233
Psychotic disorders 233–270
  delusional disorder 262–265
  schizoaffective disorder 260–261
  schizophrenia 235–257
  schizophreniform disorder 258–260
  shared psychotic disorder 265–267
Psychotropic medications
  older adults and 113
  pregnancy and 118
  risks of 118–119
  teratogenic nature of 118–119
  weight gain and 83
Public health principles 103–104
Purging 348
p value 54

Q
Qualitative hierarchy 53
Quality improvement 55
Quality of care 56
Quantitative hierarchy 53

R
Rapid cycling 177
Rapid eye movement (REM) 361
Reflective practice 52
Reflexes 80
Reflexology 132, 135
Reminiscence therapy 129
Repolarization 68
Research
  dissemination of 53–54
  donabedian model 55
  ethical considerations in 54–55
  interpretation of 54
  quality improvement 55
  utilization of 52–53
Reticular formation system (of brain) 67–68
Rett syndrome 344–346
  assessment of 344
  clinical management of 346

demographics of 344
description of 344
differential diagnosis of 346
etiology of 344
history of 345
incidence of 344
mental status exams for 345
nonpharmacological management of 346
pharmacological management of 346
physical exams for 345
prevention of 344
risk factors for 344
screening for 344
Reuptake pumps 71, 113
Reversibility 44
Right hemisphere (of brain) 65
Rights of clients 58
Risk assessment 23, 28
Risk factors 103–104
Risk management 23
Rogers, Carl 126

S

Sadness 139–140. *See also* Depression
Sam-e 134
Satir, Virginia 130
Schedules for controlled substances 118
Schizoaffective disorder 260–261
  assessment of 260–261
  clinical management of 261
  demographics of 260
  description of 260
  diagnostic and laboratory findings 261
  etiology of 260
  follow-up for 261
  mental status exams for 261
  nonpharmacological management of 261
  pharmacological management of 261
  physical exams for 261
  prevalence of 260
  prevention of 260
  risk factors for 260
  screening for 260
  symptoms of 261
Schizophrenia 233, 235–257
  abnormalities and 236
  assertive community treatment (ACT)
      for 254–255
  assessment of 238–240
  atypical antipsychotics for 248–249
  clinical management of 243
  comorbidities of 255
  delusions and 238
  demographics of 236–237
  description of 235
  diagnostic and laboratory findings 242
  differential diagnosis of 242–243
  dopamine pathways and 248–249
  downdrift and 238
  DSM-5 diagnostic criteria for 238–240
  etiology of 235–236
  extrapyramidal side effects (EPSE) of 249
  follow-up for 257–258
  genetics and 235
  group therapy for 254–255
  hallucinations and 239
  health considerations of 255–256
  history of 238–240
  illness management recovery (IMR) for 255
  incidence of 236–237
  individual therapy for 254–255
  life span considerations for 256–257
  mental status exams for 241–242
  milieu therapy for 255
  neurobiological defect and 236
  neurobiological theory of 235
  neurodevelopment and 235–236
  nonpharmacological management
      of 254–255
  pharmacological management of 248–254
  physical exams for 240–241
  prevention of 237–238
  proactice crisis management planning
      for 254–255
  risk factors for 237
  screening for 237–238
  subtypes of 240
  suicide and 255–256
  symptom of 239
  typical antipsychotics for 249–250
Schizophreniform disorder 258–260
  assessment of 258–259
  clinical management of 259
  demographics for 258
  description of 258
  diagnostic and laboratory findings 259
  etiology of 258
  follow-up for 260

Schizophreniform disorder (continued)
  history of 258–259
  mental status exams for 259
  nonpharmacological management of 259
  pharmacological management of 259
  physical exams for 259
  prevention of 258
  risk factors for 258
  screening for 258
Scholarly activities 22
Scope of practice 16
Seasonal farm workers 25
Secondary prevention of mental disorders 103
Selective serotonin reuptake inhibitors
      (SSRIs) 113, 116, 152, 156, 203
  discontinuation syndrome 165–166
Self
  awareness 102
  disclosure 102
  efficacy and social learning theory 46–47
  system 45
Seligman, Martin 141
Sensorimotor stage 44
Sensory functions 82
Separation anxiety disorder 218
Serotonin
  explanation of 69
  function of 71
  psychiatric disorders and 70
Serotonin agonist and reuptake inhibitors
      (SARIs) 154
Serotonin norepinephrine reuptake inhibitors
      (SNRIs) 152–153, 159
Serotonin syndrome 165
  symptoms of 165
Sex steroid hormones 173
Sexual
  behavior 27
  identity 26
  orientation 26–27
Sexual assault and abuse
  assessment of 378
  clinical management of 379
  demographics of 377
  description of 376–377
  diagnostic and laboratory findings 379
  differential diagnosis of 379
  etiology 377
  factors of 377

incidence of 377
mental status exams for 378
nonpharmacological management
    of 379–380
pharmacological management of 379
physical exams for 378
prevention of 377–378
screening for 377–378
Sexually transmitted infections (STIs) 185
Shapiro, Francine 127
Shared psychotic disorder
  assessment of 266
  clinical management of 266
  demographics of 266
  description of 265
  diagnostic and laboratory findings 266
  etiology 266
  history of 266
  incidence of 266
  mental status exams for 266
  nonpharmacological management of 266,
      266–267
  pharmacological management of 266
  physical exams for 266
  prevention of 266
  risk factors for 266
  screening for 266
Short Michigan alcoholism screening test
    (S-MAST) 297
Single nucleotide polymorphism (SNP)
    disorder 142
Single photon emission computed tomography
    (SPECT) 73
Sinuses 84
Sleep disorders 361–368
  considerations of 361–362
  disturbances 146
  insomnia 362–367
Social anxiety disorder 214–215
  assessment of 214–215
  clinical management of 215
  description of 214–215
  history of 214–215
  mental status exams for 215
  nonpharmacological management of 215
  pharmacological management of 215
  physical exams for 215
Social preventative factors 104
Social risk factors 104

Sodium 90–91
Solution-focused therapy 131–132
Somatic nervous system 64
Special populations, culturally competent care
        and. *See* Culturally competent care
Specific phobias 211–214
    assessment of 212–213
    client history and 212–213
    clinical management of 213
    description of 211
    diagnostic and laboratory findings 213
    differential diagnosis of 213
    mental status exams for 213
    nonpharmacological management of 214
    pharmacological management of 214
    physical exams for 213
    risk factors for 211–212
Stages of human development (Erikson) 40
Stages of interpersonal development
        (Sullivan) 45
Standard deviation 54
Standards of practice 16
State legislative statutes 14–15
Statistics
    descriptive 54
    inferential 54
Statutory law 15
Steady state 112
Stem (of neuron) 64
Stevens Johnson syndrome (SJS) 83,
        184–186
    clinical management of 184–185
    comorbidities of 185
    description of 184
    follow-up for 185–186
    health considerations for 185
    life span considerations for 185
    lithium and 186
    nonpharmacological management
        of 184–185
    symptoms of 184
Stimulants 117
St Louis University Mental Status Examination
        (SLUMS) 281
Strategic therapy 131
Structural family therapy 130
Structural imaging 72–73
Structural mapping (genogram) 130
Substance 294

Substance-related disorders 293–312
    abused agents list 298
    assessment of 298–300
    biological theories of 294–296
    clinical management of 302–304
    demographics of 296
    description of 293–294
    diagnostic and laboratory findings 302
    differential diagnosis of 302
    etiology of 294–296
    history of 298–300
    incidence of 296
    intoxication 300
    life span considerations for 306–307
    mental status exams for 301–302
    nonpharmacological management
        of 305–306
    pharmacological management of 304–305
    physical exams for 301
    prevention of 297–298
    psychodynamic theory of 294
    risk factors for 296
    screening for 297–298
    withdrawal 300
Substance use disorders. *See* Substance-related
        disorders
Suicide 143, 148–149
    assessing for 149, 379–381
    clinical management of 162
    risk factors for 163, 380–381
    schizophrenia and 255–256
    signs of imminent danger 380
    traumatic brain injury and 287–288
Sulci 65
Sullivan, Harry Stack 45, 198
Superego 43
Sympathetic nervous system 64
Synapse 68, 70
Synaptic cleft 68, 69

T
Tachyphylaxis 114
Tardive dyskinesia (TD) 248, 252
Target sites 113
Team leadership model 51–52
Telehealth 17
Teleological theory 19
Temporal lobe 65–66
Tertiary prevention of mental disorders 103

Tests
  alcohol use disorders identification test (AUDIT) 297
  CAGE alcohol screening test 297
  children and adolescents under 21 years of age test (CRAFT) 297
  clinical opiate withdrawal scale (COWS) 297
  dexamethasone suppression test (DST) 143
  liver function tests (LFTs) 181
  short Michigan alcoholism screening test (S-MAST) 297
Thalamus 66
Theory of cultural care 47
Theory of self-care 47
Therapeutic index 114
Therapeutic nurse–client relationship 38–39, 39
  theory or interpersonal theory 47
Therapies
  behavioral 126
  cognitive 125–126
  complementary and alternative 132–135
  dialectical behavioral 126
  existential 126
  eye movement desensitization and reprocessing (EMDR) 127
  family 129–132
  group 127–129
  humanistic 126–127
  individual 125–127
  interpersonal 127
  psychoanalytic 125
  reminiscence 129
Thorax 85
Thought content 328
Thought process 328
Thyroid function tests 86
Thyroid-stimulating hormone 87–88
Tolerance 294
  to drugs 114
Transcranial magnetic stimulation (TMS) 160
Transference 38
Transtheoretical model of change 46
Traumatic brain injury
  assessment of 287
  clinical management of 288
  demographics of 286
  description of 285
  diagnostic and laboratory findings 287–288
  differential diagnosis of 288
  etiology of 286
  follow-up for 290
  incidence of 286
  life span considerations for 290
  mental status of 287
  military personnel and 286
  nonpharmacological management of 288–289
  pharmacological management of 288
  physical findings for 287
  prevention of 286
  psychotherapies for 289
  risk factors for 286
  screening for 286
  suicide and 287–288
  symptoms of 287
Trichotillomania 226
Tricyclic antidepressants (TCAs) 116, 152, 156, 204
Tryptophan 134
t test 54

V
Vagal nerve stimulation (VNS) 160
Valerian 135
Variance 54
Violence 382–384
  homicide 381
  intimate partner violence (IPV) 373–376
  and lethality assessment 380
  in school 380
  sexual assault and abuse 376–379
  suicide assessment 380–381
  threats of 381
Virtue ethics 19
Vital signs 83
Vitamin E 134
Voluntary admission 21–22

W
Watson, Jean 47
Weight loss 146
Weissman, Myrna M. 127
White matter 64
Withdrawal 294, 300

Y
Yalom, Irvin 128
Yoga 132, 135
Young Mania Rating Scale (YMRS) 186

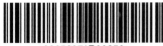

Made in the USA
Middletown, DE
08 November 2018